Spinal Deformity Update

Editors

SIGURD H. BERVEN
PRAVEEN V. MUMMANENI

NEUROSURGERY
CLINICS OF NORTH AMERICA

www.neurosurgery.theclinics.com

Consulting Editors
RUSSELL R. LONSER
DANIEL K. RESNICK

October 2023 • Volume 34 • Number 4

ELSEVIER

1600 John F. Kennedy Boulevard • Suite 1800 • Philadelphia, Pennsylvania, 19103-2899

http://www.theclinics.com

NEUROSURGERY CLINICS OF NORTH AMERICA Volume 34, Number 4
October 2023 ISSN 1042-3680, ISBN-13: 978-0-443-18250-1

Editor: Stacy Eastman
Developmental Editor: Akshay Samson

Neurosurgery Clinics of North America (ISSN 1042-3680) is published quarterly by Elsevier Inc., 360 Park Avenue South, New York, NY 10010-1710. Months of issue are January, April, July, and October. Business and Editorial Offices: 1600 John F. Kennedy Blvd., Suite 1800, Philadelphia, PA 19103-2899. Customer Service Office: 11830 Westline Industrial Drive, St. Louis, MO 63146. Periodicals postage paid at New York, NY, and additional mailing offices. Subscription prices are $451.00 per year (US individuals), $821.00 per year (US institutions), $484.00 per year (Canadian individuals), $1,019.00 per year (Canadian institutions), $562.00 per year (international individuals), $1,019.00 per year (international institutions), $100.00 per year (US students), $255.00 per year (international students), and $100.00 per year (Canadian students). International air speed delivery is included in all *Clinics* subscription prices. All prices are subject to change without notice. **POSTMASTER:** Send address changes to *Neurosurgery Clinics of North America*, Elsevier Periodicals Customer Service, 11830 Westline Industrial Drive, St. Louis, MO 63146. **Customer Service: 1-800-654-2452 (US and Canada). From outside the US and Canada, call: 1-314-453-7041. Fax: 1-314-453-5170. E-mail: JournalsCustomerService-usa@elsevier.com (for print support) and journalsonlinesupport-usa@elsevier.com (for online support).**

Reprints. For copies of 100 or more, of articles in this publication, please contact the Commercial Reprints Department, Elsevier Inc., 360 Park Avenue South, New York, NY 10010-1710. Tel. 212-633-3874; Fax: 212-633-3820; E-mail: reprints@elsevier.com.

Neurosurgery Clinics of North America is covered in *MEDLINE/PubMed (Index Medicus), EMBASE/Excerpta Medica, and Current Contents/Clinical Medicine (CC/CM).*

Printed in the United States of America.

Contributors

CONSULTING EDITORS

RUSSELL R. LONSER, MD
Professor and Chair, Department of
Neurological Surgery, The Ohio State
University Wexner Medical Center, Columbus,
Ohio, USA

DANIEL K. RESNICK, MD, MS
Professor and Vice Chairman, Program
Director, Department of Neurosurgery,
University of Wisconsin-Madison School of
Medicine and Public Health, Madison,
Wisconsin, USA

EDITORS

SIGURD H. BERVEN, MD
Professor in Residence, Chief of Spine Service,
Department of Orthopaedic Surgery, University
of California, San Francisco, San Francisco,
California, USA

PRAVEEN V. MUMMANENI, MD, MBA
Joan O'Reilly Distinguished Professor, Vice
Chair, Department of Neurological Surgery,
University of California, San Francisco, San
Francisco, California, USA

AUTHORS

MUHAMMAD M. ABD-EL-BARR, MD, PhD
Neurosurgeon, Department of Neurosurgery,
Division of Spine, Duke University, Durham,
North Carolina, USA

NITIN AGARWAL, MD
Associate Professor, Department of
Neurological Surgery, University of Pittsburgh,
Pittsburgh, Pennsylvania, USA

NOEL AKIOYAMEN, MD
Physician, Department of Orthopaedic Surgery,
Montefiore Einstein, Bronx, New York, USA

NIMA ALAN, MD
Department of Neurosurgery, Barrow
Neurological Institute, St. Joseph's Hospital
and Medical Center, Phoenix, Arizona, USA

NEEL ANAND, MD
Director of Spine Trauma, Department of
Orthopedic Surgery, Cedars-Sinai Medical
Center, Los Angeles, California, USA

AYUSH ARORA, BSE
Department of Orthopaedic Surgery, University
of California, San Francisco, San Francisco,
California, USA

OLIVER G.S. AYLING, MD, MSc
Department of Neurosurgery, Fellow,
University of Miami, Department of
Neurological Surgery, University of Miami
Miller School of Medicine, Miami, Florida, USA

STEPHEN M. BERGIN, MD, PhD
Department of Neurosurgery, Division of Spine,
Duke University, Durham, North Carolina, USA

SIGURD H. BERVEN, MD
Professor in Residence, Chief of Spine Service,
Department of Orthopaedic Surgery, University
of California, San Francisco, San Francisco,
California, USA

PETER G. CAMPBELL, MD
Attending Neurosurgeon, Spine Institute of
Louisiana, Shreveport, Louisiana, USA

LEAH Y. CARREON, MD, MSc
Clinical Research Director, Norton Leatherman
Spine Center, Louisville, Kentucky, USA

ANDREW K. CHAN, MD
Assistant Professor, Department of
Neurological Surgery, Neurological Institute of

New York, Columbia University Vagelos College of Physicians and Surgeons, The Daniel and Jane Och Spine Hospital at NewYork-Presbyterian, New York, New York, USA

DEAN CHOU, MD
Chief of the Spine Division, Department of Neurological Surgery, Neurological Institute of New York, Columbia University Vagelos College of Physicians and Surgeons, New York, New York, USA

AARON J. CLARK, MD, PhD
Department of Neurological Surgery, University of California, San Francisco, San Francisco, California, USA

TRAVIS S. CREVECOEUR, MD
Resident, Department of Neurological Surgery, Neurological Institute of New York, Columbia University Vagelos College of Physicians and Surgeons, New York, New York, USA

JAY DALTON, MD
Department of Orthopaedic Surgery, University of Pittsburgh Medical Center, Pittsburgh, Pennsylvania, USA

ANTHONY M. DIGIORGIO, DO, MHA
Assistant Professor, Department of Neurological Surgery, University of California, San Francisco, San Francisco, California, USA

JOHN R. DIMAR II, MD
Clinical Professor, Norton Leatherman Spine Center, Department of Orthopaedic Surgery, University of Louisville School of Medicine, Louisville, Kentucky, USA

ROBERT KENNETH EASTLACK, MD
Head of Division of Spine Surgery, Department of Orthopaedic Surgery, Scripps Clinic, La Jolla, California, USA

KAI-MING FU, MD, PhD
Department of Nerosurgery, Weill Cornell Medical Center, New York, New York, USA

STEVEN D. GLASSMAN, MD
Norton Leatherman Spine Center, Louisville, Kentucky, USA

JACOB L. GOLDBERG, MD
Chief Resident, Department of Nerosurgery, Weill Cornell Medical Center, New York, New York, USA

C. RORY GOODWIN, MD, PhD
Assistant Professor, Director of Spine Oncology, Department of Neurosurgery, Division of Spine, Duke University, Durham, North Carolina, USA

OREN N. GOTTFRIED, MD
Clinical Vice Chair of Quality, Department of Neurosurgery, Division of Spine, Duke University, Durham, North Carolina, USA

JASON J. HASELHUHN, DO
Research Fellow, Department of Orthopedic Surgery, University of Minnesota, Minneapolis, Minnesota, USA

IBRAHIM HUSSAIN, MD
Department of Nerosurgery, Weill Cornell Medical Center, New York, New York, USA

EVAN F. JOINER, MD
Chief Resident, Department of Neurological Surgery, Columbia University/NewYork-Presbyterian Hospital, New York, New Year, USA

KRISTEN E. JONES, MD
Assistant Professor, Department of Neurosurgery, University of Minnesota, Minneapolis, Minnesota, USA

MICHAEL LABAGNARA, MD
University of Tennessee, Semmes-Murphey Clinic, Memphis, Tennessee, USA

VIRGINIE LAFAGE, PhD
Assistant Vice President, Department of Orthopaedic Surgery, Lenox Hill Hospital, Northwell Health, New York, New York, USA

AMBER LAMAE PRICE, MD
San Diego Spine Foundation Fellow, Department of Spine Surgery, Scripps Clinic, La Jolla, California, USA

RONALD A. LEHMAN, MD
Chief of Degenerative and Minimally Invasive Spine Surgery, The Daniel and Jane Och Spine Hospital at New York-Presbyterian/Allen, New York, New York, USA

LAWRENCE G. LENKE, MD
Chief of the Division of Spinal Surgery, The Daniel and Jane Och Spine Hospital at NewYork-Presbyterian/Allen, New York, New York, USA

JOCK LILLARD, MD
University of Tennessee, Semmes-Murphey
Clinic, Memphis, Tennessee, USA

JOSEPH R. LINZEY, MD, MS
Resident, Department of Neurosurgery,
University of Michigan, Ann Arbor, Michigan,
USA

MOHAMED MACKI, MD, MPH
Department of Neurosurgery, University of
California, San Francisco, San Francisco,
California, USA

GERARD F. MARCIANO, MD
Department of Orthopedics, Resident,
Columbia University Medical Center, New
York, New York, USA

AYMAN MOHAMED, MD
Research Fellow, Department of Orthopaedic
Surgery, Lenox Hill Hospital, Northwell Health,
New York, New York, USA

PRAVEEN V. MUMMANENI, MD, MBA
Joan O'Reilly Distinguished Professor, Vice
Chair, Department of Neurological Surgery,
University of California, San Francisco, San
Francisco, California, USA

GREGORY M. MUNDIS JR, MD
Fellowship Director, San Diego Spine
Fellowship, Chief of Spine Trauma Scripps
Memorial La Jolla, Department of Spine
Surgery, Scripps Clinic, La Jolla, California,
USA

KOSEI NAGATA, MD, PhD
Spine Surgeon, Norton Leatherman Spine
Center, Louisville, Kentucky, USA

PIERCE D. NUNLEY, MD
Director, Spine Institute of Louisiana,
Shreveport, Louisiana, USA

KARI ODLAND, DAT, ATC, LAT
Researcher, Department of Orthopedic
Surgery, University of Minnesota, Minneapolis,
Minnesota, USA

CHRISTINE PARK, MS
Department of Neurological Surgery, University
of California, San Francisco, San Francisco,
California, USA

PAUL PARK, MD
Professor, University of Tennessee, Semmes-
Murphey Clinic, Memphis, Tennessee, USA

DAVID W. POLLY JR, MD
Chief of Spine Surgery, Professor,
Departments of Orthopedic Surgery and
Neurosurgery, University of Minnesota,
Minneapolis, Minnesota, USA

JERRY E. ROBINSON III, MD
Orthopedic Spine Surgeon, University of
Pittsburg Medical Center (UPMC), Harrisburg,
Pennsylvania, USA

FRANK J. SCHWAB, MD
Department of Orthopaedic Surgery, Lenox Hill
Hospital, Northwell Health, New York, New
York, USA

SAMAN SHABANI, MD
Department of Neurological Surgery, Medical
College of Wisconsin, Milwaukee, Wisconsin,
USA

CHRISTOPHER I. SHAFFREY, MD
Professor, Departments of Neurosurgery and
Orthopaedic Surgery, Division of Spine, Duke
University, Durham, North Carolina, USA

ZACHARY T. SHARFMAN, MD
Department of Orthopaedic Surgery, University
of California, San Francisco, San Francisco,
California, USA

MATTHEW E. SIMHON, MD
Department of Orthopedics, Resident,
Columbia University Medical Center, New
York, New York, USA

PAUL BRIAN O. SORIANO, MD, MBA
Department of Orthopedic Surgery, University
of Minnesota, Minneapolis, Minnesota, USA

OMAR SOROUR, MD
Department of Neurosurgery, University of
California, San Francisco, San Francisco,
California, USA

COLIN P. SPERRING, BS
Department of Neurological Surgery,
Neurological Institute of New York, Columbia
University Vagelos College of Physicians and
Surgeons, New York, New York, USA

LEE TAN, MD
Associate Professor of Neurological Surgery,
Department of Neurosurgery, University of
California, San Francisco, San Francisco,
California, USA

TEERACHAT TANASANSOMBOON, MD
Department of Orthopedic Surgery, Board of
Governors Regenerative Medicine Institute,
Cedars-Sinai Medical Center, Los Angeles,
California, USA; Department of Orthopedics,
Center of Excellence in Biomechanics and
Innovative Spine Surgery, Faculty of
Medicine, Chulalongkorn University, Bangkok,
Thailand

KHOI D. THAN, MD
Professor, Department of Neurosurgery,
Division of Spine, Duke University, Durham,
North Carolina, USA

ALEKOS A. THEOLOGIS, MD
Assistant Professor, Department of
Orthopaedic Surgery, University of California,
San Francisco, San Francisco, California, USA

JUAN S. URIBE, MD
Chief, Professor, Vice Chair, Division of Spinal
Disorders, Department of Neurosurgery,
Barrow Neurological Institute, St. Joseph's

Hospital and Medical Center, Phoenix, Arizona,
USA

MICHAEL S. VIRK, MD, PhD
Department of Nerosurgery, Weill Cornell
Medical Center, New York, New York, USA

MICHAEL Y. WANG, MD
Department of Neurosurgery, Professor of
Neurological Surgery and Rehabilitation
Medicine, University of Miami, Department of
Neurological Surgery, University of Miami
Miller School of Medicine, Miami, Florida,
USA

MICHAEL D. WHITE, MD
Department of Neurosurgery, Barrow
Neurological Institute, St. Joseph's Hospital
and Medical Center, Phoenix, Arizona,
USA

HANCI ZHANG, MD
Spine Fellow, Norton Leatherman Spine
Center, Louisville, Kentucky, USA

Contents

Section I: Preoperative Planning and Goals of Surgery

Adult spinal deformity (ASD) is common and the complication rate in ASD surgery is high due to its invasiveness. There are several factors that increase the risk of complications with ASD surgery. These include age, past medical history, frailty, osteoporosis, or operative invasiveness. Risk factors for perioperative complications can be categorized as modifiable and non-modifiable. The purpose of this article is to present the current available evidence on risk factors for perioperative complications, with a focus on frailty, osteoporosis, surgical site infection prevention, and hip-spine syndrome. In addition, we present the latest evidence for patient-specific surgical risk assessment and surgical planning.

Sagittal spinal malalignment can lead to pain, decreased function, dynamic imbalance, and compromise of patient-reported health status. The goal of reconstructive spine surgery is to restore spinal alignment parameters, and an understanding of appropriate patient-specific alignment is important for surgical planning and approaches. Radiographic spinopelvic parameters are strongly correlated with pain and function. The relationship between spinopelvic parameters and disability in adult spinal deformity patients is well-established, and optimal correction of sagittal alignment results in improved outcomes regarding patient health status and mechanical complications of surgery.

Adult Spinal Deformity (ASD) is a complex pathologic condition with significant impact on quality of life, including pain, loss of function, and fatigue. Achieving realignment goals is crucial for long-term results. Reliable preoperative planning strategies, including nomograms, measurement tools, and level selection, are key to maximizing the likelihood of achieving a good outcome following ASD corrective surgery. This review covers recent literature on such strategies, including review of the different targets for realignment and their association with outcomes (both patients-reported outcomes and complications), selection of upper and lower instrumented vertebrae, and the latest innovation in preoperative planning for deformity surgery.

Section II: Open Approaches for Deformity

Peter G. Campbell and Pierce D. Nunley

Spine surgeons are often faced with a profoundly difficult challenge in surgically treating adult degenerative scoliosis. Deformity correction surgery is complicated by the difficulty in offering extensive surgical corrections to the elderly, complication-prone population it commonly affects. As spine surgeons attempt to offer minimally invasive solutions to this disease process, the need for fusion of the fractional curve at L4, L5, and S1 may be discounted. A treatment strategy to identify, address, and treat the fractional curve with either open or minimally invasive techniques can lead to improved patient outcomes and decrease revision rates in this complicated pathologic process.

Hanci Zhang, Leah Y. Carreon, and John R. Dimar II

There are a range of anterior-based approaches to address flexible adult spinal deformity from the thoracic spine to the sacrum, with each approach offering access to a range of vertebral levels. It includes the transperitoneal (L5–S1), paramedian anterior retroperitoneal (L3–S1), oblique retroperitoneal (L1–2 to L5–S1), the thoracolumbar transdiaphragmatic approach (T9–10 to L4–5), and thoracotomy approach (T4–T12). The lumbar and lumbosacral spine is especially favorable for anterior-based approaches given the relative mobility of the peritoneal organs and position of the vasculature.

Evan F. Joiner, Praveen V. Mummaneni, Christopher I. Shaffrey, and Andrew K. Chan

Posterior-based osteotomies are crucial to the restoration of lordosis in adult spinal deformity. Posterior-column osteotomies are suited for patients with an unfused anterior column and non-focal sagittal deformity requiring modest correction in lordosis. When performed on multiple levels, posterior-column osteotomy may provide significant harmonious correction in patients who require more extensive correction. Pedicle subtraction osteotomy and vertebral column resection are appropriate for patients with a fused anterior column and more severe deformity, particularly focal and/or multiplanar deformity. The power of pedicle subtraction osteotomy and vertebral column resection to provide greater correction and to address multiplanar deformity comes at the cost of higher complication rates than posterior-column osteotomy.

David W. Polly Jr., Jason J. Haselhuhn, Paul Brian O. Soriano, Kari Odland, and Kristen E. Jones

The Meyerding classification grades the degree of slippage in the sagittal plane on lateral standing neutral imaging: 0% to 25% Grade I, 25% to 50% Grade II, 50% to 75% Grade III, 75% to 100% Grade IV, and greater than 100% Grade V (Spondyloptosis). Grades I and II are considered low-grade and Grades III-V are considered high-grade. There are several etiologies of spondylolisthesis. A classification system of the most common causes: Type I – Dysplastic, Type II – Isthmic (including subtypes: A – Lytic, B – Elongation, and C – Acute fracture), Type III – Degenerative, Type IV – Traumatic, Type V – Pathologic, and Type VI – Iatrogenic. Dysplastic spondylolisthesis is a type of spondylolisthesis that occurs at L5-S1 when dysplastic lumbosacral anatomy is present, and is associated with high-grade slip and spina bifida occulta.

Proximal junctional kyphosis (PJK) and proximal junctional failure/fractures (PJF) are common complications following long-segment posterior instrumented fusions for adult spinal deformity. As progression to PJF involves clinical consequences for patients and requires costly revisions that may undermine the utility of surgery and are ultimately unsustainable for health care systems, preventative strategies to minimize the occurrence of PJF are of tremendous importance. In this article, the authors present a detailed outline of PJK and PJF with a focus on surgical strategies aimed at preventing their occurrence.

Distal junctional pathology remains an unsolved issue in spine surgery. Distal junctional pathology can occur on a spectrum from asymptomatic radiographic finding to catastrophic distal construct failure. It is significant to address as postoperative sagittal balance has been shown to be correlated with patient-reported outcomes. Current literature and clinical experience suggest there are techniques that can be implemented regardless of setting to avoid distal junctional pathology. Much of the avoidant strategy relies on understanding the deformity pathology, selection of the lowest instrumented vertebra (LIV), health of the segments caudal to the LIV, and methods of fixation.

Section III: MIS Approaches for Deformity

Evidenced-based data-driven decision-making algorithms guide patient and approach selection for adult spinal deformity surgery. Algorithms are continually refined as surgical goals and intraoperative technology evolve.

The lateral transpsoas approach has become fundamental to minimally invasive spine surgery. The large interbody grafts that can be placed through this approach allow for robust arthrodesis of the anterior column, indirect decompression, and restoration of lordosis without disrupting the posterior musculature or ligamentous structures. The lateral decubitus position has traditionally been used for this approach but the prone position has gained popularity because it can reduce operating times for patients who also require posterior pedicle screw fixation. The transpsoas approach can be effectively performed in either position but surgeons should know the nuances that distinguish them.

Deformity surgery is advancing quickly with the use of three-dimensional navigation and robotics. In spinal fusion, the use of robotics improves screw placement accuracy and reduces radiation, complications, blood loss, and recovery time. Currently, there is limited evidence showing that robotics is better than traditional freehand techniques. Most studies favoring robotics are small and retrospective due to the novelty of the technology in deformity surgery. Using these systems can also be expensive and time-consuming. Surgeons should use these advancements as tools, but not rely on them to replace surgical experience, anatomy knowledge, and good judgment.

Section IV: Postoperative Optimization

Adult spinal deformity (ASD) is a complex disease that can result in significant disability. Although surgical treatment has been shown to be of benefit, the complication rate in the perioperative and postoperative periods can be as high as 70%. Some of the most common complications of ASD surgery include intraoperative cerebrospinal fluid leak, high blood loss, new neurologic deficit, hardware failure, proximal junctional kyphosis/failure, pseudarthrosis, surgical site infection, and medical complications. For each of these complications, one or more strategies can be utilized to avoid and/or minimize the consequences.

The authors outline a review of preoperative, intraoperative, and postoperative considerations surrounding adult spinal deformity. Preoperative management topics include imaging, hemoglobin A1c levels before spine surgery, osteoporotic management, and prehabilitation. Topics surrounding intraoperative management include the use of antibiotics, liposomal bupivacaine, and Foley catheters. The authors also discuss postoperative questions surrounding analgesia, nausea and vomiting, thromboembolic prophylaxis, and early mobilization. Throughout their discussion, the authors incorporate enhanced recovery after surgery protocols to hopefully lead to future discussions regarding optimizing complex spinal patients.

Outcome assessment in adult spinal deformity has evolved from radiographic analysis of curve correction to patient-centered perception of health-related quality-of-life. Oswestry Disability Index and the Scoliosis Research Society-22 Patient Questionnaire are the predominantly used patient-reported outcome (PRO) measurements for deformity surgery. Correction of sagittal alignment correlates with improved PRO. Functional outcomes and accelerometer measurements represent newer methods of measuring outcomes but have not yet been widely adopted or validated. Further adoption of a minimum set of core outcome domains will help facilitate international comparisons and benchmarking, and ultimately enhance value-based healthcare.

NEUROSURGERY CLINICS OF NORTH AMERICA

FORTHCOMING ISSUES

January 2024
Epilepsy Surgery: Paradigm Shifts
Jimmy Yang and R. Mark Richardson, *Editors*

April 2024
New Technologies in Spine Surgery
Adam S. Kanter and Nicholas Theodore, *Editors*

July 2024
**Disorders and Treatment of the Cerebral
Venous System**
Shahid M. Nimjee, *Editor*

RECENT ISSUES

July 2023
Meningioma
Randy L. Jensen and Gabriel Zada, *Editors*

April 2023
Ablative Therapies in Neurosurgery
Peter Nakaji and Oliver Bozinov, *Editors*

January 2023
Chiari I Malformation
David D. Limbrick and Jeffrey Leonard, *Editors*

SERIES OF RELATED INTEREST

Neurologic Clinics
https://www.neurologic.theclinics.com/
Neuroimaging Clinics
https://www.neuroimaging.theclinics.com/

Preface
Spinal Deformity Update

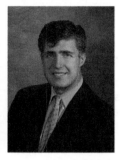
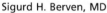
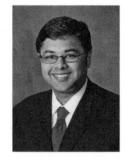

Sigurd H. Berven, MD   Praveen V. Mummaneni, MD, MBA

Editors

The management of spinal deformity is characterized by significant variability between providers. An evidence-based approach to care requires systems-based optimization across the continuum of care from preoperative optimization to intraoperative standardization through postoperative rehabilitation. Prospective, multicenter research efforts have led to significant advances in our evidence-based approach to the management of spinal deformity. The purpose of this issue of *Neurosurgery Clinics of North America* is to provide an update on information regarding the management of spinal deformity that will guide an optimal, evidence-based approach to care.

The readers will find that the issue comprises four sections with the intention of providing the reader with a comprehensive update on important topics along the continuum of care. Section 1 is focused on preoperative considerations, including identification and optimization of the patient prior to surgery, surgical planning, and defining the goals of alignment for surgical reconstructions. Preoperative optimization, including recognition and modification of risk factors, has an important impact on safety and quality of care and complication avoidance. Understanding alignment goals and achieving those goals with surgery have a measurable impact on avoiding complications, including implant failure and junctional pathology.

Sections 2 and 3 are focused on operative strategies for specific pathologies and include open and minimally invasive approaches to care. The operative management of spinal deformity encompasses a broad range of options regarding surgical invasiveness, choice of fusion levels, and reconstructive strategies. The development of innovative approaches for mobilization and stabilization of spinal deformity provides the surgeon with alternative approaches to care, each of which has specific expected outcomes and risks. The authors of the 19 articles on surgical approaches to spinal deformity provide valuable information on the indications, techniques, and risks of each approach. Understanding the approaches discussed will empower the reader to make an informed choice regarding the appropriate approach for a specific patient.

The final section addresses postoperative considerations. Early recovery after surgery pathways, evidence-based postoperative protocols, and standard care pathways have a significant and measurable impact on postoperative complication avoidance. Measuring outcomes of spinal deformity surgery is the metric of accountability for care. Adult spinal deformity has a significant and measurable impact on self-reported health status, and a sustained improvement of patient health is a critical goal in a value-based health economy.

The optimal management of spinal deformity requires system-based reforms across the continuum of care. This issue of *Neurosurgery Clinics of North America* provides the reader with important updates regarding an evidence-based approach to optimal care. The evolution of our understanding of appropriate goals of reconstruction, surgical strategies, and postoperative pathways is dynamic and ongoing. This issue is intended to provide updates based upon the best available current evidence. Ongoing innovations and outcomes assessment will require a

Neurosurg Clin N Am 34 (2023) xiii–xiv
https://doi.org/10.1016/j.nec.2023.06.017
1042-3680/23/© 2023 Published by Elsevier Inc.

neurosurgery.theclinics.com

continual reassessment of appropriate and optimal care.

Sigurd H. Berven, MD
Department of Orthopaedic Surgery
UC San Francisco
500 Parnassus Avenue, MU320W
San Francisco, CA 94143, USA

Praveen V. Mummaneni, MD, MBA
UCSF Department of Neurosurgery
505 Parnassus Avenue, M780
San Francisco, CA 94143, USA

E-mail addresses:
Sigurd.Berven@ucsf.edu (S.H. Berven)
Praveen.mummaneni@ucsf.edu
(P.V. Mummaneni)

Section I: Preoperative planning and Goals of Surgery

Preoperative Optimization
Risk Factors for Perioperative Complications and Preoperative Modification

Kosei Nagata, MD, PhD, John R. Dimar II, MD, Leah Y. Carreon, MD, MSc*,
Steven D. Glassman, MD

KEYWORDS

- Adult spinal deformity • Complications • Frailty • Osteoporosis • Surgical site infection
- Hip-spine syndrome • Planning

KEY POINTS

- Corrective surgery for adult spinal deformity (ASD) typically requires complex invasive procedures and the complication rate for complex, multilevel fusion surgery is high.
- Identification of risk factors for complications and preoperative intervention to change modifiable risk factors are important to medically optimize patients undergoing ASD corrective surgery and to reduce complication rates.
- Spinal deformity surgeons should be aware that almost half of surgical site infections can be prevented by adhering to protocols including appropriate antimicrobial prophylaxis and control of blood sugar levels.
- Spine surgeons must develop a preoperative surgical plan to achieve the ideal spinal alignment for each patient, considering the patient's age, global sagittal and coronal alignment, pelvic parameters as well as the presence of any hip and knee pathology.

INTRODUCTION

Adult spinal deformity (ASD) is a common and important disorder,[1,2] and is associated with disability similar to that of other chronic conditions such as diabetes mellitus and rheumatoid arthritis. Patients with symptomatic ASD have several treatment options, including non-operative care and surgeries with variable invasiveness.[3] One of the major concerns regarding invasive surgery for ASD is its high rate of complications.

Corrective surgery for ASD provides favorable outcomes but also poses a substantial risk for major complications, which deteriorate outcomes in both the perioperative and long-term postoperative periods.[4] Surgery for ASD typically requires extensive dissection, spinal fusion over several segments, osteotomies, blood transfusion, and extended hospitalization.[5] These factors all lead to a higher complication rate in ASD surgery compared to short-level spine surgery.[6] Members of the Scoliosis Research Society (SRS) are required to submit complication data annually and that data constitute the annual Morbidity and Mortality (M&M) report. A review of 4980 cases from the SRS registry revealed a 13.4% surgeon-reported complication rate in 2011.[7] Previous studies reported that the incidence of complications in ASD surgery ranged from 24% to 62%, and notably a major complication rate of 8% to 38%.[7–14]

When surgical management has been selected, effective preoperative planning requires the creation of an individualized surgical plan and the consideration of patient-specific risk factors that

Norton Leatherman Spine Center, 210 East Gray Street, Suite 900, Louisville, KY 40202, USA
* Corresponding author.
E-mail address: leah.carreon@nortonhealthcare.org

Neurosurg Clin N Am 34 (2023) 505–517
https://doi.org/10.1016/j.nec.2023.06.015
1042-3680/23/© 2023 Elsevier Inc. All rights reserved.

might affect the postoperative course.[6] Several factors, including age, past medical history, frailty, osteoporosis, or operative invasiveness, have been shown in previous studies to increase the risk of complications in patients undergoing surgery for ASD (**Table 1**).[7–9,11,12,14,15] These are categorized as modifiable and non-modifiable factors; that is, patient's age cannot be changed but it is possible to optimize the patient's medical condition and adjust the surgical plan. In this article, we present specific important risk factors for perioperative complications and preoperative strategies to mitigate the risk factors of ASD surgery based on the latest evidence.

FRAILTY
Epidemiology of Frailty

Frailty is a measure of physiologic age with a global prevalence estimated to be 10.7%. The prevalence is expected to rise to 26% in those older than age 85 by 2050.[16] Frailty is as an independent predictor of morbidity and mortality in patients undergoing spine surgery.[5,15] A recent systematic review[17] showed that the presence of frailty doubled the odds ratio for any complication. Particularly in ASD, significantly frail patients had high odds ratios compared with non-frail patients for proximal junctional kyphosis (PJK), ranging from 3.1 to 7.0.[17] Optimization of a patient's frailty status and efforts to restore their physiologic strength have the potential to improve outcomes in corrective spinal surgery.

Evaluation of Frailty

There are 2 major frailty models that are widely described in the literature[18]: the Frailty Index (FI)[19] and the Fried's frailty phenotype (FP).[20] The FI considers frailty as an accumulation of deficits, which includes both physical and psychosocial aspects of frailty, with a higher number of deficits indicating a worse frailty score.[19] For preoperative evaluation, the use of the 5-item modified frailty index (mFI-5) and/or the conventional 11-item modified frailty index (mFI-11) have been described.[15,21,22] An increase of 2 points in mFI-5 resulted in a 2.2-fold increase in the risk ratio for serious complications in spinal surgery.[15] Alternatively, the FP[20] defines frailty as a distinct clinical syndrome when more than 3 of 5 phenotypic criteria are met.[20] These phenotypes include weakness (grip strength), self-reported exhaustion, slow walking speed, low levels of physical activity, and unintentional weight loss. In addition to these 2 methods, the following measures had the strongest clinimetric properties in risk stratification tools: the FRAIL scale, Frailty Index of Accumulative Deficits, Comprehensive Geriatric Assessment, adult spinal deformity frailty index , and Edmonton Frailty Scale.[18,23]

Compared with accumulated knowledge of frailty measurements to date, complementary molecular biomarkers of frailty have not yet been identified.[24] Based on the theory that the immune system is involved in aging, inflammatory markers such as interleukin-6, C-reactive protein, and tumor necrosis factor alpha have all been shown to be elevated in the frail population.[25] Another review article introduced interleukin-6, C-X-C motif chemokine ligand 10 (CXCL10), and C-X3-C motif chemokine ligand 1 (CX3CL1) as a *core* panel of frailty biomarkers.[24] Telomere length, one of the candidates for genetic age biomarkers, has also been found to be associated with risk of complications in ASD for certain ethnic groups.[26]

Table 1
Risk factors with the most significant reference for each listed

Risk Factors	Related Important References	Number of Patients Analyzed	Complication Rate
Age	Yamato Y, J Orthop Sci 2017:22:237–242	1192	14.5%
Past medical history[a]	Yoshida G, Spine 2018:43:562–570	304	35.5%
Frailty	Yagi M, Spine 2019:44:E1083–E1091	281	39.1%
Osteoporosis	Bjerke BT, Global Spine J 2018:8:563–569	140	32.1%
Operative invasiveness	Sansur CA, Spine 2011:20:E593-E597	4980	13.4%

[a] In this reference, past medical history was analyzed as the Charlson Comorbidity Index and American Society of Anesthesiologists physical status.

Recommendations for Frailty

Many pharmacologic strategies are currently under investigation with respect to addressing frailty. Hormonal replacement therapies, such as testosterone, estrogen, or growth hormone, have an unacceptable side effect profile and limited proven clinical efficacy.[24] The benefit of daily vitamin D supplements on gait and posture has been proposed.[27] Protein supplementation is a potentially appealing strategy to prevent muscle loss.[28] Generally, an average daily intake of protein of at least 1.0 to 1.2 g per kg body weight per day in older adults has been recommended, and still higher amounts (1.2–1.5 g per kg body weight per day) can be recommended in patients with marked malnutrition.[28] However, research on nutritional supplementation as an intervention for frailty has yielded mixed results and evidence supporting its efficacy is lacking.[18]

Although a range of interventions have been explored, no single evidence-based exercise intervention to address frailty has been identified.[29] Additionally, there is a lack of a standardized exercise protocol throughout the literature.[18] A multidisciplinary discussion system that included anesthetists, critical care, and palliative care teams for frail patients scheduled for major noncardiac surgery has been evaluated.[30] When perioperative plans were modified based on a patient's frailty status, a reduction in mortality from 12.2% to 3.8% was observed among frail patients ($P < .001$).[30] In the field of spine surgery, cases that are discussed and evaluated at multidisciplinary committees where surgical risk and adjust treatment plans are debated have fewer complications than those who are not.[31] These findings suggest the efficacy of patient-specific planning in decreasing complications.

OSTEOPOROSIS
Epidemiology of Osteoporosis

Osteoporosis globally affects approximately 6.3% of men and 21.2% of women over the age of 50.[32] In the United States, the estimated prevalence of osteoporosis increases following the age categories; 5.1%, 8.0%, 16.4%, and 26.2% in 50s, 60s, 70s, and 80s and older, respectively.[33] However, osteoporosis is frequently undiagnosed in patients undergoing spine surgery.[34] Jain and colleagues reported that only 14.3% of patients with osteoporosis undergoing multilevel spinal fusion had received preoperative osteoporosis treatment yet osteoporosis is associated with a significant complication profile in ASD corrective surgery.[34] Patients with poor bone health are at an increased risk of instrumentation failure, pseudarthrosis, vertebral fractures, PJK, and revision surgery.[35,36] A meta-analysis showed that osteoporosis doubled the odds ratio for PJK.[37] Bjerke and colleagues reported that the incidence of osteoporosis-related complications was 23%, 33%, and 50.0% for patients who are considered normal, osteopenic, and osteoporotic, respectively.[38]

Evaluation of Osteoporosis

The preoperative evaluation of a patient's bone health is crucial for surgical planning and preoperative medical optimization.[38–40] To measure bone mineral density (BMD), dual-energy X-ray absorptiometry (DEXA) is presently used as the gold standard[41,42] However, DEXA has limited access and reliability.[40] Some studies have shown that plain computed tomography (CT) axial images can be substituted for DEXA by measuring Hounsfield unit (HU) in an elliptical region of interest in the lumbar vertebral body.[40,43–45] The HU threshold for osteoporosis is proposed as a range between 80 and 135,[43–45] and a difference of 50 HU in plain CT corresponds to a 1.0 T-score difference in DEXA.[43] DEXA is recommended for further evaluation when the HU of lumbar CT is less than or equal to 150.[34]

Recommendations for Osteoporosis

Treatment of osteoporosis consists of physical and pharmacologic therapies.[18] Weight-bearing exercises such as walking, running, and resistance training appear beneficial in maintaining and improving bone strength, although the optimum frequency and duration have yet to be determined.[46] Pharmacologic treatment should be started with an anabolic agent along with adequate calcium and vitamin D intake[47] Recommendations by the National Osteoporosis Foundation suggest a total calcium intake of 1000 mg/d for men aged 50 to 70, or 1200 mg/d for women over 50 and men over 70 years, as well as vitamin D intake of 800 to 1000 IU/day.[46] However, an ancillary study of the Vitamin D and Omega-3 Trial showed that vitamin D3 supplementation did not result in a significantly lower risk of fractures than placebo among generally healthy midlife and older adults who did not have vitamin D deficiency, low bone mass, or osteoporosis.[48] A recent meta-analysis argued that neither intermittent nor daily dosing with standard doses of vitamin D alone was associated with reduced risk of fracture, but daily supplementation with both vitamin D and calcium was a more promising strategy.[49] Based on these data, an individualized pretreatment evaluation is recommended for each patient.

Parathyroid hormone receptor agonists, teriparatide and abaloparatide, are recommended as first-line treatment prior to ASD surgery if no contraindications are present.[34,36] Teriparatide use has been shown to reduce the time to interbody fusion by 3 months compared to no treatment or bisphosphonate alone.[50,51] Teriparatide use for osteopenia has also been shown to be cost-effective; associated with a mean incremental net monetary benefit of $3948 in patients undergoing ASD surgery.[52] Approximately 50% improvement in lumbar BMD can be expected at 3 months and 75% at 6 months after the start of teriparatide administration.[53] When teriparatide was administrated less than 2 months preoperatively or less than 8 months postoperatively, the benefit was limited and the dose was considered insufficient.[54,55] Therefore, in patients on teriparatide, ASD surgery requires a waiting period of 3 months for patients with osteopenia and 6 months for patients with severe osteoporosis.[34] Treatment with teriparatide is limited to a lifetime maximum duration of 18 or 24 months.[34,36] A new treatment, romosozumab, an antisclerostin monoclonal antibody that stimulates bone formation and inhibits resorption,[56] followed by alendronate has been shown to be as effective in preventing vertebral fractures as teriparatide.[56] Although there are currently guidelines on how long romosozumab can be administered, transition from romosozumab to antiresorptive drugs is required. The optimal strategy for cycling anabolics to antiresorptives remains to be determined.[56]

Medication history should be checked carefully because treatment sequence matters.[47] If antiresorption drugs (bisphosphonates or anti-receptor activator of nuclear factor kappa beta [RANL] inhibitors) were used for a long period beforehand, use of teriparatide risks a temporary decrease in BMD, requiring 18 to 24 months for recovery.[47] Combined therapy can be an option in selected cases; denosumab was combined with teriparatide and found to be more effective than teriparatide alone in achieving interbody fusion.[57]

SURGICAL SITE INFECTIONS
Epidemiology of Surgical Site Infections After Adult Spinal Deformity Surgery

Multilevel corrective surgery for ASD has a higher infection rate than short spinal fusion.[58] From the SRS M&M database, the rates of postoperative surgical site infection (SSI) after spinal instrumentation surgery were 1.2% in 2012, 1.3% in 2015, and 0.95% in 2020.[58,59] Specifically,

postoperative SSI rates were 4.2% for adult kyphosis, 2.1% for adult spondylolisthesis, and 3.7% for adult scoliosis.[58] In a more recent prospective study, SSI rate reported was 12% to13% for multilevel thoracolumbar spine surgery.[60] The implant preservation rate after SSI is 85% at 1 year and 73% at 2 years,[61] making it all the more important for spine surgeons to properly understand the risks of SSI and implement preventive measures. Implant removal may result in progressive deformity,[62] loss of correction, or pseudoarthrosis requiring reinstrumentation in 23% to 40% of cases.[61,62]

Current Evidence of Antimicrobial Prophylaxis and Glycemic Control

Antimicrobial prophylaxis choice
Antimicrobial prophylaxis (AMP) administration is an evidence-based SSI prevention strategy. The choice of AMP should be based on their antimicrobial activity against the indigenous flora of the surgical site.[63] The American Society of Health-System Pharmacists (ASHP) guideline recommends that 2 g or 3 g (for patients weighted more than 120 kg) cefazolin be the first choice and the optimal time for administration of preoperative doses is within 60 minutes before surgical incision.[64] Avoidance of cefazolin in patients with penicillin allergy was grounded in evidence from more than 40 years ago that the cross-reactivity rate between penicillins and cephalosporins was 8%.[65] However, a recent meta-analysis revealed a frequency of 0.7% of dual allergy, indicating that most patients with a penicillin allergy may safely receive cefazolin.[65] Clindamycin and vancomycin are acceptable alternatives for patients with a true beta-lactam allergy.[64] For patients colonized with methicillin-resistant Staphylococcus aureus (MRSA), vancomycin should not be used alone but be administered with cefazolin.[64] The SRS M&M database showed that the administration of vancomycin alone paradoxically increased the proportion of MRSA among SSIs.[58]

Antimicrobial prophylaxis duration
The new World Health Organization (WHO)[66] and Centers for Disease Control and Prevention (CDC)[67] guidelines recommended no additional AMP dose after wound closure. However, a detailed analysis of the WHO guidelines[66] showed that the pooled risk ratio of postoperative AMP use was 0.51 ($P < .001$) when limited to clean orthopedic and cardiovascular surgeries.[63] This indicates that postoperative administration was still preferable.[63] The CDC guideline also focused on general surgery procedures with only 6 orthopedic-related studies (4 on fracture surgery and 2 on

arthroplasty).[63,67] The ASHP guideline recommends that AMP be discontinued within 24 h after closure for spine surgeries with instrumentation.[64] Unnecessary prolongation of the AMP should be discouraged because of the potential risk of adverse events and antibiotic resistance.[68] Two randomized control trials revealed that the use of AMP more than 24 h after spinal instrumentation surgery had no effect on SSI prevention.[60,68] However, in almost half of the cases with SSI in the SRS M&M database, AMP was used more than 24 h after skin closure.[58]

Glycemic control

Glycosylated hemoglobin (HbA1c) is a biomarker to assess long-term glycemic control in diabetic patients. Keeping HbA1c levels below 7.0 is currently recommended by the American Diabetes Association prior to elective surgery for optimal reduction of postoperative complications.[69] In the field of spine surgery, a recent systematic review showed that patients with an HbA1c of 6.5 to 6.9 had a higher risk of postoperative complications.[70] Another study showed that HbA1c levels above 7.8 were associated with less improvement of patient-reported outcome measures after elective lumbar surgery.[71]

Recommendations for Surgical Site Infection Prevention with/Without Vancomycin Powder

Some institutions introduced a standardized infection reduction protocol and succeeded in reducing SSI rates.[72,73] Poe-Kochert, et al.[72] introduced a protocol including (1) preoperative screening for nasal MRSA colonization 2 weeks preoperatively, and treatment with intranasal mupirocin when positive, (2) a preoperative chlorohexidine scrub, (3) timing of standardized AMP administration, (4) standardized intraoperative redosing of antibiotics, (5) limiting operating room traffic, and (6) standardized postoperative wound care. Intrawound vancomycin powder was introduced during the middle of the study and succeeded in decreasing SSI rates from 7.5% to 2.5% (P = .01).[72] Yamada and colleagues adopted evidence-based protocols including (1) additional vancomycin prophylaxis, (2) diluted povidone-iodine irrigation, and (3) nasal and body decontamination for high-risk patients through nasal MRSA screening.[73] Even without the use intrawound vancomycin powder, the SSI rate still decreased significantly from 3.8% to 0.7% (P < .01) after the intervention.[73]

Considering these 2 studies, the use of intrawound vancomycin powder is optional. One meta-analysis[74] revealed that the pooled estimate from 8 observational studies from the United States

indicated that the use of intrawound vancomycin statistically significantly reduced the odds of SSI. Another meta-analysis[75] of 3 prospective randomized studies showed that the overall risk ratio was 1.22 (95% CI = 0.62–2.40, P = .48), indicating no significant difference in SSI rates between cohorts with or without vancomycin powder use. A recent fourth randomized trial also found vancomycin powder to be ineffective.[76] A meta-analysis showed that vancomycin powder might also increase the rate of gram-negative and polymicrobial SSI.[77] Surgeons should be cautious before widely adopting this intervention and should be vigilant in monitoring for adverse effects including anaphylactoid reaction.[78] Almost half of SSIs can be preventable by the institution of an evidence-based infection prevention protocol.[67]

HIP-SPINE SYNDROME
Etiology of Hip-Spine Syndrome

Almost 40 years have passed since the concept of hip-spine syndrome was introduced by Offierski and MacNab.[79] Originally, "secondary hip-spine syndrome" was defined as spine symptoms, which were associated with or aggravated by deformity of the hips, or vice versa.[79] Hip joints, as the adjacent joints of the spine, can be affected by spinal corrective fusion surgery, and increased forces at the hip joint may lead to progression of hip arthritis.[80] Similarly, decreased hip joint mobility from osteoarthritis or leg length discrepancies have an impact on spine alignment.[80]

The pelvic incidence (PI) is a constant morphologic parameter that enables surgeons to predict the baseline individual sagittal alignment. This is a static anatomic parameter that does not change with positioning of the spine or pelvis. In contrast, sacral slope (SS), pelvic tilt (PT), and lumbar lordosis (LL) are variable parameters, with values dependent on body position. For planning ASD corrective spinal fusion, LL should be proportional to the PI,[81] and this is based on the theory that PI is an individual-specific parameter that changes little. A recent study has shown that total hip arthroplasty (THA) alone in patients (mean 40 year old) with high-grade developmental dysplasia of the hip increased the PI by 20°[82] without changing the SS and LL, possibly due to their relatively young age and flexibility of the lumbar spine.[82] On the other hand, in older patients (mean 61 year old) with osteoarthritis, the PI did not change before and after THA.[83] Kleeman-Forsthuber, et al. analyzed 9414 patients (mean 65 year old) and concluded that the PI alone was not indicative of either spinal or pelvic mobility.[84] This study also showed that patients with spinal deformities in the sagittal plane had increased spinopelvic stiffness, which may be the mechanism by which PI affects the risk of dislocation after THA.[84] Whether THA improves the ability of the hip joint to contribute to compensation should be evaluated and further studies are required.[84]

Current Evidence of Hip-Spine Syndrome

Kawai and colleagues retrospectively studied (retrospective means review) data in patients without hip degeneration who underwent lumbar spinal fusion and found that the rate of narrowing of the hip joint was 0.06 mm/y for single-level fusions, and 0.31 mm/y in patients with 7 or more fusion levels.[80] Interestingly, the rate of joint narrowing did not significantly change over time through 4 years postoperatively.[80] These results and previous reports indicate that long spinal fusion is associated with worsening of at least 1 Kellgren-Lawrence grade of hip osteoarthritis.

Dislocation is one of the most serious complications of THA. Patients with a history of both THA and a lumbar spinal fusion have increased risk of dislocation and hip revision.[85] The risk of THA dislocation and revision increased in patients who also had concurrent sagittal plane deformities compared with those without.[86] The incidence of THA dislocation in patients with prior lumbosacral fusion was higher at 1 year (3% vs 0.4%) and at 2 years (7.5% vs 2.1%) after surgery than in patients who have not had a fusion.[86] Decreased spinopelvic motion is compensated for by increased femoral anteversion with hip joint flexion when lumbar spinal corrective fusion is performed for adult spinal deformity.[81,87] The ensuing clinical consequence includes a risk of THA impingement or dislocation.[87] Additionally, the consequence of this inverse relationship, decreased cup motion and increased femoral motion, is the potential for cup positioning outside the functional safe zone despite positioning within the accepted anatomic Lewinnek zone.[86]

Recommendations for Reducing the Effect of Hip-Spine Syndrome

For patients with concomitant degenerative hip joints and lumbar spine disorders, the optimal order of treatment remains controversial even for experienced surgeons.[88] Treating the hip first may decrease additional or unnecessary spine procedures because eliminating hip pain has also been found to eliminate lower back pain.[87,89] However, THA surgeons (members of the North American Hip Society) and spine surgeons [Scoliosis Research Society (SRS) members] agree that patients with hip osteoarthritis and myelopathy or weakness should undergo spine surgery first.[88]

Some have suggested that deformity correction could decrease the risk of THA dislocation.[90] Lumbar osteotomy decreases pelvic tilt (PT), as a function of increased structural similarity (SS), but also causes a decrease in anteversion at the acetabulum. Every 5° reduction in PT decreases acetabular anteversion by 2.5° to 5°.[91] Sitting position decreases SS and LL by 20° compared with standing position,[92,93] and long spinal fusion to pelvis prevents such compensation mobility, resulting in anterior impingement.[92] The predictable impact of sagittal imbalance correction on acetabular anteversion warrants consideration in patients with sagittal imbalance and an existing THA. Lumbar osteotomy could place the pelvis in a more anatomic position or correct retroversion, and in turn decrease the risk of dislocation after subsequent THA.[90] There is "fair evidence" that correcting the spinal deformity first has the potential to decrease hip dislocation following THA as it allows proper positioning of the acetabular component in patients with ASD and concurrent hip abnormality.[94] Three-dimensional modeling of implant impingement after spinal corrective fusion surgery in patients with previous THA can be feasible tool for planning.[95] A recent review recommended the use of THA dual mobility cup to increase the stability for patients with lower lumbar spine fusions.[92]

In summary, long instrumented fusion is a potential risk factor for hip joint degeneration and of THA dislocation/revision. Preoperative planning for deformity correction and the use of advanced imaging systems or patient-specific implants may improve precision in achieving ideal parameters.[87] Spine surgeons can utilize guidelines from hip surgeons[86] for patients who may need ASD corrective fusion and THA simultaneously. Bridging the gap between hip and spine surgeons with an up-to-date analysis of the best available evidence is still needed.

SURGICAL PLANNING FOLLOWING PATIENT'S RISK ASSESSMENT
Nature of the Problem of Surgical Planning Following Patient's Risk Assessment

The ASD population is extremely heterogeneous presenting many challenges in establishing an appropriate individualized risk assessment for surgical planning.[96] After obtaining accurate individualized risk assessment and modifying each preoperative risk factor, the appropriate surgical plan for each patient is of utmost importance for shared surgical decision-making among the surgeon, the patient, and the patient's family. Such risk evaluation based on surgical planning should be simplified and standardized to provide a balanced risk-benefit assessment and define the patient's needs and appropriate use of medical resources (**Table 2**).

It is important to assess surgical risk during surgery. In posterior spinal surgery, an increase in estimated blood loss by 500 mL and prolongation of operative time by 1 hour have similar odds ratios (1.18–1.19) for major complication.[97] Simple sliding scales are also introduced based on patients' age with the preliminary estimated blood loss and operation time.[8,97] These pieces of evidence allow the spine surgeon to adjust the

---

Table 2
Strategy for adult spine deformity correction surgery planning

First step: plan an ideal correction following the patient status

Deformity patterns	Correction	Fusion levels
Thoracic kyphosis	Correction of kyphosis to predicted value	From T2 to sagittal stable vertebra
Thoracolumbar kyphosis	Correction of the kyphosis to neutral T11–L2	If segmental, the minimum needed for stability If regional, all the thoracolumbar junction
Lumbar kyphosis	Correction of lumbar kyphosis to its predicted lordosis value	If segmental, short fusion of the diseased levels If regional, extend cranially to L2 or T10
Lower lumbar kyphosis	Correction of lower lumbar kyphosis to the predicted lordosis value	L4–S1 or longer, as needed to restore LL
Global kyphosis	Correction of thoracic kyphosis and lumbar lordosis to predicted values	T2–ilium

High-grade[a] osteotomy is considered in rigid, iatrogenic, revision (fused), or high PI cases.

More than 10 levels fusion surgery (overcome apex) is considered in coronal imbalance or neuromuscular diseases like Parkinson disease.

Second step: Estimate each patient's risk considering age, comorbidities, operation time (OPT), estimated blood loss (EBL), and whether high-grade osteotomy or long fusion is required or not.

Third step: Following the Sliding Scale,[8] one or multiple-stage is determined.

Class	Age w/wo comorbidities	Acceptable OPT (maximum)	Acceptable EBL (maximum)
1	< 70 (ASA<3 and CCI<2)	6 h	2000 (40 mL/kg)
2	<70 (ASA$\geq$3 or CCI$\geq$2) 70–74 (ASA<3 and CCI<2)	5 h	1500 (30 mL/kg)
3	70–74 (ASA$\geq$3 or CCI$\geq$2) 75–79 (ASA<3 and CCI<2)	4 h	1000 (20 mL/kg)
4	75–79 (ASA$\geq$3 or CCI$\geq$2) <80	3 h	500 (10 mL/kg)

High-grade osteotomy or fusion segments >10 is not recommended if patients aged 80 or older or 75–79 with ASA$\geq$3 or CCI$\geq$2.

Fourth step: Finalize your plan for adult spinal deformity correction surgery.

Abbreviations: ASA, American Society of Anesthesiologists (ASA) physical status classification system; CCI, the Charlson Comorbidity Index; EBL, estimated blood loss; LL, lumbar lordosis; OPT, operation time; PI, pelvic incidence.
[a] Schwab grade 1 or 2 osteotomy can correct LL by 5 to 10° per level and Schwab grade 3 or higher osteotomy can change LL by 20 to 30° per level. Fusion levels are introduced following the European classifications.[106,107]

surgical plan both preoperatively and intraoperatively based on the surgeon's skill, the extent and number of osteotomies required, and the number of operative levels needed to achieve correction.

Current Evidence of Surgical Planning Following Patient's Risk Assessment

Efforts are ongoing to standardize patients' or surgical factors. Yoshida and colleagues introduced the adaptation and limitation of corrective osteotomy based on patients' age, current medication, and degenerative pathology.[8] Deibo and colleagues analyzed 10,912 patients with ASD and produced the risk score system, including cardiopulmonary disorder, drug abuse, congestive heart failure, neurologic disorder, alcohol abuse, renal failure, age >65, coagulopathy, treating spinal level more than 9, revision, and osteotomy.[98] The score for each element is set from 1 to 14, with the total points ranging 0 to 50.[98] They argued that surgical invasiveness should be determined following the 3 risk thresholds they proposed: mild (0–10), moderate (10–20), and severe >20 points.[98]

Predictive models have substantial potential to improve surgical outcomes for patients with ASD. In 2017, Buchlak and colleagues published the first ASD-specific on-line risk calculator.[99] They developed a decision support system tool that was able to provide a numeric probabilistic likelihood statistical representing an individual patient's risk of developing a complication within the first 30 days after surgery. In 2019, Pellisé and colleagues[100] and Ames and colleagues[101] published and validated ASD-specific on-line risk calculators based on machine learning models predicting 2-year follow-up complications.

Recommendations for Surgical Planning

Clinical benefit of a staged approach is still controversial. Theoretic benefits of staged procedures include preservation of patient endurance through 2 short procedures, reassessment of alignment, and other surgical goals following the conduct of the initial procedure, and minimization of surgeon fatigue.[4] Despite these initial advantages proposed by some deformity surgeons, staged surgery for ASD correction was reported to be an independent risk factor for venous thrombosis or respiratory distress syndrome.[102] These concerns over perioperative risk coupled with a negative impact on cost-efficiency as well as improved posterior-based techniques have resulted in controversy over the benefits of a staged approach in ASD surgery.[4,103] Large randomized control studies are needed because retrospective studies

cannot completely adjust for patient background and alignment.

Reduction of intraoperative blood loss is also another important concern. Several blood conservation strategies had been used to reduce intraoperative blood loss, including autologous blood transfusion, cell salvage, and the use of various pharmacologic agents, that is, esmolol, tranexamic acid, amicar, and aprotinin.[104] Having 2 attending surgeons instead of having 1 attending surgeon and 1 fellow or assistant can also mitigate the risk of complications.[104,105] The use of 2 surgeons at an experienced spine deformity center decreases the operative time and estimated blood loss in pedicle subtraction osteotomies.[105] An evaluation based on cost-efficacy would be necessary. The surgical planning, including medical resources, should be determined by weighing the preliminary optimized patient complications against the surgical invasiveness required for each patient's ideal spinal alignment.

DISCUSSION

Surgical treatment of ASD has advanced significantly over the past 30 years.[3] Historically, patients over 65 years were often considered too old for any fusion procedure, much less a significant ASD correction. Recent advancements in minimally invasive surgical techniques facilitate surgical treatment in the elderly. With this change in approach to ASD, deformity spine surgeons overcame some complications and faced new ones.

Avoiding complications is an important aspirational goal. We previously introduced modifiable risk factors and current evidence; however, there are many unmodifiable factors. Advanced age, male sex, and increased American Society of Anesthesiologists (ASA) class place patients at risk for delay of ASD surgery and patients experiencing surgical delay are at higher risk for postoperative complications, including a 7-fold increase in mortality.[108] These finding perhaps suggest that ASD surgery should be avoided in those with substantial non-modifiable risk factors.[108] Such decisions would require the same determination as making the decision for surgery. More importantly, spine deformity surgeons need to be aware of uncommon but devastating events; that is, superior mesenchymal artery occlusion after ASD correction can be avoidable by examining angle and calcification of the mesenchymal artery.[109] It should also be taken into consideration that spine surgeons tend to overestimate the risk of major complications and reinterventions in the first 72 h and severely underestimate the same risks at

90 days and 2 years postop when compared to the probabilities predicted by the risk calculator.[96]

A system-based approach to ASD surgery is important to identify and modify risks of complications. Early recovery pathways[110] and standardized perioperative care[31] can contribute to subsequent reduction in perioperative complication rates. To enhance safety in patients undergoing complex spinal reconstructions for ASD, the role of spine surgeon as a manager of risk is needed in the next decade.

CLINICS CARE POINTS

- Identification of pathology and appropriate surgical planning.
- Identification of modifiable risk factors for complications.
- Addressing all modifiable risk factors for complications prior to surgery.

DISCLOSURE

The article submitted does not contain information about medical device(s)/drug(s). No funds were received in support of this work. Relevant financial activities outside the submitted work.

REFERENCES

1. Kebaish KM, Neubauer PR, Voros GD, et al. Scoliosis in adults aged forty years and older: prevalence and relationship to age, race, and gender. Spine (Phila Pa 1976) 2011;36(9):731–6.
2. Schwab F, Dubey A, Gamez L, et al. Adult scoliosis: prevalence, SF-36, and nutritional parameters in an elderly volunteer population. Spine (Phila Pa 1976) 2005;30(9):1082–5.
3. Bess S, Line B, Fu KM, et al. The Health Impact of Symptomatic Adult Spinal Deformity: Comparison of Deformity Types to United States Population Norms and Chronic Diseases. Spine (Phila Pa 1976) 2016;41(3):224–33.
4. Passias PG, Poorman GW, Jalai CM, et al. Outcomes of open staged corrective surgery in the setting of adult spinal deformity. Spine J 2017; 17(8):1091–9.
5. Yagi M, Michikawa T, Hosogane N, et al. Treatment for Frailty Does Not Improve Complication Rates in Corrective Surgery for Adult Spinal Deformity. Spine (Phila Pa 1976) 2019;44(10):723–31.
6. Diebo BG, Shah NV, Boachie-Adjei O, et al. Adult spinal deformity. Lancet 2019;394(10193):160–72.
7. Sansur CA, Smith JS, Coe JD, et al. Scoliosis research society morbidity and mortality of adult scoliosis surgery. Spine (Phila Pa 1976) 2011; 36(9):E593–7.
8. Yoshida G, Hasegawa T, Yamato Y, et al. Predicting Perioperative Complications in Adult Spinal Deformity Surgery Using a Simple Sliding Scale. Spine (Phila Pa 1976) 2018;43(8):562–70.
9. Schwab FJ, Hawkinson N, Lafage V, et al. Risk factors for major peri-operative complications in adult spinal deformity surgery: a multi-center review of 953 consecutive patients. Eur Spine J 2012; 21(12):2603–10.
10. Glassman SD, Hamill CL, Bridwell KH, et al. The impact of perioperative complications on clinical outcome in adult deformity surgery. Spine (Phila Pa 1976) 2007;32(24):2764–70.
11. Yamato Y, Matsuyama Y, Hasegawa K, et al. A Japanese nationwide multicenter survey on perioperative complications of corrective fusion for elderly patients with adult spinal deformity. J Orthop Sci 2017;22(2):237–42.
12. Smith JS, Klineberg E, Lafage V, et al. Prospective multicenter assessment of perioperative and minimum 2-year postoperative complication rates associated with adult spinal deformity surgery. J Neurosurg Spine 2016;25(1):1–14.
13. Fu KM, Rhagavan P, Shaffrey CI, et al. Prevalence, severity, and impact of foraminal and canal stenosis among adults with degenerative scoliosis. Neurosurgery 2011;69(6):1181–7.
14. La Maida GA, Luceri F, Gallozzi F, et al. Complication rate in adult deformity surgical treatment: safety of the posterior osteotomies. Eur Spine J 2015;24(Suppl 7):879–86.
15. Yagi M, Michikawa T, Hosogane N, et al. The 5-Item Modified Frailty Index Is Predictive of Severe Adverse Events in Patients Undergoing Surgery for Adult Spinal Deformity. Spine (Phila Pa 1976) 2019;44(18):E1083–91.
16. Walston J, Buta B, Xue QL. Frailty Screening and Interventions: Considerations for Clinical Practice. Clin Geriatr Med 2018;34(1):25–38.
17. Laverdiere C, Georgiopoulos M, Ames CP, et al. Adult Spinal Deformity Surgery and Frailty: A Systematic Review. Global Spine J 2022;12(4):689–99.
18. McCarthy L, Haran E, Ahern DP, et al. Preoperative Considerations for the Frail Patient. Clin Spine Surg 2021. https://doi.org/10.1097/BSD.000000000000 1283.
19. Rockwood K, Song X, MacKnight C, et al. A global clinical measure of fitness and frailty in elderly people. CMAJ (Can Med Assoc J) 2005;173(5): 489–95.
20. Fried LP, Tangen CM, Walston J, et al. Frailty in older adults: evidence for a phenotype. J Gerontol A Biol Sci Med Sci 2001;56(3):M146–56.

21. Kitamura K, van Hooff M, Jacobs W, et al. Which frailty scales for patients with adult spinal deformity are feasible and adequate? A systematic review. Spine J 2022;22(7):1191–204.

22. Akbik OS, Al-Adli N, Pernik MN, et al. A Comparative Analysis of Frailty, Disability, and Sarcopenia With Patient Characteristics and Outcomes in Adult Spinal Deformity Surgery. Global Spine J 2022. https://doi.org/10.1177/219256 82221082053. 21925682221082053.

23. Moskven E, Charest-Morin R, Flexman AM, et al. The measurements of frailty and their possible application to spinal conditions: a systematic review. Spine J 2022;22(9):1451–71.

24. Cardoso AL, Fernandes A, Aguilar-Pimentel JA, et al. Towards frailty biomarkers: Candidates from genes and pathways regulated in aging and age-related diseases. Ageing Res Rev 2018;47:214–77.

25. Soysal P, Stubbs B, Lucato P, et al. Inflammation and frailty in the elderly: a systematic review and meta-analysis. Ageing Res Rev 2016;31:1–8.

26. Araujo Carvalho AC, Tavares Mendes ML, da Silva Reis MC, et al. Telomere length and frailty in older adults-A systematic review and meta-analysis. Ageing Res Rev 2019;54:100914. https://doi.org/10.1016/j.arr.2019.100914.

27. Yoshikawa TT. Changes for the Journal of the American Geriatrics Society effective January 1, 2012. J Am Geriatr Soc 2011;59(12):2199–200.

28. Bauer J, Biolo G, Cederholm T, et al. Evidence-based recommendations for optimal dietary protein intake in older people: a position paper from the PROT-AGE Study Group. J Am Med Dir Assoc 2013;14(8):542–59.

29. Kidd T, Mold F, Jones C, et al. What are the most effective interventions to improve physical performance in pre-frail and frail adults? A systematic review of randomised control trials. BMC Geriatr 2019;19(1):184.

30. Hall DE, Arya S, Schmid KK, et al. Association of a Frailty Screening Initiative With Postoperative Survival at 30, 180, and 365 Days. JAMA Surg 2017; 152(3):233–40.

31. Sethi RK, Pong RP, Leveque JC, et al. The Seattle Spine Team Approach to Adult Deformity Surgery: A Systems-Based Approach to Perioperative Care and Subsequent Reduction in Perioperative Complication Rates. Spine Deform 2014;2(2):95–103.

32. Kanis JA, McCloskey EV, Johansson H, et al. A reference standard for the description of osteoporosis. Bone 2008;42(3):467–75.

33. Wright NC, Looker AC, Saag KG, et al. The Recent Prevalence of Osteoporosis and Low Bone Mass in the United States Based on Bone Mineral Density at the Femoral Neck or Lumbar Spine. J Bone Miner Res 2014;29(11):2520–6.

34. Sardar ZM, Coury JR, Cerpa M, et al. Best Practice Guidelines for Assessment and Management of Osteoporosis in Adult Patients Undergoing Elective Spinal Reconstruction. Spine (Phila Pa 1976) 2022; 47(2):128–35.

35. Karikari IO, Metz LN. Preventing Pseudoarthrosis and Proximal Junctional Kyphosis: How to Deal with the Osteoporotic Spine. Neurosurg Clin N Am 2018;29(3):365–74.

36. Seki S, Hirano N, Kawaguchi Y, et al. Teriparatide versus low-dose bisphosphonates before and after surgery for adult spinal deformity in female Japanese patients with osteoporosis. Eur Spine J 2017;26(8):2121–7.

37. Kim JS, Phan K, Cheung ZB, et al. Surgical, radiographic, and patient-related risk factors for proximal junctional kyphosis: a meta-analysis. Global Spine J 2018;9(1):32–40.

38. Bjerke BT, Zarrabian M, Aleem IS, et al. Incidence of osteoporosis-related complications following posterior lumbar fusion. Global Spine J 2018;8(6): 563–9.

39. Jain N, Labaran L, Phillips FM, et al. Prevalence of osteoporosis treatment and its effect on postoperative complications, revision surgery and costs after multi-level spinal fusion. Global Spine J 2022;12(6):1119–24.

40. Ahern DP, McDonnell JM, Riffault M, et al. A meta-analysis of the diagnostic accuracy of Hounsfield units on computed topography relative to dual-energy X-ray absorptiometry for the diagnosis of osteoporosis in the spine surgery population. Spine J 2021;21(10):1738–49.

41. Bone HG, Hosking D, Devogelaer JP, et al. Ten years' experience with alendronate for osteoporosis in postmenopausal women. N Engl J Med 2004;350(12):1189–99.

42. Cauley JA, Lui LY, Ensrud KE, et al. Bone mineral density and the risk of incident nonspinal fractures in black and white women. JAMA 2005;293(17): 2102–8.

43. Choi MK, Kim SM, Lim JK. Diagnostic efficacy of Hounsfield units in spine CT for the assessment of real bone mineral density of degenerative spine: correlation study between T-scores determined by DEXA scan and Hounsfield units from CT. Acta Neurochir 2016;158(7):1421–7.

44. Hendrickson NR, Pickhardt PJ, Del Rio AM, et al. Bone mineral density t-scores derived from ct attenuation numbers (hounsfield units): clinical utility and correlation with dual-energy x-ray absorptiometry. Iowa Orthop J 2018;38:25–31.

45. Zou D, Li W, Deng C, et al. The use of CT Hounsfield unit values to identify the undiagnosed spinal osteoporosis in patients with lumbar degenerative diseases. Eur Spine J 2019;28(8):1758–66.

46. Cosman F, de Beur SJ, LeBoff MS, et al. Clinician's Guide to Prevention and Treatment of Osteoporosis. Osteoporos Int 2014;25(10):2359–81.

47. Cosman F, Nieves JW, Dempster DW. Treatment Sequence Matters: Anabolic and Antiresorptive Therapy for Osteoporosis. J Bone Miner Res 2017;32(2):198–202.

48. LeBoff MS, Chou SH, Ratliff KA, et al. Supplemental Vitamin D and Incident Fractures in Midlife and Older Adults. N Engl J Med 2022;387(4):299–309.

49. Yao P, Bennett D, Mafham M, et al. Vitamin D and Calcium for the Prevention of Fracture: A Systematic Review and Meta-analysis. JAMA Netw Open 2019;2(12):e1917789.

50. Ohtori S, Inoue G, Orita S, et al. Teriparatide accelerates lumbar posterolateral fusion in women with postmenopausal osteoporosis: prospective study. Spine (Phila Pa 1976) 2012;37(23):E1464–8.

51. Ohtori S, Inoue G, Orita S, et al. Comparison of teriparatide and bisphosphonate treatment to reduce pedicle screw loosening after lumbar spinal fusion surgery in postmenopausal women with osteoporosis from a bone quality perspective. Spine (Phila Pa 1976) 2013;38(8):E487–92.

52. Raad M, Ortiz-Babilonia C, Hassanzadeh H, et al. Cost-utility Analysis of Neoadjuvant Teriparatide Therapy in Osteopenic Patients Undergoing Adult Spinal Deformity Surgery. Spine (Phila Pa 1976) 2022;47(16):1121–7.

53. Leder BZ, Tsai JN, Uihlein AV, et al. Denosumab and teriparatide transitions in postmenopausal osteoporosis (the DATA-Switch study): extension of a randomised controlled trial. Lancet 2015;386(9999):1147–55.

54. Jespersen AB, Andresen ADK, Jacobsen MK, et al. Does systemic administration of parathyroid hormone after noninstrumented spinal fusion surgery improve fusion rates and fusion mass in elderly patients compared to placebo in patients with degenerative lumbar spondylolisthesis? Spine (Phila Pa 1976) 2019;44(3):157–62.

55. Oba H, Takahashi J, Yokomichi H, et al. Weekly teriparatide versus bisphosphonate for bone union during 6 months after multi-level lumbar interbody fusion for osteoporotic patients: a multicenter, prospective, randomized study. Spine (Phila Pa 1976) 2020;45(13):863–71.

56. Reid IR, Billington EO. Drug therapy for osteoporosis in older adults. Lancet 2022;399(10329):1080–92.

57. Ide M, Yamada K, Kaneko K, et al. Combined teriparatide and denosumab therapy accelerates spinal fusion following posterior lumbar interbody fusion. Orthop Traumatol Surg Res 2018;104(7):1043–8.

58. Shillingford JN, Laratta JL, Reddy H, et al. Postoperative surgical site infection after spine surgery:

59. Bivona LJ, France J, Daly-Seiler CS, et al. Spinal deformity surgery is accompanied by serious complications: report from the Morbidity and Mortality Database of the Scoliosis Research Society from 2013 to 2020. Spine Deform 2022. https://doi.org/10.1007/s43390-022-00548-y.

60. Takemoto RC, Lonner B, Andres T, et al. Appropriateness of twenty-four-hour antibiotic prophylaxis after spinal surgery in which a drain is utilized: a prospective randomized study. J Bone Joint Surg Am 2015;97(12):979–86.

61. Nunez-Pereira S, Pellise F, Rodriguez-Pardo D, et al. Implant survival after deep infection of an instrumented spinal fusion. Bone Joint Lett J 2013;95-B(8):1121–6.

62. Hedequist D, Haugen A, Hresko T, et al. Failure of attempted implant retention in spinal deformity delayed surgical site infections. Spine (Phila Pa 1976) 2009;34(1):60–4.

63. Nagata K, Yamada K, Shinozaki T, et al. Non-inferior comparative study comparing one or two day antimicrobial prophylaxis after clean orthopaedic surgery (NOCOTA study): a study protocol for a cluster pseudo-randomized controlled trial comparing duration of antibiotic prophylaxis. BMC Musculoskelet Disord 2019;20(1):533.

64. Bratzler DW, Dellinger EP, Olsen KM, et al. Clinical practice guidelines for antimicrobial prophylaxis in surgery. Am J Health Syst Pharm 2013;70(3):195–283.

65. Sousa-Pinto B, Blumenthal KG, Courtney L, et al. Assessment of the Frequency of Dual Allergy to Penicillins and Cefazolin: A Systematic Review and Meta-analysis. JAMA Surg 2021;156(4):e210021.

66. Organization WH. Global guidelines for the prevention of surgical site infection. 2016.

67. Berrios-Torres SI, Umscheid CA, Bratzler DW, et al. Centers for Disease Control and Prevention Guideline for the Prevention of Surgical Site Infection. JAMA Surg 2017;152(8):784–91.

68. Nagata K, Yamada K, Shinozaki T, et al. Effect of Antimicrobial Prophylaxis Duration on Health Care-Associated Infections After Clean Orthopedic Surgery: A Cluster Randomized Trial. JAMA Netw Open 2022;5(4):e226095.

69. American Diabetes A. 6. glycemic targets: standards of medical care in diabetes-2020. Diabetes Care 2020;43(Suppl 1):S66–76.

70. Suresh KV, Wang K, Sethi I, et al. Spine surgery and preoperative hemoglobin, hematocrit, and hemoglobin A1c: a systematic review. Global Spine J. Jan 2022;12(1):155–65.

71. Gupta R, Chanbour H, Roth SG, et al. The ideal threshold of hemoglobin a1c in diabetic patients

undergoing elective lumbar decompression surgery. Clin Spine Surg 2022. https://doi.org/10.1097/BSD.0000000000001399.

72. Poe-Kochert C, Shimberg JL, Thompson GH, et al. Surgical site infection prevention protocol for pediatric spinal deformity surgery: does it make a difference? Spine Deform 2020;8(5):931–8.

73. Yamada K, Abe H, Higashikawa A, et al. Evidence-based care bundles for preventing surgical site infections in spinal instrumentation surgery. Spine (Phila Pa 1976) 2018;43(24):1765–73.

74. Evaniew N, Khan M, Drew B, et al. Intrawound vancomycin to prevent infections after spine surgery: a systematic review and meta-analysis. Eur Spine J 2014;24(3):533–42.

75. Shan S, Tu L, Gu W, et al. A meta-analysis of the local application of vancomycin powder to prevent surgical site infection after spinal surgeries. J Int Med Res 2020;48(7). https://doi.org/10.1177/0300060520920057.

76. Salimi S, Khayat Kashani HR, Azhari S, et al. Local vancomycin therapy to reduce surgical site infection in adult spine surgery: a randomized prospective study. Eur Spine J 2022;31(2):454–60.

77. Gande A, Rosinski A, Cunningham T, et al. Selection pressures of vancomycin powder use in spine surgery: a meta-analysis. Spine J. Jun 2019;19(6):1076–84.

78. Mariappan R, Manninen P, Massicotte EM, et al. Circulatory collapse after topical application of vancomycin powder during spine surgery. J Neurosurg Spine. Sep 2013;19(3):381–3.

79. Offierski CM, MacNab I. Hip-spine syndrome. Spine (Phila Pa 1976) 1983;8(3):316–21.

80. Kawai T, Shimizu T, Goto K, et al. Number of levels of spinal fusion associated with the rate of joint-space narrowing in the hip. J Bone Joint Surg Am 2021;103(11):953–60.

81. Schwab F, Patel A, Ungar B, et al. Adult spinal deformity—postoperative standing imbalance. Spine 2010;35(25):2224–31.

82. Can A, Erdogan F, Yontar NS, et al. Spinopelvic alignment does not change after bilateral total hip arthroplasty in patients with bilateral Crowe type-IV developmental dysplasia of the hip. Acta Orthop Traumatol Turc 2020;54(6):583–6.

83. Blondel B, Parratte S, Tropiano P, et al. Pelvic tilt measurement before and after total hip arthroplasty. Orthop Traumatol Surg Res 2009;95(8):568–72.

84. Kleeman-Forsthuber L, Vigdorchik JM, Pierrepont JW, et al. Pelvic incidence significance relative to spinopelvic risk factors for total hip arthroplasty instability. Bone Joint Lett J 2022;104-B(3):352–8.

85. Rodkey DL, Lundy AE, Tracey RW, et al. Hip-spine syndrome: which surgery first? Clin Spine Surg 2022;35(1):1–3.

86. Sultan AA, Khlopas A, Piuzzi NS, et al. The impact of spino-pelvic alignment on total hip arthroplasty outcomes: a critical analysis of current evidence. J Arthroplasty. May 2018;33(5):1606–16.

87. Chavarria JC, Douleh DG, York PJ. The hip-spine challenge. J Bone Joint Surg Am 2021;103(19):1852–60.

88. Liu N, Goodman SB, Lachiewicz PF, et al. Hip or spine surgery first?: a survey of treatment order for patients with concurrent degenerative hip and spinal disorders. Bone Joint Lett J 2019;101-B(6_Supple_B):37–44.

89. Parvizi J, Pour AE, Hillibrand A, et al. Back pain and total hip arthroplasty: a prospective natural history study. Clin Orthop Relat Res 2010;468(5):1325–30.

90. Grammatopoulos G, Gofton W, Jibri Z, et al. 2018 Frank Stinchfield Award: Spinopelvic Hypermobility Is Associated With an Inferior Outcome After THA: Examining the Effect of Spinal Arthrodesis. Clin Orthop Relat Res 2019;477(2):310–21.

91. Hu J, Qian BP, Qiu Y, et al. Can acetabular orientation be restored by lumbar pedicle subtraction osteotomy in ankylosing spondylitis patients with thoracolumbar kyphosis? Eur Spine J 2017;26(7):1826–32.

92. Ike H, Dorr LD, Trasolini N, et al. Spine-pelvis-hip relationship in the functioning of a total hip replacement. J Bone Joint Surg Am 2018;100(18):1606–15.

93. Hey HW, Wong CG, Lau ET, et al. Differences in erect sitting and natural sitting spinal alignment-insights into a new paradigm and implications in deformity correction. Spine J 2017;17(2):183–9.

94. Wright JG. Revised grades of recommendation for summaries or reviews of orthopaedic surgical studies. J Bone Joint Surg Am 2006;88(5):1161–2.

95. Yamato Y, Furuhashi H, Hasegawa T, et al. Simulation of Implant Impingement After Spinal Corrective Fusion Surgery in Patients with Previous Total Hip Arthroplasty: A Retrospective Case Series. Spine (Phila Pa 1976) 2021;46(8):512–9.

96. Pellise F, Vila-Casademunt A, Nunez-Pereira S, et al. Surgeons' risk perception in ASD surgery: The value of objective risk assessment on decision making and patient counselling. Eur Spine J 2022;31(5):1174–83.

97. Nagata K, Shinozaki T, Yamada K, et al. A sliding scale to predict postoperative complications undergoing posterior spine surgery. J Orthop Sci 2020;25(4):545–50.

98. Diebo BG, Jalai CM, Challier V, et al. Novel Index to Quantify the Risk of Surgery in the Setting of Adult Spinal Deformity: A Study on 10,912 Patients From the Nationwide Inpatient Sample. Clin Spine Surg 2017;30(7):E993–9.

99. Buchlak QD, Yanamadala V, Leveque JC, et al. The Seattle spine score: Predicting 30-day complication risk in adult spinal deformity surgery. J Clin Neurosci 2017;43:247–55.

100. Pellise F, Serra-Burriel M, Smith JS, et al. Development and validation of risk stratification models for adult spinal deformity surgery. J Neurosurg Spine 2019;28:1–13.

101. Ames CP, Smith JS, Pellise F, et al. Development of deployable predictive models for minimal clinically important difference achievement across the commonly used health-related quality of life instruments in adult spinal deformity surgery. Spine (Phila Pa 1976) 2019;44(16):1144–53.

102. Passias PG, Ma Y, Chiu YL, et al. Comparative safety of simultaneous and staged anterior and posterior spinal surgery. Spine (Phila Pa 1976) 2012;37(3):247–55.

103. Yamato Y, Hasegawa T, Yoshida G, et al. Planned two-stage surgery using lateral lumbar interbody fusion and posterior corrective fusion: a retrospective study of perioperative complications. Eur Spine J 2021;30(8):2368–76.

104. Kwan MK, Chiu CK, Chan CY. Single vs two attending senior surgeons: assessment of intraoperative blood loss at different surgical stages of posterior spinal fusion surgery in Lenke 1 and 2 adolescent idiopathic scoliosis. Eur Spine J 2017;26(1):155–61.

105. Ames CP, Barry JJ, Keshavarzi S, et al. Perioperative outcomes and complications of pedicle subtraction osteotomy in cases with single versus two attending surgeons. Spine Deform 2013;1(1):51–8.

106. Lamartina C, Berjano P. Classification of sagittal imbalance based on spinal alignment and compensatory mechanisms. Eur Spine J 2014;23(6):1177–89.

107. Obeid I, Berjano P, Lamartina C, et al. Classification of coronal imbalance in adult scoliosis and spine deformity: a treatment-oriented guideline. Eur Spine J 2018;28(1):94–113.

108. Wade SM, Fredericks DR Jr, Elsenbeck MJ, et al. The Incidence, Risk Factors, and Complications Associated With Surgical Delay in Multilevel Fusion for Adult Spinal Deformity. Global Spine J 2022;12(3):441–6.

109. Khanna K, Berven SH. Mesenteric ischemia following the correction of adult spinal deformity: case report. J Neurosurg Spine 2017;26(4):426–9.

110. Kim HJ, Steinhaus M, Punyala A, et al. Enhanced recovery pathway in adult patients undergoing thoracolumbar deformity surgery. Spine J 2021;21(5):753–64.

Spinopelvic Alignment
Importance in Spinal Pathologies and Realignment Strategies

Christine Park, MS[a],*, Nitin Agarwal, MD[b],
Praveen V. Mummaneni, MD, MBA[a], Sigurd H. Berven, MD[c]

KEYWORDS

- Spinopelvic alignment • Lumbopelvic parameters • Quality of life outcomes • Spinal pathologies
- Realignment • Complications

KEY POINTS

- Sagittal spinal alignment is associated with patient-reported health status.
- Postoperative malalignment of the spine is associated with mechanical complications, morbidity and disability.
- The lumbopelvic parameters define the goals of lumbosacral reconstruction.
- Surgical techniques to change lumbopelvic parameters include a spectrum of posterior column osteotomies for mobilization of the spine.
- For realignment strategies, identifying and achieving patient-specific radiographic parameter goals may lead to more reliable and durable surgical outcomes.

INTRODUCTION

The spinal column in humans has evolved to accommodate upright posture and bipedalism. Sagittal alignment is established by pelvic incidence (PI) and the resultant lumbar lordosis (LL), thoracic kyphosis (TK), and cervical lordosis (CL) that support a balanced upright posture in stance. There is a close correlation between alignment of adjacent regions of the spine based on the subjacent regional alignment, beginning with PI.[1] The concept of the cone of economy, introduced by Dubousset, posits that there is a range of postures that allows for balance and movement with minimal effort.[2] As an individual moves outside of the boundaries of this cone, additional energy is required to maintain balance, leading to accelerated degeneration and ultimately pain as well as instability. It follows that deformity of the spinal column can lead to increased strain on the intrinsic musculature of the back, compromised stability, and decreased function. Spinopelvic alignment is the foundation of dynamic balance and function of the spinal column. An understanding of spinopelvic alignment is important for restoration of balance, economical stance, and function in the spine with deformity.[3-10]

Sagittal spinal malalignment is associated with morbidity and disability.[3,11-15] The role of reconstructive surgery in restoring sagittal alignment parameters of the spine and pelvis in the treatment of spinal deformities is important for improving health status of patients and avoiding mechanical complications of surgery.[16,17] Radiographic parameters of sagittal spinal alignment include global, regional, and segmental metrics. Global parameters include the sagittal vertical axis (SVA), T1 spinopelvic inclination (T1SPI), T9 spinopelvic inclination (T9SPI), and T1 pelvic angle (TPA) (**Fig. 1**). Regional parameters include CL, cervical SVA (CSVA), TK, and LL (**Fig. 2**). Lumbopelvic parameters include PI, pelvic tilt (PT), and sacral slope (SS) (**Fig. 3**). The

[a] Department of Neurological Surgery, University of California, San Francisco, 505 Parnassus Avenue, San Francisco, CA 94143, USA; [b] Department of Neurological Surgery, University of Pittsburgh, Pittsburgh, PA, USA; [c] Department of Orthopaedic Surgery, University of California, San Francisco, CA, USA

* Corresponding author.

E-mail address: christine.park@ucsf.edu

Neurosurg Clin N Am 34 (2023) 519–526
https://doi.org/10.1016/j.nec.2023.05.001
1042-3680/23/Published by Elsevier Inc.

neurosurgery.theclinics.com

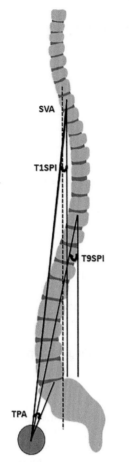

Fig. 1. Global parameters.

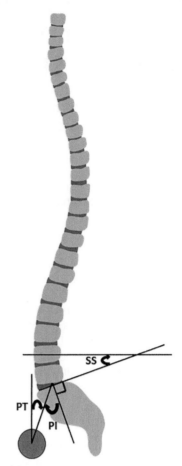

Fig. 3. Pelvic parameters.

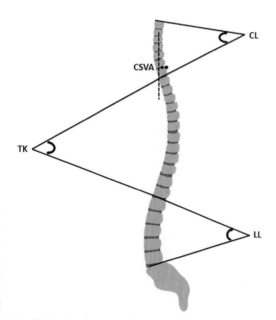

Fig. 2. Regional parameters.

descriptions of the parameters are summarized in **Table 1**. Common patterns of sagittal malalignment include loss of LL, increase in TK with resulting increase in sacrospinal angle, anterior displacement of the C7 plumb line, and pelvic retroversion compensatory (increase in PT). There are important correlations between alignment of different regions of the normal spine, and deformity in one region of the spine will result in compensatory changes in other regions.[1] Mathematical relationships between sagittal parameters are based both on direct geometric relationships (PI=SS + PT) and on correlations that are associated with health status (LL = PI ± 10°).[12,16]

The goal of reconstructive spine surgery is to restore spinal alignment parameters to measures that existed before the development of spinal deformity or to an age-appropriate alignment pattern. Mobilization of the spine with posterior-based osteotomies is a powerful tool for realignment of the spine with deformity. Schwab and colleagues[18] classified spinal osteotomy techniques into 6 anatomic grades according to the

Table 1
Summary of spinopelvic parameters

Parameters	Description
Global parameters	
SVA	Vertical line from the middle of body of C7 that passes <5 cm from the posterior superior endplate of S1
T1SPI	Angle formed between the line extending from the bicoxofemoral axis to the center of T1 and a vertical reference line from the center of T1
T9SPI	Angle formed between the line extending from the bicoxofemoral axis to the center of T9 and a vertical reference line from the center of T9
TPA	Angle between the line from the femoral head axis to the center of T1 and the line from femoral head axis to the midpoint of S1 endplate
Regional parameters	
CL	Normal inward curvature of the cervical spine: 2/3 of CL at occiput to C2; 1/3 of CL in the subaxial cervical spine
CSVA	Distance from C2 plumb line to upper posterior corner of C7, <4 cm
TK	Normal outward curvature of the thoracic spine between 10° and 40°
LL	Normal inward curvature of the lumbar spine from the rostral L1 endplate to the caudal L5 or rostral S1 endplate; LL-PI mismatch <10°
Lumbopelvic parameters	
SS	Angle between S1 endplate and a horizontal reference line
PT	Angle between a vertical reference line and a line from the midpoint of the S1 endplate to the center axis of the femoral head
PI	A line subtended from the femoral head to a reference line perpendicular to the midpoint of the rostral S1 endplate. A fixed parameter, approximated by the summation of SS and PT.

degree of destabilization of the spine: grade 1 is partial facet joint resection; grade 2 is complete facet joint resection; grade 3 is pedicle and partial body resection; grade 4 is pedicle, partial body, and supra-adjacent disc resection; grade 5 is complete vertebra and disc resection, such as vertebral column resection and anterior column resection; and grade 6 is multiple adjacent vertebrae and disc resection. The surgical approach should be determined based on patient and anatomic characteristics and the extent of the needed deformity correction.

Measuring Lumbopelvic Parameters

The major classifications for adult spinal deformity include considerations of spinal shape, and spinal regional and global sagittal alignment. The Roussouly sagittal classification system was developed in 2005 and groups the standing spine into four types.[19] Types I and II have SS < 35°, type III has 35° < SS < 45°, and type IV has SS > 45°. PI is generally low in types I and II and high in types III and IV. The apex of the LL increases with increasing type grade. The SRS-Schwab classification system was developed in 2012, which correlates radiographic deformity with patient-reported outcomes and also considers the relevant radiographic spinopelvic parameters such as PI, LL, PT, and SVA, which were shown to be strongly correlated to pain and functional outcomes.[20] This was a significant improvement from the previous versions of the adult deformity classification systems which were largely descriptive and did not take clinical parameters into account.[21–23] There are 2 parts to the SRS-Schwab classification system: 4 coronal curve types and the sagittal modifiers (PI-LL mismatch, SVA, PT). The coronal curve types are classified as follows: type T (thoracic major curve > 30°, apical level of T9 or higher), type L (lumbar or thoracolumbar major curve > 30°, apical level of T10 or lower), type D (double major curve with each curve > 30°), and type N (normal or no coronal curve < 30°). Each of the sagittal modifiers is grouped as follows: PI-LL (0: within 10°, +: moderate 10°-20°, ++: marked > 20°), SVA (0: < 4 cm, +: 4 to 9.5 cm, ++: > 9.5 cm), PT (0 < 20°, +: 20°-30°, ++: > 30°).

Lumbopelvic Parameters and Disability

In the surgical treatment of symptomatic adult spinal deformity, restoration of sagittal alignment is important to optimize clinical outcomes and to improve the durability of treatment.[24–26] There is a well-established correlation between spinopelvic alignment and patient-reported health status in spinal deformity (pain, function, and quality of life).[27,28] Specifically, several parameters, including PT, PI-LL mismatch, and SVA, have been correlated with health status measures, including the Oswestry Disability Index and the Short Form 12. Optimal spinopelvic alignment goals should consist of PT < 20°, a PI-LL mismatch ± 10°, and an SVA ≤ 6 cm.[12,29–36] Compensatory mechanisms such as pelvic retroversion and knee flexion can also be a source of major discomfort, fatigue, and disability.[31,37,38] Based on correlation studies, it has been presumed that achieving these optimal postoperative alignment parameter goals is necessary to obtain clinical improvement.[39,40] However, it is well known that a correlation does not necessarily equate to a causal relationship. Although a correlation between spinopelvic alignment with pain and function has been established, the exact nature of this relationship has not been completely defined, and the observed correlations are low, indicating that sagittal parameters alone only account for a minor amount of the patient's health status. Metrics that include general health, mental health, and social determinants of health are important factors that contribute to self-reported health status. Sagittal alignment, while a minor factor, is a factor that can be optimized with appropriate surgical planning and execution.

A single set of parameters for radiographic alignment, such as the generally acknowledged optimal radiographic thresholds of PT < 20°, a PI-LL mismatch ± 10°, and an SVA ≤ 6 cm, are not adequate to define the appropriate alignment for every patient. Patient-specific alignment must consider other factors, including age, gender, body habitus, and Roussouly type.[7,41] Aging is a physiological process that results in loss of lordosis and increase in SVA.[18–21] Asai and colleagues[15] studied 1461 patients aged 19-94 years and found an increase in SVA, TK, PT, and PI-LL mismatch with age (also loss of LL with age). While the mean SVA was not high, ranging from 4.7 mm to 13.9 mm in the 50- to 59-year-old and 70- to 79-year-old groups, respectively, the standard deviation was large for each age group. This showed that an SVA > 5 cm was present and was present more frequently in the older individuals. In another study of 50 asymptomatic volunteers aged 70 to 85 years, the average SVA measured 40.4 mm, but the range of SVA values was −37 to 139 mm, which also confirms that a higher SVA can occur in the elderly and is not necessarily associated with increased pain and disability. Acknowledging the changes that occur with aging, the authors of a more recent study have proposed age-specific spinopelvic parameters with graded changes in thresholds for SVA, PT, and PI-LL mismatch from −4.0 mm, 15.5°, and −6.2° for

35- to 44-year-old patients to 79.9 mm, 28.8°, and 13.7° for ≥74-year-old patients, respectively.

Beyond age, sex differences in spinopelvic alignment have been investigated. Asai and colleagues[15] found statistically significant differences in the SVA, PT, LL, and PI between males and females in certain age groups. However, the amount of difference in the various radiographic parameters was not excessive. Yukawa and colleagues[41] also found significant sex differences in PT and, to a lesser extent, LL in different age groups.

Taken together, these results suggest that a similar degree of meaningful clinical improvement can be obtained without achieving the proposed optimal spinopelvic radiographic thresholds. It is possible that age and sex among other patient characteristics could have factored into the amount of radiographic correction needed in each patient to achieve a meaningful improvement. In other words, although a patient may not have achieved optimal spinopelvic alignment, this "suboptimal" postoperative spinal alignment was adequate for that particular individual. Rather than a single set of optimal spinopelvic parameters applied to all patients, a graded or individualized set of radiographic alignment goals based on factors such as age may be a more accurate predictor of clinical improvement. Further investigation of patient-specific alignment goals will enable surgeons to apply techniques of precision medicine to develop alignment goals that are optimized for the individual patient.

Association Between Pelvic Incidence and Spinal Pathologies

PI is the foundational anatomic parameter that defines the sagittal alignment profile of the spine. Although PI is usually a fixed value unaffected by pelvic position and age, it may be altered by motion in the sacroiliac joint due to degeneration, trauma, or iatrogenic injury. Because PI strongly correlates with LL, PI is considered the key parameter in determining the mechanisms of different degenerative diseases of the lumbar spine, including developmental pathologies such as spondylolisthesis and degenerative pathologies including symptomatic disc degeneration.[42,43] Reconstruction strategies for the lumbopelvic region of the spine to match lordosis to PI are important in both deformity surgery and surgery for degenerative pathology. Inadequate restoration of lordosis, even in short-segment surgeries, is associated with a high rate of adjacent segment degeneration and revision surgery.[44]

PI is associated with the development of spinal pathologies including spondylolisthesis, scoliosis, disc degeneration, disc herniation, and facet joint arthritis.[45,46] Sacropelvic morphology is an important determinant of shear and stress forces at the lumbosacral region and etiologic in the development of common spinal disorders. An increase in PI correlates results in increased shear forces at the lumbopelvic junction and developmental spondylolisthesis. In contrast, low PI results in more stress on the anterior column of the spine and is associated with a higher risk of low back pain, intervertebral disc degeneration, and sagittal imbalance.[47] Patients with low PI have less capacity to adapt to sagittal imbalance and are more prone to femoroacetabular impingement at the femoral neck due to hip overextension.[47] Those with high PI, in contrast, have less significant acetabular version angle and have better ability to compensate with a greater capacity for hip extension. However, they are at higher risk of anterior dislocation of the hip joint as well as hip osteoarthritis because of the anterior uncovering of the femoral heads. Hence, both high and low PI can be a risk factor for spinal and hip developmental and degenerative pathologies.

Junctional Pathology and Mechanical Failure with Postoperative Pelvic Incidence-Lumbar Lordosis (PI-LL) Mismatch

Among the sagittal spinopelvic parameters, PI-LL is commonly used as a key reference value for planning in deformity surgical correction for estimating the ideal LL to match the PI for optimal alignment.[25,48] PI-LL within ±10° should be the aim of the surgery to achieve optimal clinical outcomes.[12,20,49] With increasing sagittal malalignment, patients develop compensatory pelvic retroversion (as noted by a PT ≥ 20°) to maintain an upright posture. In patients undergoing fusion surgery for spinal deformity, restoration of these spinopelvic parameters to normative values is an important surgical goal and has been suggested to represent a primary determinant of health-related quality of life.[29] Despite the recognized importance, the optimal PI-LL for corrective surgery remains controversial.[40,50–53] To date, ideal range of PI-LL remains unknown for the individual patient.

One of the important and common complications of lumbopelvic reconstructive surgery is the development of proximal junctional kyphosis (PJK). PJK is defined as kyphosis at the segment above the upper instrumented vertebra of a construct greater than 10° more than the preoperative alignment. PJK can lead to progressive decompensation in the sagittal plane, neurological compromise, and compromise of clinical outcomes.[54] Radiographic PJK is apparent in 10% to 40% of long fusions

from the thoracolumbar spine to the sacrum, and risk factors for its development include fixation to the sacrum, the magnitude of increased of LL, instrumentation techniques including pedicle screws at the upper instrumented vertebra, integrity of the posterior soft tissue tension band, combined anterior/posterior spine surgery, pedicle subtraction osteotomies, postoperative alignment, and patient-specific factors including bone quality.[55,56] In order to reduce the rate of PJK postoperatively, care should be taken to thoroughly evaluate the clinical and radiographic characteristics of the patient and consider taking preventative measures such as soft tissue protection, choice of level and instrumentation, vertebral augmentation, and age-appropriate spinopelvic alignment goals. Optimal postoperative alignment may reduce the risk of mechanical complications and improve the durability of reconstructive surgery.

Postoperative alignment is an important determinant of mechanical complications of surgery, including implant failure and junctional pathology. The Global Alignment and Proportion (GAP) Score is a scoring system proposed by the European Spine Study Group (ESSG) and designed to predict risk for mechanical complications after adult spinal deformity surgery. It is based on global alignment parameters in relation to PI, notably including the morphologic parameter Lumbar Distribution Index (LDI).[57] The scoring system was designed to predict risk for mechanical complications after adult spinal deformity surgery. Kwan and colleagues[58] in an external validation study done by the AO Spine and SRS, however, did not demonstrate increased risk of mechanical complications with higher GAP scores at 2 years. The authors did, however, find some association between lower GAP scores and improved health-related quality of life outcomes. Im and colleagues[59] concluded in a retrospective review of 228 consecutive cases of 8-segment T10-S1 PSF with PSO or multilevel SPO that postoperative PI-LL was the sole parameter significantly associated with achieving postoperative "balance" (SVA ≤ 6 cm) at a mean follow-up of 45.3 months. Specifically, they did not find an association between lumbar morphologic parameters (proximal LL, distal LL, and lordosis distribution index) and sagittal alignment. Overall, postoperative alignment is related to health status and durability of outcomes, but the ideal alignment for the individual patient is incompletely defined.

SUMMARY

Lumbopelvic parameters are associated with the development of lumbar pathology and strongly correlated with important clinical and health-related quality of life outcomes. Surgeons should strongly consider them in their planning for surgical reconstruction to avoid postoperative pathologies, including mechanical failure and junctional pathology, as well as optimize postoperative outcomes in the adult spinal deformity population.

CLINICS CARE POINTS

- There are 2 major classification systems for spinal deformity: Roussouly sagittal classification and the SRS-Schwab classification.

- PI is fixed and unique to each patient, and the spine has compensatory implications for high and low PI values. Because of the relationship between PI and other pelvic measurements (PI=PT + SS), the overall balance relies on the match between PI and LL.

- Although the optimal spinopelvic alignment goals for patients with adult spinal deformity generally consist of PT < 20°, a PI-LL mismatch ± 10°, and an SVA ≤ 6 cm, different patient characteristics may impact clinical improvement observed postoperatively.

DISCLOSURE

C. Park: None; N. Agarwal: None; P.V. Mummaneni: DePuy Spine, Globus, Nuvasive, Brainlab, BK Medical, Thieme Publishing, Springer Publishing, Spinicity/ISD, AO Spine, ISSG, NREF, PCORI, Alan and Jacqueline Stuart Spine Outcomes Center, Joan O'Reilly Endowed Professorship, NIH/NIAMS; S.H. Berven: NIH, NSF, AO Spine, Medtronic, Stryker, Globus, Camber, Kuros, Innovasis, Accelus, Elsevier, Medtronic, Stryker, Green Sun, Novapproach.

REFERENCES

1. Lee SH, Son ES, Seo EM, et al. Factors determining cervical spine sagittal balance in asymptomatic adults: correlation with spinopelvic balance and thoracic inlet alignment. Spine J 2015;15(4):705–12.

2. Dubousset J. Three-dimensional analysis of the scoliotic deformity. Weinstein SL: The Pediatric Spine. Raven Press; 1994. p. 479–96.

3. Schwab F, Lafage V, Patel A, et al. Sagittal plane considerations and the pelvis in the adult patient. Spine 2009;34(17):1828–33.

4. Bernhardt M, Bridwell KH. Segmental analysis of the sagittal plane alignment of the normal thoracic and lumbar spines and thoracolumbar junction. Spine 1989;14(7):717–21.

5. Berthonnaud E, Dimnet J, Roussouly P, et al. Analysis of the sagittal balance of the spine and pelvis using shape and orientation parameters. J Spinal Disord Tech 2005;18(1):40–7.

6. During J, Goudfrooij H, Keessen W, et al. Toward standards for posture. Postural characteristics of the lower back system in normal and pathologic conditions. Spine 1985;10(1):83–7.

7. Gelb DE, Lenke LG, Bridwell KH, et al. An analysis of sagittal spinal alignment in 100 asymptomatic middle and older aged volunteers. Spine 1995;20(12):1351–8.

8. Vaz G, Roussouly P, Berthonnaud E, et al. Sagittal morphology and equilibrium of pelvis and spine. Eur Spine J 2002;11(1):80–7.

9. Schwab F, Lafage V, Boyce R, et al. Gravity line analysis in adult volunteers: age-related correlation with spinal parameters, pelvic parameters, and foot position. Spine 2006;31(25):E959–67.

10. Jackson RP, Kanemura T, Kawakami N, et al. Lumbopelvic lordosis and pelvic balance on repeated standing lateral radiographs of adult volunteers and untreated patients with constant low back pain. Spine 2000;25(5):575–86.

11. Vedantam R, Lenke LG, Keeney JA, et al. Comparison of standing sagittal spinal alignment in asymptomatic adolescents and adults. Spine 1998;23(2):211–5.

12. Schwab F, Patel A, Ungar B, et al. Adult spinal deformity-postoperative standing imbalance: how much can you tolerate? An overview of key parameters in assessing alignment and planning corrective surgery. Spine 2010;35(25):2224–31.

13. Jackson RP, McManus AC. Radiographic analysis of sagittal plane alignment and balance in standing volunteers and patients with low back pain matched for age, sex, and size. A prospective controlled clinical study. Spine 1994;19(14):1611–8.

14. Bridwell KH. Decision making regarding Smith-Petersen vs. pedicle subtraction osteotomy vs. vertebral column resection for spinal deformity. Spine 2006;31(19 Suppl):S171–8.

15. Asai Y, Tsutsui S, Oka H, et al. Sagittal spino-pelvic alignment in adults: the Wakayama Spine Study. PLoS One 2017;12(6):e0178697.

16. Ames CP, Smith JS, Scheer JK, et al. Impact of spinopelvic alignment on decision making in deformity surgery in adults: a review. J Neurosurg Spine 2012;16(6):547–64.

17. Bodin A, Roussouly P. Sacral and pelvic osteotomies for correction of spinal deformities. Eur Spine J 2015;24(Suppl 1):S72–82.

18. Schwab F, Blondel B, Chay E, et al. The comprehensive anatomical spinal osteotomy classification. Neurosurgery 2014;74(1):112–20 [discussion: 120].

19. Roussouly P, Gollogly S, Berthonnaud E, et al. Classification of the normal variation in the sagittal

alignment of the human lumbar spine and pelvis in the standing position. Spine 2005;30(3):346–53.

20. Schwab F, Ungar B, Blondel B, et al. Scoliosis research society-schwab adult spinal deformity classification: a validation study. Spine 2012; 37(12):1077–82.

21. Aebi M. The adult scoliosis. Eur Spine J 2005; 14(10):925–48.

22. Schwab F, Farcy JP, Bridwell K, et al. A clinical impact classification of scoliosis in the adult. Spine 2006;31(18):2109–14.

23. Lowe T, Berven SH, Schwab FJ, et al. The SRS classification for adult spinal deformity: building on the King/Moe and Lenke classification systems. Spine 2006;31(19 Suppl):S119–25.

24. Duval-Beaupère G, Schmidt C, Cosson P. A Barycentremetric study of the sagittal shape of spine and pelvis: the conditions required for an economic standing position. Ann Biomed Eng 1992; 20(4):451–62.

25. Legaye J, Duval-Beaupère G, Hecquet J, et al. Pelvic incidence: a fundamental pelvic parameter for three-dimensional regulation of spinal sagittal curves. Eur Spine J 1998;7(2):99–103.

26. Lafage V, Schwab F, Vira S, et al. Spino-pelvic parameters after surgery can be predicted: a preliminary formula and validation of standing alignment. Spine 2011;36(13):1037–45.

27. Glassman SD, Berven S, Bridwell K, et al. Correlation of radiographic parameters and clinical symptoms in adult scoliosis. Spine 2005;30(6):682–8.

28. Lafage V, Schwab F, Patel A, et al. Pelvic tilt and truncal inclination: two key radiographic parameters in the setting of adults with spinal deformity. Spine 2009;34(17):E599–606.

29. Schwab FJ, Blondel B, Bess S, et al. Radiographical spinopelvic parameters and disability in the setting of adult spinal deformity: a prospective multicenter analysis. Spine 2013;38(13):E803–12.

30. Joseph SA Jr, Moreno AP, Brandoff J, et al. Sagittal plane deformity in the adult patient. J Am Acad Orthop Surg 2009;17(6):378–88.

31. Glassman SD, Bridwell K, Dimar JR, et al. The impact of positive sagittal balance in adult spinal deformity. Spine 2005;30(18):2024–9.

32. Lee JS, Youn MS, Shin JK, et al. Relationship between cervical sagittal alignment and quality of life in ankylosing spondylitis. Eur Spine J 2015;24(6): 1199–203.

33. Tang JA, Scheer JK, Smith JS, et al. The impact of standing regional cervical sagittal alignment on outcomes in posterior cervical fusion surgery. Neurosurgery 2012;71(3):662–9 [discussion: 669].

34. Wang K, Deng Z, Li Z, et al. The Influence of Natural Head Position on the Cervical Sagittal Alignment. J Healthc Eng 2017;2017. https://doi.org/10.1155/2017/2941048.

35. Ames CP, Blondel B, Scheer JK, et al. Cervical radiographical alignment: comprehensive assessment techniques and potential importance in cervical myelopathy. Spine 2013;38(22 Suppl 1): S149–60.

36. Hyun SJ, Kim KJ, Jahng TA, et al. Relationship between T1 slope and cervical alignment following multilevel posterior cervical fusion surgery: impact of T1 slope minus cervical lordosis. Spine 2016; 41(7):E396–402.

37. Schwab FJ, Smith VA, Biserni M, et al. Adult scoliosis: a quantitative radiographic and clinical analysis. Spine 2002;27(4):387–92.

38. Roussouly P, Nnadi C. Sagittal plane deformity: an overview of interpretation and management. Eur Spine J 2010;19(11):1824–36.

39. Pellise F, Vila-Casademunt A, Ferrer M, et al. Impact on health related quality of life of adult spinal deformity (ASD) compared with other chronic conditions. Eur Spine J 2015;24(1):3–11.

40. Smith JS, Klineberg E, Schwab F, et al. Change in classification grade by the SRS-Schwab Adult Spinal Deformity Classification predicts impact on health-related quality of life measures: prospective analysis of operative and nonoperative treatment. Spine 2013;38(19):1663–71.

41. Yukawa Y, Kato F, Suda K, et al. Normative data for parameters of sagittal spinal alignment in healthy subjects: an analysis of gender specific differences and changes with aging in 626 asymptomatic individuals. Eur Spine J 2018;27(2):426–32.

42. Roussouly P, Pinheiro-Franco JL. Biomechanical analysis of the spino-pelvic organization and adaptation in pathology. Eur Spine J 2011;20(Suppl 5): 609–18.

43. Lee JH, Na KH, Kim JH, et al. Is pelvic incidence a constant, as everyone knows? Changes of pelvic incidence in surgically corrected adult sagittal deformity. Eur Spine J 2016;25(11):3707–14.

44. Di Martino A, Quattrocchi CC, Scarciolla L, et al. Estimating the risk for symptomatic adjacent segment degeneration after lumbar fusion: analysis from a cohort of patients undergoing revision surgery. Eur Spine J 2014;23(Suppl 6):693–8.

45. Cho KJ, Suk SI, Park SR, et al. Risk factors of sagittal decompensation after long posterior instrumentation and fusion for degenerative lumbar scoliosis. Spine 2010;35(17):1595–601.

46. Hong JY, Suh SW, Modi HN, et al. Correlation of pelvic orientation with adult scoliosis. J Spinal Disord Tech 2010;23(7):461–6.

47. Chen H-F, Zhao C-Q. Pelvic incidence variation among individuals: functional influence versus genetic determinism. J Orthop Surg Res 2018;13(1): 59.

48. Diebo BG, Henry J, Lafage V, et al. Sagittal deformities of the spine: factors influencing the outcomes

and complications. Eur Spine J 2015;24(Suppl 1): S3–15.

49. Berven S, Wadhwa R. Sagittal Alignment of the Lumbar Spine. Neurosurg Clin N Am 2018;29(3):331–9.

50. Yamada K, Abe Y, Yanagibashi Y, et al. Mid- and long-term clinical outcomes of corrective fusion surgery which did not achieve sufficient pelvic incidence minus lumbar lordosis value for adult spinal deformity. Scoliosis 2015;10(Suppl 2):S17.

51. Inami S, Moridaira H, Takeuchi D, et al. Optimum pelvic incidence minus lumbar lordosis value can be determined by individual pelvic incidence. Eur Spine J 2016;25(11):3638–43.

52. Aoki Y, Nakajima A, Takahashi H, et al. Influence of pelvic incidence-lumbar lordosis mismatch on surgical outcomes of short-segment transforaminal lumbar interbody fusion. BMC Musculoskelet Disord 2015;16:213.

53. Ha KY, Jang WH, Kim YH, et al. Clinical relevance of the SRS-Schwab classification for degenerative lumbar scoliosis. Spine 2016;41(5):E282–8.

54. Hyun SJ, Lee BH, Park JH, et al. Proximal junctional kyphosis and proximal junctional failure following adult spinal deformity surgery. Korean J Spine 2017;14(4):126–32.

55. Wang H, Ma L, Yang D, et al. Incidence and risk factors for the progression of proximal junctional kyphosis in degenerative lumbar scoliosis following long instrumented posterior spinal fusion. Medicine 2016;95(32):e4443.

56. Kim HJ, Bridwell KH, Lenke LG, et al. Patients with proximal junctional kyphosis requiring revision surgery have higher postoperative lumbar lordosis and larger sagittal balance corrections. Spine 2014;39(9):E576–80.

57. Yilgor C, Sogunmez N, Boissiere L, et al. Global alignment and proportion (GAP) score: development and validation of a new method of analyzing spinopelvic alignment to predict mechanical complications after adult spinal deformity surgery. J Bone Joint Surg Am 2017;99(19):1661–72.

58. Kwan KYH, Lenke LG, Shaffrey CI, et al. Are higher global alignment and proportion scores associated with increased risks of mechanical complications after adult spinal deformity surgery? an external validation. Clin Orthop Relat Res 2021;479(2):312–20.

59. Im SK, Lee KY, Lim HS, et al. Optimized surgical strategy for adult spinal deformity: quantitative lordosis correction versus lordosis morphology. J Clin Med 2021;10(9). https://doi.org/10.3390/jcm10091867.

PreOperative Planning for Adult Spinal Deformity Goals
Level Selection and Alignment Goals

Jay Dalton, MD[a], Ayman Mohamed, MD[b], Noel Akioyamen, MD[c],
Frank J. Schwab, MD[b], Virginie Lafage, PhD[b],*

KEYWORDS

- Adult spinal deformity • Upper instrumented vertebra • Lower instrumented vertebra
- Age-adjusted alignment • Preoperative planning

KEY POINTS

- Age-related alignment goals have been associated with fewer junctional complications compared with fixed alignment goals.
- Upper and lower instrumented vertebra selection has unique benefits and drawbacks. Although smaller constructs create less morbidity for the patient, there are clear risk factors that would indicate the use of a higher upper instrumented vertebra and a lower instrumented vertebra.
- Three-dimensional printed models, rods, and implants have the potential to revolutionize individualized deformity care, allowing for the most precise translation of a preoperative plan into the operating room.

INTRODUCTION

Spinal alignment is essential to a well-functioning musculoskeletal system. Normal standing orientation as defined by Dubousset[1] is with the skull positioned roughly over the femoral heads within the "cone of economy." Maintenance of this position allows for minimal energy expenditure, performance of activities of daily living, and retention of horizontal gaze.[1] Spinal deformity can occur in the coronal and sagittal planes and result in chronic pain, fatigue, loss of function, and decreased quality of life.[2]

Although the adverse effects of adult spinal deformity (ASD) on quality of life have been well documented,[3–6] deformity overcorrection and undercorrection have also been associated with the development of junctional complications, adjacent segment changes, and persistently poor quality-of-life scores.[7–9] Achieving specific realignment goals is therefore critical to long-term outcome.[10]

Reliable preoperative planning strategies, including nomograms, measurement tools, and level selection, are key to maximizing the likelihood of achieving a good outcome following ASD corrective surgery. Recent literature regarding such strategies is addressed in this review.

PLANNING FOR SPINAL DEFORMITY CORRECTION

Sagittal plane correction is the cornerstone to ASD surgical treatment, as association between global sagittal malalignment and decreased quality of life has been demonstrated.[11–14] Key parameters of sagittal alignment include the mismatch between

Conflicts of Interest: None related to this work.
[a] Department of Orthopaedic Surgery, University of Pittsburgh Medical Center, 3471 Fifth Avenue, Pittsburgh, PA 15213, USA; [b] Department of Orthopaedic Surgery, Lenox Hill Hospital, 130 East 77th Street, 11th Floor, New York, NY 10075, USA; [c] Department of Orthopaedic Surgery, Monteriore Medical Center, 1250 Waters Place, Tower 1, 11th Floor, Bronx, NY 10461, USA
* Corresponding author. Department of Orthopaedic Surgery, Lenox Hill Hospital, 130 East 77th Street, 11th Floor, New York, NY 10075.
E-mail address: Virginie.lafage@gmail.com

Neurosurg Clin N Am 34 (2023) 527–536
https://doi.org/10.1016/j.nec.2023.06.016
1042-3680/23/© 2023 Elsevier Inc. All rights reserved.

pelvic incidence (PI) and L1-S1 lumbar lordosis (LL), pelvic tilt (PT), and sagittal vertical axis (SVA) (**Fig. 1**). The Scoliosis Research Society (SRS) and Schwab and colleagues published a hybrid classification system in 2012 to correlate radiographic spinal deformity parameters in the sagittal and coronal planes, pelvic parameters, and patient-reported outcomes.[15] The SRS-Schwab classification defined a main coronal curve (>30°) type based on anatomic region and included the sagittal modifiers: PI-LL mismatch to characterize lumbar regional deformity, PT as a key compensatory mechanism, and SVA as a global alignment metric.[7,16,17] Threshold values associated with the limit of severe disability used for this system when defining preoperative ASD correction goals include a PI-LL mismatch of less than 10°, a PT of less than 20°, and an SVA less than 4 cm.[16] T1 pelvic angle (TPA), originally described by Protopsaltis and colleagues,[17] is a parameter of more recent interest that can also be used to define global alignment.

A growing body of research suggests that age-related changes should be taken into consideration when correcting sagittal plane deformity.[18,19] Health-related quality of life (HRQOL), as measured with the SRS-30, the Short Form-36 physical and mental component scores, and the Oswestry Disability Index, declines with aging owing to a multitude of complex factors, including medical comorbidities, muscle atrophy, and neurosensory degeneration.[20–22] A recent study by Lafage and colleagues[23] performed a multilinear regression analysis using age and HRQOL scores as independent factors and radiographic parameters as dependent factors in order to establish age-specific alignment values in line with HRQOL. As illustrated in **Table 1**, recommendation from this study was that alignment goals in patients with ASD should account for the age of the patient.[23] Such age-related targets were associated with improved outcomes compared with fixed alignment targets in older patients. A retrospective study by Lafage and colleagues[24] with a total of 679 patients reported that patients overcorrected with respect to age-adjusted sagittal alignment targets were more likely to develop proximal junctional kyphosis (PJK). These findings have been externally validated in a 2022 study on 78 patients with ASD.[25]

A larger body of radiographic and outcomes data has permitted the development of more comprehensive scoring systems. The combined Global Alignment and Proportion (GAP) system used normative data to address the overall shape of the spine using PI as its essential parameter.[26] However, subsequent cohort studies were unable to validate the GAP scoring system in isolation.[27] Lafage and colleagues[28] combined the methodologies used for the development of the SRS-Schwab classification, GAP score, and age-adjusted alignment parameters to produce the Sagittal Age-Adjusted Score (SAAS) with the hope of predicting outcomes following ASD surgery more reliably. The SAAS system uses 3 sagittal parameters from the previous systems (PI-LL, PT, and TPA) as surrogates for lumbar deformity, pelvic compensation,

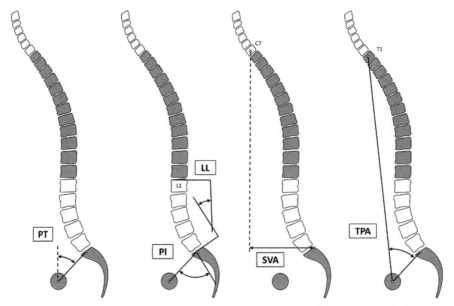

Fig. 1. The common radiographic parameters applied in quantifying spinopelvic alignment: PT, PI minus LL, SVA as well as TPA.

Table 1
Alignment targets associated with age-adjusted US-normative health-related quality of life[23]

Age Group (y)	PT	PI-LL	SVA	TPA
<35	11.1	−11.3	−29.1	4.4
35–44	15.5	−6.2	−4.0	10.0
45–54	18.9	−1.7	16.5	14.5
55–64	22.1	3.3	37.0	18.8
65–74	25.2	7.5	55.6	22.8
>74	28.8	13.7	79.9	27.8

Adapted from Lafage R, Schwab F, Challier V, Henry JK, Gum J, Smith J, Hostin R, Shaffrey C, Kim HJ, Ames C, Scheer J, Klineberg E, Bess S, Burton D, Lafage V; International Spine Study Group. Spine (Phila Pa 1976). 2016 Jan;41(1):62-8. doi: 10.1097/BRS.0000000000001171.

and global sagittal malalignment, respectively, and assigns points according to age-adjusted targets.[28] SAAS correlated with both PJK and HRQOL differences at 2-year follow-up, supporting its utility in the establishment of preoperative goals for sagittal ASD correction.[28]

Although outcome studies following the surgical correction of ASD often focus on the sagittal plane, coronal malalignment can also be a significant source of pain and impairment.[29] The indications for coronal deformity correction have generally been defined as a Cobb angle greater than 30° or a coronal balance (CVA) greater than 3 cm causing cosmetic deformity, pain, disability, or neuromuscular dysfunction.[30] The Qiu classification characterized coronal deformity using coronal balance distance (CBD), the horizontal distance between a C7 plumb line (C7PL), and the central sacral vertical line.[31] This classification system subdivided patients with degenerative scoliosis into 3 groups—type A with CBD ≤ 3 cm, type B with CBD greater than 3 CM and a C7PL shifted to the concave side of the curve, and type C with CBD greater than 3 cm and C7PL shifted toward the convex side of the curve (Fig. 2).[31] Glassman and colleagues[32] reported that patients with a CBD greater than 4 cm had significantly improved pain and function HRQOL scores after corrective surgery compared with unoperated patients.

DEFINING UPPER LOWER INSTRUMENTED VERTEBRA IN DEFORMITY SURGERY
Upper Instrumented Vertebra

A central tenet of upper instrumented vertebra (UIV) level selection for patients with ASD is to fuse to a stable and neutral vertebra in order to maintain overall alignment.[33–35] The stable vertebra in a patient with ASD is frequently defined as the level that is bisected by the center sacral vertical line in the coronal plane, but consideration of sagittal plane alignment is also important.[36] A link has been demonstrated between UIV selection and complications, including PJK and proximal junctional failure (PJF).[10,37–39]

UIV selection in long construct fusions for ASD is divided into upper thoracic and lower thoracic proximal fusion end points.[40] This distinction has several clinical, radiographic, and quality-of-life implications. Ending a long fusion construct in the upper thoracic spine has the potential to provide more powerful deformity correction for larger curves, may enhance the long-term maintenance of correction, and may avoid PJK and PJF.[41–45] However, fusion to the upper thoracic region may negatively impact patient-reported outcomes[46] owing to increased stiffness restricting certain activities of daily living, such as personal hygiene.[46] The benefits of ending a long fusion construct in the lower thoracic spine include decreased postoperative stiffness, decreased operative time, decreased blood loss, and decreased surgical cost.[47–49]

There is still substantial controversy and a lack of large prospective data regarding the ideal UIV for different presentations of ASD. A recent work presented a series of 11 patients with ASD to 14 experienced spinal deformity surgeons, who were asked what UIV they would select and why in order to develop a level selection algorithm.[40] The most favored vertebrae for a lower thoracic UIV was T10, and for an upper thoracic UIV was T3. T10 has been identified as the lowest static region in the thoracic spine, which likely contributes to it being a preferred lower thoracic UIV.[50,51] Overall, the amount of kyphosis in the thoracic spine was a key determinant of UIV selection.[40] Coronal curves greater than 20° and hyperkyphosis greater than 50° both favor a UIV in the upper thoracic spine (Fig. 3).[40] A recent large, multicenter ASD database retrospective review reported that a greater preoperative deformity and/or the need for a three-column osteotomy both increased the likelihood of the operating surgeon choosing an upper thoracic UIV.[52] Despite both a longer operative time and greater blood loss, patients with an upper thoracic UIV had better sagittal correction and lower PJK rates at 2-year follow-up.[52] Junctional and apical regions have classically been avoided when selecting the UIV owing to their relative hypermobility and large biomechanical lever arm. A large body of prior work indicates that selecting a UIV at the thoracolumbar junction, especially between T11 and L1, is associated with PJF.[53–57]

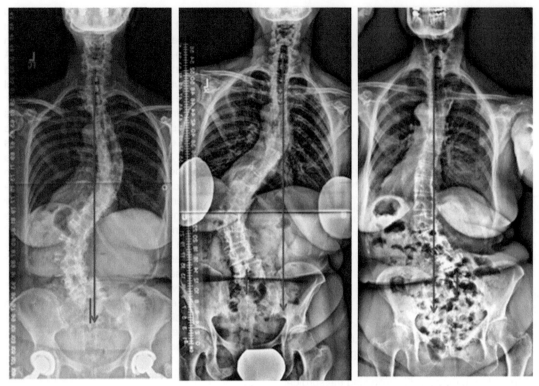

Fig. 2. Qiu classification for coronal deformity: type A (*left*) CBD <3 cm; type B (middle) CBD >3 cm toward concave side; type C (*right*) CBD >3 cm toward convex side. For each x-ray, the short (*line*) represents the center of the sacrum, the (*arrow*) represents the C7 plumbline.

In addition to radiographic considerations, it is important to factor in the increased invasiveness of longer fusion constructs when considering ASD correction in medically complex patients. A recent large study noted that patients with ASD undergoing surgery who sustained at least one medical complication had a significantly longer operative time compared with patients who did not experience complications.[58] The number of instrumented vertebra has also been identified as

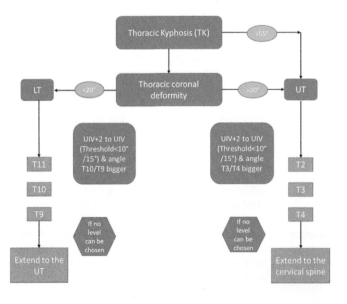

Fig. 3. Decision algorithm for UIV selection based on Virk and colleagues.[40] LT, lower thoracic spine; UT, upper thoracic spine.

a risk factor for mechanical or neurologic complications after ASD surgery.[59] Thus, whether a patient can sustain the morbidity of a larger fusion and a longer surgery is an important preoperative and intraoperative consideration when deciding between a lower versus upper thoracic UIV. Local anatomy, including stenosis and osteoporosis, should also be considered when selecting the UIV in order to avoid complications such as instrumentation failure and PJK.[60]

Lower Instrumented Vertebra

Similar to the UIV, lower instrumented vertebra (LIV) selection is for the fusion construct to end at a stable and neutral vertebra. The ideal LIV avoids the hypermobility of the thoracolumbar junction and extends at least past the apex of lumbar lordosis, which typically exists at L3-L4.[61] The choice of extending the LIV past this region is important owing to several patient outcome differences after fusion to the lower lumbar spine, sacrum, and pelvis. Fusions to S1 and/or the ilium have been associated with sacral insufficiency, increased estimated blood loss, increased operating time, and a higher incidence of PJK and pseudoarthrosis.[62–64] However, the benefits of extending the LIV to this level include increased construct stability and better restoration of sagittal alignment.[64–67]

Several foundational studies have indicated that regional deformity at the lower lumbar segments, including an L5-S1 spondylolisthesis, more severe sagittal misalignment, and lumbar hypolordosis, should influence surgeons to consider extension of the LIV past L5.[67,68] Extension of the LIV via iliac or S2 alar-iliac screws has been shown to improve the correction of multiple sagittal parameters and decrease the lumbosacral failure rate.[69] These benefits are likely related to greater biomechanical construct strength compared with those with a more proximal LIV. Concordantly, data from a recent large, propensity-matched study comparing the clinical and radiographic results of LIVs at L4/L5 versus S1/ilium reported superior correction of sagittal parameters in the S1/ilium LIV group.[64] However, it should be noted that several prior works have commented on the drawbacks of iliac screws, which include pain, prominent screw heads, and iliac screw breakage owing to a prominence that is particularly prevalent in smaller, thinner patients.[65,70]

In addition to deformity considerations, degenerative changes, such as stenosis or severe disc degeneration, are factors that should influence the extension of LIV past L5.[34] Patients with ASD with LIVs ending at L5 who had disc collapse at L5-S1 were at increased risk of distal junctional kyphosis and sagittal alignment decompensation.[71] Despite the biomechanical and alignment benefits of a more distal LIV, a significantly higher total revision rate in patients with distal fixation to the sacrum compared with patients with LIVs at L5 was reported.[72,73] Prior work has suggested that patients undergoing sacral fixation, especially those with poor bone quality, may benefit from interbody fusion support and rigid sacropelvic fixation in order to decrease lumbosacral pseudoarthrosis and screw loosening.[65–67,69,71] There is also some evidence that extension to the pelvis at a later point after an index surgery with an LIV at L5 yields equivalent outcomes.[74] Sparing L5-S1 may therefore be advantageous in younger patients who want to preserve motion or in medically frail patients who cannot tolerate the prolonged surgery and dissection needed for pelvic fixation. However, these patients should understand that additional surgery may be necessary in the future.

THE FUTURE OF PREOPERATIVE PLANNING IN DEFORMITY SURGERY
Imaging/Software

Although ASD was historically assessed using imaging in the coronal plane, it is now common practice to obtain a sagittal film from at least C7 to the pelvis. Advanced imaging modalities, such as EOS imaging (ATEC Spine Group), now permit whole body anteroposterior and lateral imaging to be obtained. This in turn can be used to construct a three-dimensional (3D) image of the spine in a weight-bearing position. These images are unique from those obtained using computed tomography (CT) scans and MRI, which are typically performed in a supine position.[75] Computer software has begun to revolutionize preoperative decision making, in particular, the precision of alignment measurements.[76] Lafage and colleagues[77] reported on the use of novel software to calculate PT, PI, LL, PI-LL mismatch, thoracic kyphosis, T1 spinopelvic inclination (T1SPI), and SVA. They reported excellent interrater reliabilities and that their analysis required only 75 seconds on average to complete.[77] This technology has since been demonstrated to yield more reliable measurements than those obtained by surgeons using PACS.[78] More recently, deep learning–based algorithms and software solutions have emerged and permit the automatic analysis of coronal and sagittal radiographs.[79–81]

Artificial Intelligence

Artificial intelligence (AI) has the potential to revolutionize and standardize preoperative planning.

Machine learning algorithms are a step beyond simple statistical analyses, such as linear and logistic regressions, which traditionally provide averages across entire populations and compare user-defined outcomes of interest. Machine learning can process large amounts of data and uncover and make sense of relationships between seemingly unrelated data points. AI has become more relevant as we move toward the age of personalized medicine because of its ability to provide specific information centered on each patient's care goals.[82] When used in predictive analytics for ASD surgery, AI can help foreshadow potential complications at various points of care and remove subjectivity when identifying relevant variables.[42,44,83–91] AI has also been used to predict large unforeseen costs after ASD.[92] Although machine learning can process large amounts of data and accurately predict specific outcomes, it is not without fault. Immense data sets are a prerequisite to training machine learning models, the acquisition of which may be unfeasible given the paucity of large prospective data sets in spine surgery.

Three-Dimensional Printing and Custom Rods

3D printing of spine models allows for the real-life models that permit the identification of anatomic details that would be otherwise difficult to appreciate on CT scan or MRI.[28] Preoperative planning with 3D printed models has been associated with decreased operative time, decreased blood loss, decreased radiation exposure, and decreased health care costs.[93–97] 3D printed drill guide templates have been shown to significantly improve the accuracy of screw placement compared with traditional screws placement.[97] Increased screw placement accuracy during spine deformity surgery using such templates has been found to decrease operative time, decrease blood loss, and decrease screw misplacement.[98] Finally, prebent custom rods provide patient-specific instrumentation without intraoperative bending and can significantly improve PT, sacral slope, LL, and SVA.[99]

SUMMARY

Preoperative planning is critical to the long-term success and outcome of ASD surgery. Improved understanding of ASD as a pathologic condition and the greater ability to predict postoperative outcomes have led to increasingly sophisticated modalities for planning, predicting, and executing ASD corrections. The advent of patient-specific instrumentation for ASD surgery has the potential

to maximize the reliability of properly executing a preoperative plan.

CLINICS CARE POINTS

- Preoperative goal setting of ASD correction is a key factor in improving quality of life and avoiding postoperative complications.
- Age adjusted values in sagittal plane correction had significantly improved pain and HRQOL.
- UIV level selection is determined by the amount of thoracic kyphosis and the degree of thoracic coronal deformity

REFERENCES

1. Dubousset J. Reflections of an orthopaedic surgeon on patient care and research into the condition of scoliosis. J Pediatr Orthop 2011;31(1 Suppl):S1–8.
2. Haddas R, Sambhariya V, Kosztowski T, et al. Cone of economy classification: evolution, concept of stability, severity level, and correlation to patient-reported outcome scores. Eur Spine J 2021;30(8): 2271–82.
3. Jackson RP, Simmons EH, Stripinis D. Incidence and severity of back pain in adult idiopathic scoliosis. Spine (Phila Pa 1976) 1983;8(7):749–56. Available at: http://www.ncbi.nlm.nih.gov/pubmed/6229884. Accessed August 22, 2013.
4. Robin GC, Span Y, Steinberg R, et al. Scoliosis in the elderly: a follow-up study. Spine (Phila Pa 1976) 1982;7(4):355–9.
5. Lowe T, Berven SH, Schwab FJ, et al. The SRS classification for adult spinal deformity: building on the King/Moe and Lenke classification systems. Spine (Phila Pa 1976) 2006;31(19 Suppl):S119–25.
6. Terran J, Schwab FJ, Shaffrey CI, et al. The SRS-Schwab Adult Spinal Deformity Classification: Assessment and Clinical Correlations Based on a Prospective Operative and Nonoperative Cohort. Neurosurgery 2013;73(4):559–68.
7. Lafage V, Schwab FJ, Patel A, et al. Pelvic tilt and truncal inclination: two key radiographic parameters in the setting of adults with spinal deformity. Spine (Phila Pa 1976) 2009;34(17):E599–606.
8. Rothenfluh DA, Mueller DA, Rothenfluh E, et al. Pelvic incidence-lumbar lordosis mismatch predisposes to adjacent segment disease after lumbar spinal fusion. Eur Spine J 2014;24(6):1251–8.
9. Lafage R, Passias P, Sheikh Alshabab B, et al. Patterns of Lumbar Spine Malalignment Leading to Revision Surgery for Proximal Junctional Kyphosis: A Cluster Analysis of Over- Versus Under-Correction.

Global Spine J 2022. https://doi.org/10.1177/21925 682211047461.

10. Bhagat S, Vozar V, Lutchman L, et al. Morbidity and mortality in adult spinal deformity surgery: Norwich Spinal Unit experience. Eur Spine J 2013;22(Suppl 1):S42–6.

11. Blondel B, Schwab FJ, Ungar B, et al. Impact of magnitude and percentage of global sagittal plane correction on health-related quality of life at 2-years follow-up. Neurosurgery 2012;71(2):341–8 [discussion: 348].

12. Diebo BG, Varghese JJ, Lafage R, et al. Sagittal alignment of the spine: What do you need to know? Clin Neurol Neurosurg 2015;139:295–301.

13. Glassman SD, Coseo MP, Carreon LY. Sagittal balance is more than just alignment: why PJK remains an unresolved problem. Scoliosis Spinal Disord 2016;11(1):1.

14. Obeid I, Hauger O, Aunoble SSSS, et al. Global analysis of sagittal spinal alignment in major deformities: correlation between lack of lumbar lordosis and flexion of the knee. Eur Spine J 2011;20(Suppl 5):681–5.

15. Schwab FJ, Ungar B, Blondel B, et al. Scoliosis Research Society-Schwab adult spinal deformity classification: a validation study. Spine (Phila Pa 1976) 2012;37(12):1077–82.

16. Slattery C, Verma K. Classification in Brief: SRS-Schwab Classification of Adult Spinal Deformity. Clin Orthop Relat Res 2018;476(9):1890–4.

17. Protopsaltis T, Schwab F, Bronsard N, et al. TheT1 pelvic angle, a novel radiographic measure of global sagittal deformity, accounts for both spinal inclination and pelvic tilt and correlates with health-related quality of life. J Bone Joint Surg Am 2014; 96(19):1631–40.

18. Larsson L, Li X, Frontera WR. Effects of aging on shortening velocity and myosin isoform composition in single human skeletal muscle cells. Am J Physiol 1997;272(2 Pt 1):C638–49. http://www.ncbi.nlm.nih.gov/pubmed/9124308.

19. Lord SR, Clark RD, Webster IW. Postural stability and associated physiological factors in a population of aged persons. J Gerontol 1991;46(3):M69–76.

20. Baldus C, Bridwell K, Harrast J, et al. The Scoliosis Research Society Health-Related Quality of Life (SRS-30) age-gender normative data: an analysis of 1346 adult subjects unaffected by scoliosis. Spine (Phila Pa 1976) 2011;36(14):1154–62.

21. Ware JE. SF-36 health survey update. Spine (Phila Pa 1976) 2000;25(24):3130–9. Available at: http://www.ncbi.nlm.nih.gov/pubmed/11124729. Accessed July 7, 2015.

22. Fairbank JC, Pynsent PB. The Oswestry Disability Index. Spine (Phila Pa 1976) 2000;25(22):2940–52 [discussion: 2952].

23. Lafage R, Schwab F, Challier V, et al, International Spine Study Group. Defining Spino-Pelvic Alignment Thresholds: Should Operative Goals in Adult Spinal Deformity Surgery Account for Age? Spine (Phila Pa 1976) 2016;41(1):62–8.

24. Lafage R, Schwab F, Glassman S, et al. Age-Adjusted Alignment Goals Have the Potential to Reduce PJK. Spine (Phila Pa 1976) 2017;42(17): 1275–82.

25. Byun CW, Cho JH, Lee CS, et al. Effect of overcorrection on proximal junctional kyphosis in adult spinal deformity: analysis by age-adjusted ideal sagittal alignment. Spine J 2022;22(4):635–45.

26. Yilgor C, Sogunmez N, Boissiere L, et al. Global Alignment and Proportion (GAP) Score. J Bone Joint Surg 2017;99(19):1661–72.

27. Bari TJ, Ohrt-Nissen S, Hansen LV, et al. Ability of the Global Alignment and Proportion Score to Predict Mechanical Failure Following Adult Spinal Deformity Surgery—Validation in 149 Patients With Two-Year Follow-up. Spine Deform 2019;7(2):331–7.

28. Lafage R, Smith JS, Elysee J, et al. Sagittal age-adjusted score (SAAS) for adult spinal deformity (ASD) more effectively predicts surgical outcomes and proximal junctional kyphosis than previous classifications. Spine Deform 2022;10(1):121–31.

29. Ploumis A, Simpson AK, Cha TD, et al. Coronal Spinal Balance in Adult Spine Deformity Patients with Long Spinal Fusions: A Minimum 2-5 Year Follow-up Study. J Spinal Disord Tech 2013;28(9):341–7.

30. Zuckerman SL, Cerpa M, Lai CS, et al. Coronal Alignment in Adult Spinal Deformity Surgery: Definitions, Measurements, Treatment Algorithms, and Impact on Clinical Outcomes. Clin Spine Surg 2022;35(5):196–203.

31. Bao H, Yan P, Qiu Y, et al. Coronal imbalance in degenerative lumbar scoliosis. Bone Joint Lett J 2016;98-B(9):1227–33.

32. Glassman SD, Berven S, Bridwell K, et al. Correlation of radiographic parameters and clinical symptoms in adult scoliosis. Spine (Phila Pa 1976) 2005; 30(6):682–8.

33. Kuklo TR. Principles for selecting fusion levels in adult spinal deformity with particular attention to lumbar curves and double major curves. Spine (Phila Pa 1976) 2006;31(19 Suppl):S132–8.

34. Bridwell KH. Selection of instrumentation and fusion levels for scoliosis: where to start and where to stop. Invited submission from the Joint Section Meeting on Disorders of the Spine and Peripheral Nerves, March 2004. J Neurosurg Spine 2004;1(1):1–8.

35. Kim YJ, Bridwell KH, Lenke LG, et al. Is the T9, T11, or L1 the more reliable proximal level after adult lumbar or lumbosacral instrumented fusion to L5 or S1? Spine (Phila Pa 1976) 2007;32(24):2653–61.

36. Blondel B, Wickman AM, Apazidis A, et al. Selection of fusion levels in adults with spinal deformity: an update. Spine J 2013;13(4):464–74.

37. Kim HJ, Iyer S, Zebala LP, et al. Perioperative Neurologic Complications in Adult Spinal Deformity Surgery: Incidence and Risk Factors in 564 Patients. Spine (Phila Pa 1976) 2017;42(6):420–7.

38. Smith JS, Klineberg E, Lafage V, et al. Prospective multicenter assessment of perioperative and minimum 2-year postoperative complication rates associated with adult spinal deformity surgery. J Neurosurg Spine 2016;25(1):1–14.

39. Soroceanu A, Diebo BG, Burton D, et al. Radiographical and Implant-Related Complications in Adult Spinal Deformity Surgery: Incidence, Patient Risk Factors, and Impact on Health-Related Quality of Life. Spine (Phila Pa 1976) 2015;40(18):1414–21.

40. Virk S, Platz U, Bess S, et al. Factors influencing upper-most instrumented vertebrae selection in adult spinal deformity patients: qualitative case-based survey of deformity surgeons. J Spine Surg 2021;7(1):37–47.

41. Zou L, Liu J, Lu H. Characteristics and risk factors for proximal junctional kyphosis in adult spinal deformity after correction surgery: a systematic review and meta-analysis. Neurosurg Rev 2019;42(3):671–82.

42. Yagi M, Fujita N, Okada E, et al. Fine-tuning the Predictive Model for Proximal Junctional Failure in Surgically Treated Patients With Adult Spinal Deformity. Spine (Phila Pa 1976) 2018;43(11):767–73.

43. Luo M, Wang P, Wang W, et al. Upper Thoracic versus Lower Thoracic as Site of Upper Instrumented Vertebrae for Long Fusion Surgery in Adult Spinal Deformity: A Meta-Analysis of Proximal Junctional Kyphosis. World Neurosurg 2017;102:200–8.

44. Scheer JK, Osorio JA, Smith JS, et al. Development of Validated Computer-based Preoperative Predictive Model for Proximal Junction Failure (PJF) or Clinically Significant PJK With 86% Accuracy Based on 510 ASD Patients With 2-year Follow-up. Spine (Phila Pa 1976) 2016;41(22):E1328–35.

45. Scheer JK, Lafage V, Smith JS, et al. Maintenance of radiographic correction at 2 years following lumbar pedicle subtraction osteotomy is superior with upper thoracic compared with thoracolumbar junction upper instrumented vertebra. Eur Spine J 2015; 24(Suppl 1):121–30.

46. Sciubba DM, Scheer JK, Smith JS, et al. Which daily functions are most affected by stiffness following total lumbar fusion: comparison of upper thoracic and thoracolumbar proximal endpoints. Spine (Phila Pa 1976) 2015;40(17):1338–44.

47. Kim HJ, Boachie-Adjei O, Shaffrey CI, et al. Upper Thoracic versus Lower Thoracic Upper Instrumented Vertebrae Endpoints have Similar Outcomes and Complications in Adult Scoliosis. Spine (Phila Pa 1976) 2014;39(13):E795–9.

48. Banno T, Hasegawa T, Yamato Y, et al. Prevalence and Risk Factors of Iliac Screw Loosening After Adult Spinal Deformity Surgery. Spine (Phila Pa 1976) 2017;42(17):E1024–30.

49. Fujimori T, Inoue S, Le H, et al. Long fusion from sacrum to thoracic spine for adult spinal deformity with sagittal imbalance: upper versus lower thoracic spine as site of upper instrumented vertebra. Neurosurg Focus 2014;36(5):E9.

50. Cho KJ, Suk SI, Park SR, et al. Selection of proximal fusion level for adult degenerative lumbar scoliosis. Eur Spine J 2013;22(2):394–401.

51. Hey HWD, Tan KA, Neo CSE, et al. T9 versus T10 as the upper instrumented vertebra for correction of adult deformity-rationale and recommendations. Spine J 2017;17(5):615–21.

52. Daniels AH, Reid DBC, Durand WM, et al. Upper-thoracic versus lower-thoracic upper instrumented vertebra in adult spinal deformity patients undergoing fusion to the pelvis: surgical decision-making and patient outcomes. J Neurosurg Spine 2019; 1–7. https://doi.org/10.3171/2019.9.spine19557.

53. Bridwell KH, Lenke LG, Cho SK, et al. Proximal junctional kyphosis in primary adult deformity surgery: evaluation of 20 degrees as a critical angle. Neurosurgery 2013;72(6):899–906.

54. Hostin R, McCarthy I, O'Brien M, et al. Incidence, mode, and location of acute proximal junctional failures after surgical treatment of adult spinal deformity. Spine (Phila Pa 1976) 2013;38(12):1008–15.

55. Kim DYK, Kim JY, Kim DYK, et al. Risk Factors of Proximal Junctional Kyphosis after Multilevel Fusion Surgery: More Than 2 Years Follow-Up Data. J Korean Neurosurg Soc 2017;60(2):174–80.

56. Park SHSJ, Lee CS, Chung SS, et al. Different Risk Factors of Proximal Junctional Kyphosis and Proximal Junctional Failure Following Long Instrumented Fusion to the Sacrum for Adult Spinal Deformity: Survivorship Analysis of 160 Patients. Neurosurgery 2017;80(2):279–86.

57. Park SJ, Lee CS, Park JS, et al. Should Thoracolumbar Junction Be Always Avoided as Upper Instrumented Vertebra in Long Instrumented Fusion for Adult Spinal Deformity?: Risk Factor Analysis for Proximal Junctional Failure. Spine (Phila Pa 1976) 2020;45(10):686–93.

58. Soroceanu A, Burton DC, Oren JH, et al. Medical Complications after Adult Spinal Deformity Surgery: Incidence, Risk factors, and Clinical Impact. Spine (Phila Pa 1976) 2016;18(5):345–52.

59. Charosky S, Guigui P, Blamoutier A, et al, Study Group on Scoliosis. Complications and risk factors of primary adult scoliosis surgery: a multicenter study of 306 patients. Spine (Phila Pa 1976) 2012; 37(8):693–700.

60. Yagi M, Fujita N, Tsuji O, et al. Low Bone-Mineral Density Is a Significant Risk for Proximal Junctional

Failure After Surgical Correction of Adult Spinal Deformity: A Propensity Score-Matched Analysis. Spine (Phila Pa 1976) 2018;43(7):485–91.

61. Roussouly P, Gollogly S, Berthonnaud E, et al. Classification of the normal variation in the sagittal alignment of the human lumbar spine and pelvis in the standing position. Spine (Phila Pa 1976) 2005; 30(3):346–53.

62. Koller H, Pfanz C, Meier O, et al. Factors influencing radiographic and clinical outcomes in adult scoliosis surgery: a study of 448 European patients. Eur Spine J 2015;25(2):532–48.

63. Cho KJ, Suk SI, Park SR, et al. Risk factors of sagittal decompensation after long posterior instrumentation and fusion for degenerative lumbar scoliosis. Spine (Phila Pa 1976) 2010;35(17):1595–601.

64. Yao YC, Kim HJ, Bannwarth M, et al. Lowest Instrumented Vertebra Selection to S1 or Ilium Versus L4 or L5 in Adult Spinal Deformity: Factors for Consideration in 349 Patients With a Mean 46-Month Follow-Up. Global Spine J 2021. https://doi.org/10.1177/21925682211009178. 21925682211009176.

65. Tsuchiya K, Bridwell KH, Kuklo TR, et al. Minimum 5-year analysis of L5-S1 fusion using sacropelvic fixation (bilateral S1 and iliac screws) for spinal deformity. Spine (Phila Pa 1976) 2006;31(3):303–8.

66. Tumialán LM, Mummaneni PV. Long-segment spinal fixation using pelvic screws. Neurosurgery 2008; 63(3 Suppl):183–90.

67. Cho KJ, Suk SI, Park SR, et al. Arthrodesis to L5 versus S1 in long instrumentation and fusion for degenerative lumbar scoliosis. Eur Spine J 2009;18(4):531–7.

68. Edwards CC, Bridwell KH, Patel A, et al. Long adult deformity fusions to L5 and the sacrum. A matched cohort analysis. Spine (Phila Pa 1976) 2004;29(18): 1996–2005.

69. Yasuda T, Hasegawa T, Yamato Y, et al. Lumbosacral Junctional Failures After Long Spinal Fusion for Adult Spinal Deformity-Which Vertebra Is the Preferred Distal Instrumented Vertebra? Spine Deform 2016;4(5):378–84.

70. Emami A, Deviren V, Berven S, et al. Outcome and complications of long fusions to the sacrum in adult spine deformity: Luque-Galveston, combined iliac and sacral screws, and sacral fixation. Spine (Phila Pa 1976) 2002;27(7):776–86.

71. Jia F, Wang G, Liu X, et al. Comparison of long fusion terminating at L5 versus the sacrum in treating adult spinal deformity: a meta-analysis. Eur Spine J 2020; 29(1):24–35.

72. Chen S, Luo M, Wang Y, et al. Stopping at Sacrum Versus Nonsacral Vertebra in Long Fusion Surgery for Adult Spinal Deformity: Meta-Analysis of Revision with Minimum 2-Year Follow-Up. World Neurosurg 2018. https://doi.org/10.1016/j.wneu.2018.12.102.

73. Pichelmann MA, Lenke LG, Bridwell KH, et al. Revision rates following primary adult spinal deformity surgery: six hundred forty-three consecutive patients followed-up to twenty-two years postoperative. Spine (Phila Pa 1976) 2010;35(2):219–26.

74. Fu KMMG, Smith JS, Burton DC, et al. Revision Extension to the Pelvis versus Primary Spinopelvic Instrumentation in Adult Deformity: Comparison of Clinical Outcomes and Complications. World Neurosurg 2013;82(3):8–13.

75. Smith JS, Shaffrey CI, Bess S, et al. Recent and Emerging Advances in Spinal Deformity. Neurosurgery 2017;80(3S):S70–85.

76. Langella F, Villafañe JH, Damilano M, et al. Predictive Accuracy of SurgimapTM Surgical Planning for Sagittal Imbalance: A Cohort Study. Spine (Phila Pa 1976) 2017;42(22):E1297–304.

77. Lafage R, Ferrero E, Henry JK, et al. Validation of a new computer-assisted tool to measure spinopelvic parameters. Spine J 2015;15(12):2493–502.

78. Gupta M, Henry JK, Schwab F, et al. Dedicated spine measurement software quantifies key spinopelvic parameters more reliably than traditional picture archiving and communication systems tools. Spine (Phila Pa 1976) 2016;41(1):E22–7.

79. Zerouali M, Parpaleix A, Benbakoura M, et al. Automatic deep learning-based assessment of spinopelvic coronal and sagittal alignment. Diagn Interv Imaging 2023. https://doi.org/10.1016/j.diii.2023.03.003.

80. Grover P, Siebenwirth J, Caspari C, et al. Can artificial intelligence support or even replace physicians in measuring sagittal balance? A validation study on preoperative and postoperative full spine images of 170 patients. Eur Spine J 2022;31(8): 1943–51.

81. Orosz LD, Bhatt FR, Jazini E, et al. Novel artificial intelligence algorithm: an accurate and independent measure of spinopelvic parameters. J Neurosurg Spine 2022;37(6):893–901.

82. Caruso JP, Kafka BR, Traylor JI, et al. Applying 3-Dimensional Printing and Modeling for Preoperative Reconstruction and Instrumentation Placement Planning in Complex Deformity Surgery. Oper Neurosurg (Hagerstown). 2022;23(6):514–22.

83. Durand WM, DePasse JM, Daniels AH. Predictive Modeling for Blood Transfusion After Adult Spinal Deformity Surgery: A Tree-Based Machine Learning Approach. Spine (Phila Pa 1976) 2018;43(15): 1058–66.

84. Safaee MM, Scheer JK, Ailon T, et al. Predictive Modeling of Length of Hospital Stay Following Adult Spinal Deformity Correction: Analysis of 653 Patients with an Accuracy of 75% within 2 Days. World Neurosurg 2018;115:e422–7.

85. Scheer JK, Daniels AH, Smith JS, et al. Development of a preoperative predictive model for major complications following adult spinal deformity surgery. J Neurosurg Spine 2017;26:1–8.

86. Joshi RS, Haddad AF, Lau D, et al. Artificial intelligence for adult spinal deformity. Neurospine 2019; 16(4):686–94.

87. Yagi M, Hosogane N, Fujita N, et al. Predictive model for major complications 2 years after corrective spine surgery for adult spinal deformity. Eur Spine J 2019;28(1):180–7.

88. Passias PG, Oh C, Jalai CM, et al. Predictive Model for Cervical Alignment and Malalignment Following Surgical Correction of Adult Spinal Deformity. Spine (Phila Pa 1976) 2016;41(18):E1096–103.

89. Oh T, Scheer JK, Smith JS, et al. Potential of predictive computer models for preoperative patient selection to enhance overall quality-adjusted life years gained at 2-year follow-up: a simulation in 234 patients with adult spinal deformity. Neurosurg Focus 2017;43(6):E2.

90. Scheer JK, Osorio JA, Smith JS, et al. Development of a Preoperative Predictive Model for Reaching the Oswestry Disability Index Minimal Clinically Important Difference for Adult Spinal Deformity Patients. Spine Deform 2018;6(5):593–9.

91. Ames CP, Smith JS, Pellisé F, et al. Development of Deployable Predictive Models for Minimal Clinically Important Difference Achievement Across the Commonly Used Health-Related Quality of Life Instruments in Adult Spinal Deformity Surgery. Spine (Phila Pa 1976) 2019;1. https://doi.org/10.1097/BRS.0000000000003031.

92. Ames CP, Smith JS, Gum JL, et al. Utilization of Predictive Modeling to Determine Episode of Care Costs and to Accurately Identify Catastrophic Cost Nonwarranty Outlier Patients in Adult Spinal Deformity Surgery. Spine (Phila Pa 1976) 2020;45(5): E252–65.

93. Parr WCH, Burnard JL, Wilson PJ, et al. 3D printed anatomical (bio)models in spine surgery: clinical benefits and value to health care providers. J Spine Surg 2019;5(4):549–60.

94. Öztürk AM, Süer O, Govsa F, et al. Patient-specific three-dimensional printing spine model for surgical planning in AO spine type-C fracture posterior long-segment fixation. Acta Orthop Traumatol Turc 2022;56(2):138–46.

95. Kabra A, Mehta N, Garg B. 3D printing in spine care: A review of current applications. J Clin Orthop Trauma 2022;35:102044.

96. Aili A, Ma Y, Sui J, et al. Application of 3D printed models in the surgical treatment of spinal deformity. Am J Transl Res 2022;14(9):6341–8.

97. Lopez CD, Boddapati V, Lee NJ, et al. Three-Dimensional Printing for Preoperative Planning and Pedicle Screw Placement in Adult Spinal Deformity: A Systematic Review. Global Spine J 2021;11(6):936–49.

98. Pan A, Ding H, Hai Y, et al. The Value of Three-Dimensional Printing Spine Model in Severe Spine Deformity Correction Surgery. Global Spine J 2023; 13(3):787–95.

99. Sadrameli SS, Boghani Z, Steele WJ Iii, et al. Utility of Patient-Specific Rod Instrumentation in Deformity Correction: Single Institution Experience. Spine Surg Relat Res 2020;4(3):256–60.

Section II: Open Approaches for Deformity

The Lumbosacral Fractional Curve in Adult Degenerative Scoliosis

Peter G. Campbell, MD*, Pierce D. Nunley, MD

KEYWORDS

- Fractional curve • Scoliosis • Fusion • Scoliosis correction • Adult degenerative scoliosis
- L5 obliquity • Adult spinal deformity

KEY POINTS

- In the setting of adult degenerative scoliosis (ADS) the compensatory curve at the level of the lumbosacral junction below the major curve is called the fractional curve.
- The L4, L5, and S1 nerve roots on the side of the concavity of the fractional curve are the most frequent radicular pain generators in the setting of ADS.
- Ending a scoliosis construct at L4 or L5 with a preexisting fractional curve places patients at high risk of adjacent segment breakdown or causing a compensatory major curve above the correction.
- Instrumentation options to address the fractional curve include anterior lateral interbody fusion (ALIF), oblique lateral interbody fusion, transforaminal lumbar interbody fusion (TLIF), and open rod reduction techniques.
- ALIF and TLIF at L4-S1 likely both can provide viable surgical options for reduction of the fractional curve in ADS long-segment constructs.

INTRODUCTION

Adult degenerative scoliosis (ADS) is a 3-dimensional spinal disorder that affects the adult spine. Typically, the major curve can be found in the mid-lumbar spine.[1] Epidemiologically, degenerative lumbar scoliosis is most frequently identified in patients in the sixth decade of life or greater, with a slight female predilection. ADS is thought to be related to osteoporotic degeneration and/or degenerative disc disease, resulting in an asymmetric degradation of the intervertebral disc and facet joints.[2,3] These distortions induce a progressive coronal imbalance of the vertebra and ultimately lead to scoliosis, a potential loss of lumbar lordosis, vertebral body translation, and rotational subluxation.[4]

In treating adult degenerative scoliosis, the main indication for surgical treatment is radiculopathy.[5] Unlike the typical adolescent scoliosis patient, the curve parameters are generally considered to be unsuitable for ending fixation at L3 or L4.[6] Oftentimes, a rotatory subluxation or a coronal imbalance is present at the L4 or L5 segments. In the setting of ADS the compensatory curve at the level of the lumbosacral junction below the major curve is called the fractional curve.[7] The nerve roots on the concave side of the fractional curve are the most frequent radicular pain generators in the ADS population.[1]

The general goals of adult deformity surgery are like those of the adolescent population. Efforts are directed to obtaining both sagittal and coronal balance, symptom relief, and solid fusion.[8,9] Unfortunately, a major difficulty of attempting to apply a minimally invasive solution to ADS curves has been in the treatment of the fractional portion of the curve.[7] Traditional approaches to deformity correction include both anterior-posterior approaches as well as posterior-only treatments. Open surgical procedures allow the surgeon to

Spine Institute of Louisiana, 1500 Line Avenue, Shreveport, LA 71101, USA
* Corresponding author.
E-mail address: pcampbell@louisianaspine.org

Neurosurg Clin N Am 34 (2023) 537–544
https://doi.org/10.1016/j.nec.2023.06.001
1042-3680/23/© 2023 Elsevier Inc. All rights reserved.

perform reduction maneuvers that allow for correction of the deformity. Minimally invasive spinal surgery offers fewer options for rigid curve manipulation at the lumbosacral junction. If the fractional curve is not addressed properly, it is unlikely coronal realignment will occur. The patient may then experience aggravation of the coronal imbalance.[1] Hence, a spinal deformity surgeon should be able to effectively evaluate the fractional curve preoperatively to ensure adherence to these established goals to prevent clinical worsening secondary to coronal and spinopelvic malalignment.

CHALLENGES IN TREATING THE FRACTIONAL CURVE

In treating ADS, full-length standing anteroposterior and lateral radiographs are always obtained to identify coronal imbalance and spinopelvic parameters. Typically ADS curves have a high lumbar apex.[10] These deformities are often concomitant with the loss of lumbar lordosis and reciprocating curves without significant scoliosis in the upper thoracic levels. A fractional curve, L4 to the sacrum, is often appreciated on anteroposterior imaging (**Fig. 1**).

Much like other degenerative conditions, pain is the typical indication for seeking treatment of more than 90% of the patient population with ADS.[11] Patients with ADS may present with back pain, radiculopathy, and/or neurogenic claudication.[12] Severe foraminal stenosis is very commonly seen in up to 97% of patients with ADS.[13] The probability of radiculopathy has been shown to increase linearly as the root level advances caudally.[14] Hence, the L4, L5, and S1 nerve roots on the

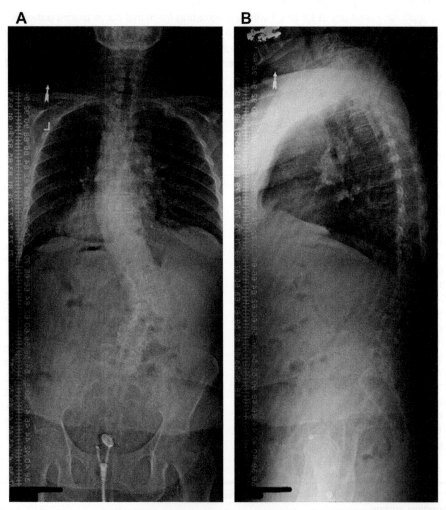

Fig. 1. (*A*) Anteroposterior and (*B*) lateral 36-inch standing radiographs demonstrating an adult degenerative scoliosis major curve with an apex at the L2/3 disc space and a fractional curve causing a rightward obliquity of L5.

side of the concavity of the fractional curve are the most frequent radicular pain generators in the setting of ADS.[3]

In treating ADS, spine surgeons must offer a weighted evaluation of the extent of surgical intervention against the directly proportional increase in complication incidence associated with lengthening surgical constructs. Although there is no consensus regarding the best available option, decompression alone, direct, or indirect decompression with short- and long-segment fusions are frequently used.[15,16] Furthermore, various techniques to correct fractional curve have been described in the literature, including anterior lumbar interbody fusion (ALIF), oblique lumbar interbody fusion (OLIF), posterior or transforaminal lumbar interbody fusion (PLIF or TLIF).[5] If a short-segment fusion is selected, degeneration can be accelerated in the remaining curve and result in adjacent segment disease.[16] Therefore, to fully reduce or avoid adjacent segment pathology, a long-segment fusion extending to the far proximal thoracic spine and sacrum should be performed. However, this option invariably increases both the major complication rate including proximal junctional kyphosis and unplanned reoperation rate in this elderly population.[17]

Ending a surgical construct before the lumbosacral junction in ADS can be performed when a surgeon is attempting to minimize the number of levels fused and thus the complication rate of spine surgery. Maintenance of motion at the L4/5 or L5/S1 segments does allow for the pelvic compensatory mobility to continue accommodate a stiff construct above the lumbosacral junction.[18] However, the most common intricacy associated with stopping an ADS fusion at L4 or L5 seems to be adjacent segment disease at the L5/S1 disc.[19] Literature reported rates of adjacent segment disease at L5-S1 after short- and long-segment ADS fusions range from 38% to 61%.[20–23] One factor potentially placing patients at high risk for adjacent segment breakdown after fusions ending at L4 or L5 is the presence of a fractional curve at L5/S1.[7] Ending a construct above a fractional curve makes subsequent spinal balance difficult to achieve, while also increasing the likelihood that any adjacent segment degeneration will reduce the cross-sectional area even further in one foramen. Postoperatively, this may lead to a clinically symptomatic L5 radiculopathy that could ultimately require a revision surgery requiring extension to the sacrum.[6] Some investigators have recommended that all fractional curves greater than 15° be corrected and included within the construct.[10]

Consideration and management of the fractional curve at L5 is of considerable importance in treating patients with ADS. If a fractional curve is present and neglected at the time of the index surgery, the patient is unlikely to obtain coronal balance.[24] If a minimally invasive solution is selected, surgeons must understand and be able to realistically gauge the degree of obtainable correction available from these techniques.[7] In ADS, rigid fractional curves are generally recommended to be included in the fusion construct and often require management with anterior or posterior interbody placement to prevent coronal decompensation[24] (**Fig. 2**).

CHALLENGES MANAGING THE LUMBOSACRAL JUNCTION

There remains considerable controversy in the literature regarding the appropriate distal fusion level in the setting of a long construct fusion.[19] However, there does seem to be a consensus on several situations whereby fixation to the sacrum is indicated. Many spine surgeons agree that indications to include the sacrum in an ADS construct include the presence of an L5/S1 spondylolisthesis, if an L5 or S1 radiculopathy is present, previous decompression at the L5/S1 segment, and the presence of a fractional curve at the lumbosacral junction.[6,18,19] Terminating a long-segment fusion at L5 when the L5/S1 segment is healthy can offer benefits such as maintaining lumbar motion, reducing operative morbidity, and decreasing the perioperative complication rates associated with lumbosacral fixation.[18] However, disadvantages to L4 or L5 construct termination include the increased potential for adjacent segment degeneration at L5/S1, loss of ability to correct sagittal plane deformities with the initial operation, and oftentimes the lack of a solid fixation endpoint for pedicle screw fixation owing to the L5 pedicular challenges.[6,18] If there is formidable degeneration at the L5/S1 disc many surgeons suggest for instrumenting to the sacrum.[6] However, considerable disagreement exists regarding the assessment of degeneration. Validated algorithms exist that score disc degeneration on radiograph by evaluating variables such as disc height, status of the end plates, spondylolisthesis, and vacuum disc phenomenon.[25] However, radiographic evaluation in ADS is quite difficult given the obliquity and opacification related to pelvic structures. The use of MRI to evaluate disc degeneration has not yet been validated for this indication.[26] Furthermore, the use of MRI to evaluate disc degeneration in this setting is beset with innate challenges such as poor correlation between mild and

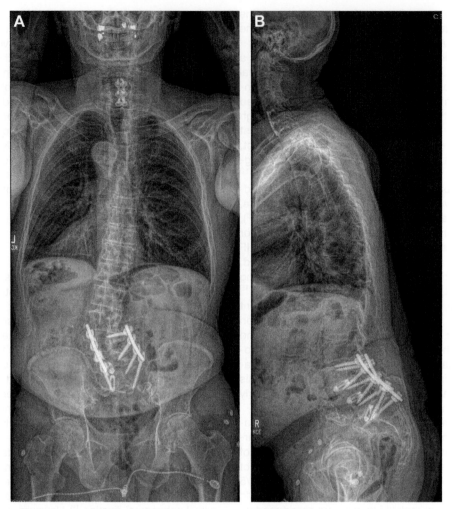

Fig. 2. (*A*) Anteroposterior and (*B*) lateral EOS standing radiographs showing an increased major curve after L3-S1 transforaminal lumbar interbody fusion without appropriate correction of the fractional curve.

moderate disc disease to pain, lack of a clear clinical correlation of Modic endplate changes to pain, and significant interobserver variability of assessing the disc itself in the setting of lumbar scoliosis.[6,27] Computed tomography scans have been used to evaluate for facet arthropathy at this level also with uncertain significance given that patients in the age range necessary to acquire ADS often have degenerative changes.[28] Even if there is only minor degeneration in the L5/S1 disc, for patients with a sagittal imbalance and lumbar hypolordosis, most investigators agree that the L5-S1 segment should be included in the fusion to attempt to correct these parameters in service of an improvement in global spinal alignment.[6,19,29]

Several clinical challenges must be managed in the patient population with ADS when a long construct fusion encompasses a fractional curve. True correction of both coronal and sagittal plane

deformity often mandates long posterior constructs from the distal thoracic spine to the sacrum. Given the long lever arms and associated cantilever forces, high amounts of stresses are placed on the base of the construct.[30] In addition, cancellous L5 and S1 pedicles coupled with osteopenia and osteoporosis in the elderly patient may lead to distal hardware failure. Common techniques to augment long segment fusions for additional sacropelvic fixation include the use of S2 alar iliac screws and iliac bolts.[31] The addition of pelvic fixation provides the attractive biomechanical benefit of being both divergent anchors from the proximal fixation points in the coronal plane as well as a stabilization point anterior to the axis of rotation of the pelvis.[31,32] Although absolute and relative indications for using this instrumentation remain undefined, these modern day pelvic fixation techniques offer an improved construct profile for long-segment fusion that reduces distal failure in at-risk patients.[30] However, proximal junctional kyphosis then becomes a significant concern associated with relatively high return to the operating room.[33]

TECHNIQUES TO CORRECT THE FRACTIONAL CURVE

The stated goals of adult deformity surgery are to obtain sagittal and coronal balance, symptom relief, and solid fusion.[8,9] Unfortunately, the population with ADS that is often elderly have poor bone substrate and are prone to higher perioperative complications. A recent multicenter prospective study conducted to assess perioperative and postoperative complication rates after open ASD procedures identified 69.8% complication rate at 2-year follow-up. Furthermore 28.2% of patients required one or more reoperation.[33] Given the high complication rates of this procedure, treatment goals are often adjusted to focus more on symptom management as an important subtext to the overall scoliosis surgical planning.[34] Hence, various techniques to combine appropriate spinal outcomes with complication avoidance have been described.[35] Decompression alone at the level of radiculopathy is occasionally used to treat severe radiculopathy. Placement of interbody cages that enhance correction of deformity and provide anterior column support and circumferential arthrodesis are also described as viable options. Furthermore, short- and long-segment posterior instrumentation with facetectomies have also been used for more extensive deformity correction. All the aforementioned strategies have been used to treat fractional curve pathology.

ADS treatment is a challenge for spine surgeons especially when treating an elderly patient population with multiple medical comorbidities. A truly corrective operation may result in prohibitively high complication rates. Oftentimes the presenting complaint is severe radiculopathy from mechanical compression from L4-S1; this often necessitates treatment to the fractional curve.[3] Various minimally invasive decompressions involving the use of microscopes, tubular retractors, and endoscopes have been used to treat this type of degenerative disease. These techniques largely focus on the preservation of the posterior elements, supraspinatus, and interspinous ligament and facet joints.[36] However, decompression alone for ADS often is not supported by robust literature in favor of good long-term outcomes.[4,37,38] However, some investigators do describe performing decompression alone as an option in certain settings. Berven and colleagues recommended a

unilateral minimally invasive surgical (MIS) decompression for patients with ADS with radicular pain only stemming from the convex side of the deformity with an intact pars interarticularis and facet joint.[39] Hansraj and colleagues reported that decompression alone could be performed in patients with central stenosis and less than 20° of coronal curvature.[40] Kato and colleagues noted poor success rates if MIS decompression is performed at a level with greater than 3° degrees coronal disc wedging or lateral listhesis at that level; this was noted to be especially severe if it occurred at the level of the L4/5 space.[36] Other investigators have also found that similar radiographic findings alone were strong predictors of degenerative scoliosis curve progression.[41] Using an MIS decompression in the fractional curve has been presented in the literature as an option in very select cases when there are no signs of asymmetrical degeneration that would predispose patients to postoperative curve progression and thus extensive reconstructive procedure.

Spine surgeons performing scoliosis operations generally pay close attention to the lumbosacral junction. ALIF is often used to address the clinical symptoms associated with a fractional curve at L4/5 and L5/S1. ALIF has been considered the gold-standard technique for achieving interbody fusion with rates up to 97%.[42] ALIF offers several benefits in ADS: (1) large graft size with significant surface area for fusion, (2) anterior load sharing with the posterior hardware, (3) indirect decompression of a narrowed neural foramen in the fractional curve, (4) sectioning of the anterior longitudinal ligament that allows for increased lordosis to be added to the final construct, and (5) improved coronal and sagittal balance.[7] An L4/5 and L5/S1 ALIF at the base of a long-segment scoliosis construct will effectively address the fractional curve treatment in its entirety. In a review by McPhee and colleagues staged anterior and posterior lumbar procedures showed better fractional curve improvement as well as sagittal balance correction in patients with ADS than posterior procedures alone.[43] Unfortunately, the addition of ALIF to a scoliosis solution is also associated with disadvantages including increased intraoperative time and anesthetic times, the risk of intra-abdominal vascular and visceral injury as well as superior hypogastric plexus injury.[35,44]

Minimally invasive techniques have recently been applied to surgical correction of ADS.[45] When treating a disease process in an aging population, the reduction of tissue dissection and perioperative complications rates is certainly paramount to some patients. Access to the L5/S1 space is currently problematic for traditional transpsoas procedures currently used for lateral access. Hence, with this traditional transpsoas approach, there is often a need for another surgical approach to fully treat the fractional curve.[46] A second lateral technique first described in 2012, called an OLIF, has been suggested as a possibly less invasive option to provide fractional curve stability at the lumbosacral junction.[47] Although this procedure will be fully discussed elsewhere in this issue in full detail, this approach has been publicized as a potential option to obtain access to multiple lumbar interspaces, including both the L4/5 and L5/S1 levels, with an anterior fusion corridor associated with fewer complications than the ALIF and transpsoas approaches.[48] The theoretic benefit to the procedure is the ability to manipulate the fractional curve in both the coronal and sagittal planes through one minimally invasive incision. However, it still shares the associated risks of the ALIF operation such as increased operative times and vascular injury. Current literature has not fully critically evaluated the indications for OLIF procedure in the setting of spinal deformity at this time.

Interbody cages placed through a posterior approach are also options when attempting to correct a fractional curve. The posterior insertion rigid cages can restore the disc height, possibly providing a mechanism for lasting decompression of the neural elements. Using a unilateral interbody cage insertion Heary and Karimi reported excellent improvements in coronal imbalance in patients with ADS when a unilateral interbody cage was inserted into the concavity of the curve.[9] Wang reported an improvement in both the coronal and sagittal alignment with unilateral insertion of an expandable mesh bag.[46] Wang suggested placement of a unilaterally inserted cage into the side of the concavity of the fractional curve to elevate and correct the curve.[46] However, posteriorly inserted interbody cages do require a more extensive bony removal than posterior surgery alone, an increased operative time for facetectomy and discectomy, and a narrow access corridor that mandates a smaller implant footprint that can lead to subsidence in the longer term.[42]

Several studies have compared the results of ALIF versus TLIF for long-segment corrections (Buell, Revella, Crandall, Doward). Crandall and Revella found similar improvements in clinical outcome measures for visual analog scores and Oswestry Disability Index (ODI) scores between patient groups undergoing long instrumented correction with TLIF versus ALIF (Crandall, Revella) although these were not specific to patients with ADS. Buell demonstrated that final ODI and physical component summary scores were inferior in the TLIF versus the ALIF group in the population with ADS.[49] These investigators also demonstrated similar fractional curve corrections of approximately 67% for L4-S1 TLIF patients and 65% for L4-S1 ALIF patients. More rod fractures were seen in the TLIF group.[49]

Unlike adolescent scoliosis, fractional curves in ASD are generally associated with a rigid spine. Hence, open surgical approaches may be more powerful in obtaining sagittal alignment but at the cost of an increased perioperative complication rate. Posterior techniques to provide a correction of the fractional curve can be used; this includes both osteotomy and rod reduction options. Rod rotation maneuvers can allow the frontal scoliotic deformity to be converted into a lumbar lordosis with a 3-dimensional correction.[50] However, these techniques are limited by anterior or lateral bridging osteophytes that can only be released by a circumferential surgical option.[51]

SUMMARY

Understanding the relationship of the lumbosacral fractional curve to degenerative scoliosis is critically important to surgical management. It is vitally important for surgeons to understand the cause and pathogenesis of this disease process, given the increasing patient age as well as the resultant associated increase in medical comorbidities experienced with large corrective operations. As more minimally invasive instrumentation solutions are applied to ADS to decrease perioperative complication rates, surgeons have realized that ending a construct at the L5 obliquity may in part be responsible for suboptimal patient outcomes.[7] Although a well-planned ALIF or TLIF procedure effectively corrects the fractional curve, other MIS and open treatment strategies may also be dependable options.

DISCLOSURE

P.G. Campbell—Consultant: Stryker, Nexus Spine. Pierce Nunley—Royalties: K2M, LDR. Speakers bureau: K2M, LDR. Consultant: K2M. Stock: Amedica, Paradigm, Spineology.

REFERENCES

1. Wang H, et al. Posterior column osteotomy plus unilateral cage strutting for correction of lumbosacral fractional curve in degenerative lumbar scoliosis. J Orthop Surg Res 2020;15(1):482.
2. Daffner SD, Vaccaro AR. Adult degenerative lumbar scoliosis. Am J Orthop (Belle Mead NJ) 2003;32(2): 77–82 [discussion: 82].

3. Ploumis A, et al. Radiculopathy in degenerative lumbar scoliosis: correlation of stenosis with relief from selective nerve root steroid injections. Pain Med 2011;12(1):45–50.

4. Aebi M. The adult scoliosis. Eur Spine J 2005; 14(10):925–48.

5. Chou D, et al. Treatment of the Fractional Curve of Adult Scoliosis With Circumferential Minimally Invasive Surgery Versus Traditional, Open Surgery: An Analysis of Surgical Outcomes. Global Spine J 2018;8(8):827–33.

6. Bridwell KH, Edwards CC, Lenke LG. The pros and cons to saving the L5-S1 motion segment in a long scoliosis fusion construct. Spine (Phila Pa 1976) 2003;28(20):S234–42.

7. Wang MY. The Importance of the Fractional Curve. In: Wang MY, et al, editors. Minimally invasive spinal deformity surgery: an Evolution of modern techniques. Springer; 2014. p. 47–52.

8. Birknes JK, et al. Adult degenerative scoliosis: a review. Neurosurgery 2008;63(3 Suppl):94–103.

9. Heary RF, Kumar S, Bono CM. Decision making in adult deformity. Neurosurgery 2008;63(3 Suppl): 69–77.

10. Silva FE, Lenke LG. Adult degenerative scoliosis: evaluation and management. Neurosurg Focus 2010;28(3):E1.

11. Winter RB, Lonstein JE, Denis F. Pain patterns in adult scoliosis. Orthop Clin North Am 1988;19(2): 339–45.

12. Schwab FJ, et al. Adult scoliosis: a quantitative radiographic and clinical analysis. Spine (Phila Pa 1976) 2002;27(4):387–92.

13. Fu KM, et al. Prevalence, severity, and impact of foraminal and canal stenosis among adults with degenerative scoliosis. Neurosurgery 2011;69(6): 1181–7.

14. Hawasli AH, et al. Interpedicular height as a predictor of radicular pain in adult degenerative scoliosis. Spine J 2016;16(9):1070–8.

15. Bridwell KH. Selection of instrumentation and fusion levels for scoliosis: where to start and where to stop. Invited submission from the Joint Section Meeting on Disorders of the Spine and Peripheral Nerves, March 2004. J Neurosurg Spine 2004;1(1):1–8.

16. Cho KJ, et al. Short fusion versus long fusion for degenerative lumbar scoliosis. Eur Spine J 2008; 17(5):650–6.

17. Akbarnia BA, Ogilvie JW, Hammerberg KW. Debate: degenerative scoliosis: to operate or not to operate. Spine (Phila Pa 1976) 2006;31(19 Suppl):S195–201.

18. Swamy G, Berven SH, Bradford DS. The selection of L5 versus S1 in long fusions for adult idiopathic scoliosis. Neurosurg Clin N Am 2007;18(2):281–8.

19. Cho KJ, et al. Arthrodesis to L5 versus S1 in long instrumentation and fusion for degenerative lumbar scoliosis. Eur Spine J 2009;18(4):531–7.

20. Edwards CC, et al. Long adult deformity fusions to L5 and the sacrum. A matched cohort analysis. Spine (Phila Pa 1976) 2004;29(18):1996–2005.

21. Edwards CC, et al. Thoracolumbar deformity arthrodesis to L5 in adults: the fate of the L5-S1 disc. Spine (Phila Pa 1976) 2003;28(18):2122–31.

22. Emami A, et al. Outcome and complications of long fusions to the sacrum in adult spine deformity: luque-galveston, combined iliac and sacral screws, and sacral fixation. Spine (Phila Pa 1976) 2002; 27(7):776–86.

23. Horton WC, Holt RT, Muldowny DS. Controversy. Fusion of L5-S1 in adult scoliosis. Spine (Phila Pa 1976) 1996;21(21):2520–2.

24. Youssef JA, et al. Current status of adult spinal deformity. Global Spine J 2013;3(1):51–62.

25. Weiner DK, et al. Does radiographic osteoarthritis correlate with flexibility of the lumbar spine? J Am Geriatr Soc 1994;42(3):257–63.

26. Pfirrmann CW, et al. Magnetic resonance classification of lumbar intervertebral disc degeneration. Spine (Phila Pa 1976) 2001;26(17):1873–8.

27. Sandhu HS, et al. Association between findings of provocative discography and vertebral endplate signal changes as seen on MRI. J Spinal Disord 2000;13(5):438–43.

28. Boos N, et al. Classification of age-related changes in lumbar intervertebral discs: 2002 Volvo Award in basic science. Spine (Phila Pa 1976) 2002;27(23): 2631–44.

29. Schwab FJ, et al. Radiographical spinopelvic parameters and disability in the setting of adult spinal deformity: a prospective multicenter analysis. Spine (Phila Pa 1976) 2013;38(13):E803–12.

30. Shen FH, et al. Pelvic fixation for adult scoliosis. Eur Spine J 2013;22(Suppl 2):S265–75.

31. Kebaish KM. Sacropelvic fixation: techniques and complications. Spine (Phila Pa 1976) 2010;35(25): 2245–51.

32. McCord DH, et al. Biomechanical analysis of lumbosacral fixation. Spine (Phila Pa 1976) 1992;17(8 Suppl):S235–43.

33. Smith JS, et al. Prospective multicenter assessment of perioperative and minimum 2-year postoperative complication rates associated with adult spinal deformity surgery. J Neurosurg Spine 2016;25(1): 1–14.

34. Turner JA, et al. Surgery for lumbar spinal stenosis. Attempted meta-analysis of the literature. Spine (Phila Pa 1976) 1992;17(1):1–8.

35. Mobbs RJ, et al. Lumbar interbody fusion: techniques, indications and comparison of interbody fusion options including PLIF, TLIF, MI-TLIF, OLIF/ ATP, LLIF and ALIF. J Spine Surg 2015;1(1):2–18.

36. Kato M, et al. Radiographic Risk Factors of Reoperation Following Minimally Invasive Decompression for Lumbar Canal Stenosis Associated With

Degenerative Scoliosis and Spondylolisthesis. Global Spine J 2017;7(6):498–505.

37. Frazier DD, et al. Associations between spinal deformity and outcomes after decompression for spinal stenosis. Spine (Phila Pa 1976) 1997;22(17):2025–9.

38. Vaccaro AR, Ball ST. Indications for instrumentation in degenerative lumbar spinal disorders. Orthopedics 2000;23(3):260–71 [quiz: 272-3].

39. Berven SH, et al. Operative management of degenerative scoliosis: an evidence-based approach to surgical strategies based on clinical and radiographic outcomes. Neurosurg Clin N Am 2007; 18(2):261–72.

40. Hansraj KK, et al. Decompression, fusion, and instrumentation surgery for complex lumbar spinal stenosis. Clin Orthop Relat Res 2001;(384):18–25.

41. Seo JY, et al. Risk of progression of degenerative lumbar scoliosis. J Neurosurg Spine 2011;15(5): 558–66.

42. Yen CP, Mosley YI, Uribe JS. Role of minimally invasive surgery for adult spinal deformity in preventing complications. Curr Rev Musculoskelet Med 2016; 9(3):309–15.

43. McPhee IB, Swanson CE. The surgical management of degenerative lumbar scoliosis. Posterior instrumentation alone versus two stage surgery. Bull Hosp Jt Dis 1998;57(1):16–22.

44. Phan K, Thayaparan GK, Mobbs RJ. Anterior lumbar interbody fusion versus transforaminal lumbar interbody fusion–systematic review and meta-analysis. Br J Neurosurg 2015;29(5):705–11.

45. Anand N, Baron EM. Minimally invasive approaches for the correction of adult spinal deformity. Eur Spine J 2013;22(Suppl 2):S232–41.

46. Wang MY. Improvement of sagittal balance and lumbar lordosis following less invasive adult spinal deformity surgery with expandable cages and percutaneous instrumentation. J Neurosurg Spine 2013;18(1):4–12.

47. Silvestre C, et al. Complications and Morbidities of Mini-open Anterior Retroperitoneal Lumbar Interbody Fusion: Oblique Lumbar Interbody Fusion in 179 Patients. Asian Spine J 2012;6(2):89–97.

48. Mehren C, et al. The Oblique Anterolateral Approach to the Lumbar Spine Provides Access to the Lumbar Spine With Few Early Complications. Clin Orthop Relat Res 2016;474(9):2020–7.

49. Buell TJ, et al. Multicenter assessment of outcomes and complications associated with transforaminal versus anterior lumbar interbody fusion for fractional curve correction. J Neurosurg Spine 2021;35(6): 729–42.

50. Matsumura A, et al. Posterior corrective surgery with a multilevel transforaminal lumbar interbody fusion and a rod rotation maneuver for patients with degenerative lumbar kyphoscoliosis. J Neurosurg Spine 2017;26(2):150–7.

51. Hsieh MK, et al. Combined anterior lumbar interbody fusion and instrumented posterolateral fusion for degenerative lumbar scoliosis: indication and surgical outcomes. BMC Surg 2015;15:26.

The Role of Anterior Spine Surgery in Deformity Correction

Hanci Zhang, MD[a], Leah Y. Carreon, MD, MSc[a,*], John R. Dimar II, MD[a,b]

KEYWORDS

- Anterior approach • Adult spine deformity • Surgical technique

KEY POINTS

- Anterior spine surgery offers an effective tool to correct spinal deformity.
- Anterior spine surgery provides an excellent alternative fusion site.
- A wide variety of lordosing cages are available in various materials/sizes.
- Various effective bone grafting materials are available to induce fusion.

INTRODUCTION

First described in the 1906 by Muller via a transperitoneal approach, anterior approaches to the spinal column have been used to address a variety of spinal pathologies.[1] This includes situations where a circumferential (360°) fusion enhancement is required, and also spondylolisthesis, fractures, tumors, infections, degenerative disc disease, and finally various adult spinal deformities.[2–6] Recent advancements in surgical techniques, implant design, and exposure techniques have dramatically expanded the potential of anterior lumbar surgeries and have allowed for the powerful correction of both flexible and short-segment fixed deformities.[2,7]

INDICATIONS

In adult spine deformity surgery, anterior spinal approaches are generally used to directly reconstruct the anterior column and restore adequate thoracic and lumbar alignment in both the coronal and sagittal planes. When considering anterior surgery for these purposes, the intrinsic mobility of the anterior column is essential. Commonly, spinal deformity results from degenerative collapse of the disc spaces (de novo deformity), which results in a degenerative scoliosis and loss of lumbar sagittal alignment (flatback), producing scoliotic and kyphotic deformities.[8–11] Such deformities are commonly relatively flexible, and anterior-based approaches offer correction via releases of the anterior longitudinal ligament (anterior releases) and interbody cages. Releasing the ligaments and discs along with reconstructive cage placement will allow for the restoration of disc height, rotation of the spine into a more normal alignment, improving both sagittal and coronal malalignment, and providing additional support for fusion.

In rigid deformities such as congenital scoliosis or post-traumatic kyphosis, simple soft tissue releases of the discs and ligaments, either from anterior or posterior approaches, are insufficient to gain adequate correction. In these cases, anterior-based resection of the fused segment or vertebral abnormality (vertebrectomy/corpectomy) is required to gain sufficient correction. Otherwise, a posteriorly based spinal osteotomy, such as a pedicle subtraction osteotomy, is required.[8,12]

For purposes of achieving and maintaining deformity correction, all anterior adult corrective surgeries

[a] Norton Leatherman Spine Center, 210 East Gray Street, Suite 900, Louisville, KY 40202, USA; [b] Department of Orthopaedic Surgery, University of Louisville School of Medicine, 550 S. Jackson St., 1st Floor ACB, Louisville, KY 40202, USA
* Corresponding author.
E-mail address: leah.carreon@nortonhealthcare.org

Neurosurg Clin N Am 34 (2023) 545–554
https://doi.org/10.1016/j.nec.2023.06.005
1042-3680/23/© 2023 Elsevier Inc. All rights reserved.

should be combined with a posterior fusion, instrumentation, and in certain circumstances additional corrective posterior column osteotomies (PCOs or Ponte). Anterior-based procedures also provide mechanical support and an increased fusion surface to supplement posterior fixation and fusion constructs and increase their likelihood of success. Such circumferential (360°) constructs are particularly important in long-segment deformity correction, which are at particular risk for pseudoarthrosis, especially at the L5–S1 level.[6,13]

OVERVIEW

There are a range of anterior-based approaches to address flexible adult spinal deformity from the thoracic spine to the sacrum, with each approach offering access to a range of vertebral levels.[2,11,14–17] These include the transperitoneal (L5–S1), paramedian anterior retroperitoneal (L3–S1), oblique retroperitoneal (L1–2 to L5–S1), the thoracolumbar trans-diaphragmatic approach (T9–10 to L4–5), and thoracotomy approach (T4–T12). The lumbar and lumbosacral spine is especially favorable for anterior-based approaches given the relative mobility of the peritoneal organs and position of the vasculature. Although left-sided approaches are generally favored due to the anatomy of the great vessels on the right side, in specific circumstances the latter 3 techniques may also be done from the right side. The discussion will also include the minimally invasive lateral lumbar interbody fusion (MIS-LLIF) technique, which is primarily limited to the L2–3 to L4–5 levels. Depending on the area of the deformity that requires realignment, the thoracic, thoracolumbar, or a combination of multiple spinal areas, the most appropriate approach(es), should be selected and matched to these areas of the spine to successfully realign the deformity.

LUMBAR APPROACHES
Anterior Transperitoneal Approach

The anterior transperitoneal approach is particularly advantageous in lumbar deformity, especially when attempting to restore lumbar lordosis, as it offers direct access to the L5–S1 disc level, where a large proportion of natural lumbar lordosis is seen.[2,14,18] The transperitoneal approach is routinely used by a general, transplant, or vascular surgeon to address intra-abdominal pathologies and but may be challenging in patients who are obese, have had prior intra-abdominal surgery with scarring and adhesions, abdominal wall hernias, or a low lying aortic and vena cava bifurcation.

The patient is positioned supine on a hyperextended table, and a kidney rest may be elevated at the level of the sacrum to introduce further lordosis. For patients with a high sacral slope, this allows for more direct visualization and instrumentation of the L5–S1 level. A Pfannenstiel or midline incision may be made through the skin followed by the identification and splitting of the midline raphe of the rectus sheath and division of the anterior peritoneum. For this approach and all abdominal approaches in general, current commercially available self-retaining retractors greatly facilitate exposure. Once the bowel is mobilized and packed away, the posterior peritoneum may be incised longitudinally to reveal the disc, middle sacral artery, and the medial margins of the great vessels overlying the lumbar/lumbosacral spine. The bifurcation of the great vessels is variable in the cephalad and caudal directions but generally lies just above the L5–S1 disc level (**Fig. 1**). The middle sacral vessels that overlie the disc should be ligated with ties and the hypogastric plexus should be mobilized out of the way with blunt dissection. Electrocautery should be avoided since it can cause direct damage to the hypogastric plexus in male patients causing an increased risk of retrograde ejaculation.[19–22] The anterior longitudinal ligament and the underlying anterior annulus may be directly incised/released, allowing for discectomy and interbody fusion. Cages with large-surface areas that are available in a wide variety of heights and widths, angulations, shapes, and materials can be inserted (see **Fig. 1**). At the conclusion of the procedure, the incised peritoneal layers may be repaired directly with suture, and the rectus sheath closed securely using a running number 2 double arm polydioxanone suture, followed by a standard subcutaneous closure.

Paramedian Anterior Retroperitoneal Approach

The paramedian retroperitoneal approach (PRA) is a versatile workhorse approach that can be applied reliably from the L3–4 level to the L5–S1 disc level with the patient in a supine position or on occasion the oblique position (see **Fig. 1**; **Figs. 2–4**). Depending on individual anatomy, L2–3 may also be accessed but from a full lateral decubitus position due to the increased trunk rotation required (see **Figs. 1–4**). A longitudinal paramedian incision is made in the rectus sheath and the rectus muscle is the mobilized laterally, and the transversalis fascia/posterior rectus sheath incised above the underlying peritoneal contents, followed by blunt finger dissection of

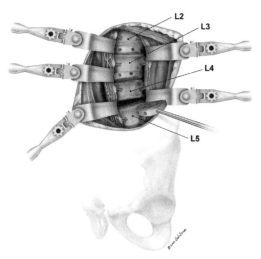

**Retroperitoneal Anterior Psoas Approach L2/L5
with Cage Insertion**

Fig. 1. Anterolateral muscle splitting anatomic view (in line incision of the external oblique, internal oblique, and transversalis muscles followed by mobilization of the retroperitoneum off of the psoas and spine and optional ligation of the segmental vessels) of L2–3 to L4–5 showing complete disc removal and preparation followed by sequential normal-lordotic cage placement in an adult left lumbar scoliosis designed to restore normal segmental lordosis and lumbar alignment. (Image courtesy: John R. Dimar II, MD)

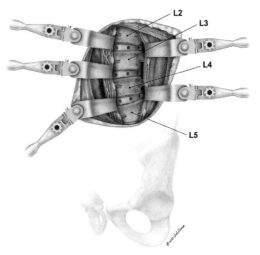

**Retroperitoneal Anterior Psoas Approach L2/L5
with All Cages Placed**

Fig. 2. Anatomic view following seating of the lordotic cages from L2–3 to L4–5 showing correction of the disc space collapse, restoration of segmental lordosis, and improvement of the lumbar alignment including the scoliosis and loss of normal lumbar overall lordosis. For all of these approaches, it is essential to have a modern multiblade, self-retaining radiolucent retractor to protect the vital structures of the chest and abdomen. (Image courtesy: John R. Dimar II, MD)

the transversalis fascia off of the retroperitoneal fat. Blunt finger dissection or scissors can be then used to separate the transversalis fascia from the lateral abdominal wall in a cephalad direction to fully expose and sweep the retroperitoneal fat off of the quadratus lumborum and iliopsoas muscles, and then expose the ureter, and the left iliac artery and vein overlying the vertebral bodies. A radiolucent self-retaining retractor is then placed to visualize the retroperitoneal space. The ipsilateral ureter overlying the psoas muscle should be identified and retracted medially along with the vessels to identify the ante-psoas interval allowing for the identification of the vertebral bodies and discs from L1–2 to L4–5. The genitofemoral nerve may also be visualized as it emerges from the anterior aspect of the psoas and should be carefully protected (see **Fig. 4**).

With further dissection inferiorly the L5–S1 disc level may be reliably accessed retroperitoneally between the aortic bifurcation to place an implant if required. Ligation of the iliolumbar vessels and others may be necessary if the vascular pedicle needs to be mobilized medially and laterally to access greater exposure to the L5 body and discs. For L2–5 levels, the interval between the psoas muscle laterally and the great vessels medially is

taken. Segmental lumbar arteries may be directly ligated, and care should be taken to avoid excessive dissection of the sympathetic chain overlying the anterolateral aspect of the vertebral bodies.[23]

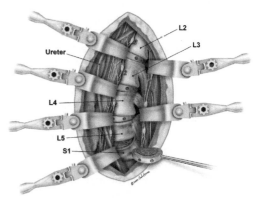

**Retroperitoneal Anterior Lateral Approach to L2/S1
with Left Iliac Vein/Artery Retracted to the Left**

Fig. 3. The extended anterolateral approach can be variably placed up and down the lateral and anterolateral abdominal wall or extended caudally into the rectus to potentially expose the L5–S1 disc space following ligation of the left iliolumbar vein(s) and mobilizing the left iliac artery/vein vascular pedicle to the midline, exposing the anterolateral disc for cage placement. (Image courtesy: John R. Dimar II, MD).

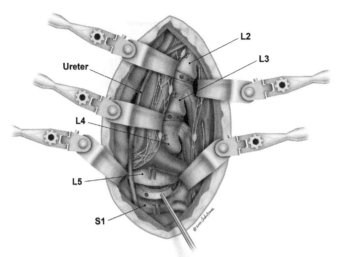

Fig. 4. Anatomic view of the paramedian rectus muscle incision following cage placement where the muscle has been mobilized laterally, the transversalis muscle tendonous portion has been released from the lateral abdominal wall, and the retroperitoneal fat and abdominal contents have been mobilized to the midline exposing the L3–4 to L5–S1 disc spaces for normal-lordotic cage placement to restore sagittal and coronal alignment. Rarely the L2–3 disc can be reached but it is generally limited by the renal artery and veins. The paramedian incision is perhaps one of the most versatile incisions for correcting lumbar deformity. (Image courtesy: John R. Dimar II, MD)

Retroperitoneal Approach Between the Bifurcation at L5/S1

As the iliolumbar or ascending lumbar vein arises from the common iliac vein at a right angle and directly over the vertebral body, medial retraction runs the risk of avulsion, leading to brisk venous bleeding. Thus, vessel ligation is critical to gaining adequate access to the L4–5 disc space.[24]

Oblique Retroperitoneal Approach

The oblique retroperitoneal (OPA) or anterolateral approach is a traditionally extensile approach from the flank that offers access from T12–L1 level to L5–S1.[2,25] The consequence of a long, single extensile incision to address multiple spinal levels through the oblique muscles and into the rectus sheath is the risk of an abdominal pseudohernia, due to transection of the T11 and T12 intercostal nerves.[26] Presently most anterolateral approaches are performed using regional muscle splitting incisions at each level directly over the disc or vertebra of interest, from the 12th rib to the iliac crest. A modification of this OPA technique is the proprietary minimally invasive open anterior antepsoas approach, which uses tubular retractors to access the same lower spinal intervals.[15] This oblique tubular approach is generally used to approach the L4–5 disc level, and an understanding of the open approach is a prerequisite since many of the same anatomic landmarks need to be identified and similar risks are present with the approach (see **Figs. 2–4**).

The patient is placed in the lateral decubitus position, with left-sided approaches most commonly preferred due to the more favorable interval between the great vessels, a longer vascular pedicle, and avoids any liver retraction, but right-sided approaches may also be performed if necessary. The leg on the approach side should be flexed slightly at the hip to relax the iliopsoas muscle and allow for better dissection/retraction. A kidney rest or table extension centered between the iliac crests, and 12th rib can be used to facilitate easier exposure to open the abdominal wall between the crest and ribs and when possible, allows for some reduction of any scoliotic deformity.

An oblique incision is made through the fascia of the external oblique, internal oblique, and transverse abdominis muscle mobilizing each muscle from the other. The incision should split in line with the muscle fibers at each layer, with care to avoid the T11 and T12 intercostal nerves, which can lay in the field. When the incision is high on the flank at the 11th or 12th rib that overlie the upper spine, it may be partially resected and harvested for autograft, a step that further increases exposure. Past the transverse abdominis muscle, the peritoneum is bluntly dissected from the lateral abdominal wall muscle and from the psoas muscle in much the same fashion as the PRA technique. The exposure of the vertebral levels of interest proceeds in the interval between the aorta and the lumbar vertebral bodies and discs is done bluntly or with electrocautery, taking care to identify and ligate the segmental arteries and veins at each level as needed. At L4–5, the iliolumbar vein is again at risk under the psoas muscle for injury with excessive retraction, and care should be taken to ligate it (see **Figs. 1** and **2**).[24,27] The lumbar spine can be commonly accessed below the diaphragm in this approach, whereas the T12–L1–L2 levels are often subdiaphragmatic. Deformities, long fusions, and patient anatomic variants can require dissection of the diaphragm. If this is needed, then the diaphragm may be incised close to its insertion on the vertebral body, the lateral chest/abdominal wall to maintain its innervation making sure a cuff of its insertion is left for repair. This avoids injury to the phrenic nerve, which travels in the more central portion of the diaphragm. After the orthopedic part of the procedure, a large bore chest tube is placed, and the diaphragm repaired with number 2 nonabosorbable sutures, and the patient followed postoperatively to rule out pneumothoraxes.

Lateral Transpsoas Approach

In contrast to the above approaches, which require a vascular surgeon to assist in the approach, the lateral transpsoas approach or lateral lumbar interbody fusion (LLIF) approach has become popular in recent years as a single-surgeon approach.[16,28] Proprietary tubular retractor systems have also been developed to allow for exposure and access through relatively smaller incisions for minimally invasive techniques. The lateral transpsoas approach offers access from T12 to L5 levels but cannot access L5/S1 level due to the iliac crests, and depending on patient anatomy or characteristics of their deformity, an overhanging crest or ribs must be considered when approaching the upper thoracic levels.

The lateral transpsoas approach uses the same retroperitoneal interval as the PRA or OPA. The patient is placed in full lateral decubitus, and the approach may be done from either the left or the right depending on surgeon preference, and the hip on the operative side should be flexed to relax the psoas. Once the levels of interest are marked and identified, a small incision either directly in line with the disc space at the skin for single level procedures or obliquely connecting multiple levels may be made. Muscle splitting dissection through the external obliques, internal obliques, and the transverse abdominis is performed, followed by finger dissection into the retroperitoneal space to locate the psoas.

Here, the most significant challenge of the transpsoas technique is encountered, which is dissection through the psoas while avoiding the lumbar plexus that runs through the psoas muscle. This step through the psoas to access the underlying disc necessitates neuromonitoring to prevent nerve injury, and understanding of the safe working zones at each level is critical for safe application of this approach.

Although the anterior column is not directly visualized from the lateral transpsoas approach, anterior column releases may be performed with careful retraction and protection of the abdominal viscera and great vessels. Intradiscal cage trials can also be used to elevate and lordose the disc space under fluoroscopic visualization. Although this technique does offer minimally invasive means to correct deformity, a comprehensive and facile understanding of its risks and the anatomy is necessary to prevent bowel, vascular, or neurologic injury. There is a significant incidence of transitory (25%) anterior thigh paresthesias postoperatively and an 8% incidence of persistent symptoms at 1 year.[29,30] Additionally, there are reports of major visceral, vascular, and urogenital injuries.[22,29,31–33]

THORACIC APPROACHES

Transthoracic approaches are well described in the literature, and a thoracotomy approach offers excellent access to the majority of the thoracic spine, from T4 to T11.[2] These can be classified based on the laterality of the approach, from either right or left and either a high or low incision. At the most proximal thoracic levels (T1–4), where the axilla and arms preclude a lateral-based approach, various types of sternotomies may be used to approach anterior-based pathology such as infection or tumors that may not be well addressed using a posterior-based approach such as costotransversectomy. Because of the close proximity of the aortic arch and superior mediastinum, a well-trained thoracic surgeon is recommended for the latter approach.

Left Thoracic Approach

A left-sided thoracotomy is the preferred means of approaching the thoracic spine anteriorly, chiefly due to the relative safety of mobilizing the aorta from the left as compared to doing so with the vena cava in the right chest cavity (**Fig. 5**).[34] The patient is positioned in the lateral decubitus position with the arms flexed out of the way of the field. A variety of high or low incisions may be chosen depending on the desired level. An oblique incision is taken through the latissimus dorsi, and in the case of proximal incisions, the serratus anterior. Because of the diagonal trajectory of the ribs, typically the rib from 2 levels proximal to the targeted level is encountered, and may be isolated and resected, and preservation of the associated intercostal vessels and nerve should be attempted, ligating it only when necessary. Preservation is especially desired at T11 and T12, where the intercostal nerves and vessels should be preserved due to their innervation of the abdominal wall musculature and risk of pseudohernia if resected.

Once the thoracic cavity is entered, the pleura may be divided, and the lung taken down by reducing ventilation and packed away from the

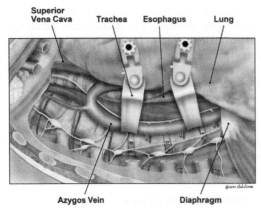

Superior
Vena Cava   Trachea   Esophagus   Lung

Azygos Vein   Diaphragm

Fig. 5. Anatomic view of a right T7 thoracotomy used to expose the thoracic spine for right scoliosis deformities to release anterior fusion and anterior interbody implants which can apply significant corrective forces, maximum care must be exercised to not over lengthen the anterior column of the thoracic spine and preserve the segmental arteries and veins if feasible. (Image courtesy: John R. Dimar II, MD)

operative field. The medial pleura is then divided longitudinally over the targeted thoracic levels. At this point the segmental vertebral arteries are encountered arising directly from the aorta. These vessels are a part of the extensive anastomotic network providing blood supply to the spinal cord and every attempt should be made to preserve them.[23] When the pathology dictates it, the involved segmental vessels are typically ligated. Unilateral ligation is generally recommended, due to the nonzero risk of spinal cord infarct despite the presence anastomotic connections.[35] A major exception is the artery of Adamkiewicz, which arises variably from the aorta but most commonly on the left from T9 to L2 and constitutes a majority of the anterior blood supply to the spinal cord via the anterior spinal artery.[23] Injury to the artery of Adamkiewicz can lead to spinal cord infarct and catastrophic neurologic injury.[23,34]

Dissection and exposure of the vertebral bodies should also be taken with consideration of the sympathetic chain, which overlays the thoracic spine from T1 to L2. Injury to the sympathetic chain risks postoperative Horner's syndrome during dissection in the more cephalad vertebra, which has been described as up to 7% of cases.[36] At the proximal levels, the thoracic duct also crosses from the right side of the spine to the left, and care should be taken to avoid injury to this structure to avoid postoperative chylothorax.[37]

Right Thoracic Approach

Although the left thoracic approach is preferred in most cases, there are instances in which the

pathology dictates it or makes a right-sided approach preferable, such as a right-sided scoliotic curve or right-sided unilateral tumor (**Fig. 6**). In such cases, positioning and superficial dissections are similar as to the left. The major caveat of the right-sided approach is the azygous vein which is prominent over the proximal ribs and spine along with a more anterior medially and vena cava on the right side of the vertebral column, which necessitates careful handling due to their fragility and lower tolerance for retraction. If sacrificed, the vessel must be securely double tied to ensure it is adequately ligated.

Trapdoor Sternotomy

The most proximal thoracic vertebrae (T1–4) are challenging to directly access from an anterior approach due to the overlying sternum and mediastinum, and posterior-based approaches, such as costotransversectomy, are most commonly used for pathologies in this region. Nevertheless, an anterior-based procedure may be indicated in cases of extensive tumor or infection where a posterior-based procedure is inadequate.[38] Given the hazards of the anatomy in this region, the assistance of a skilled cardiothoracic surgeon is needed.

The most direct and extensile approach to these vertebrae is via a sternotomy at the second and

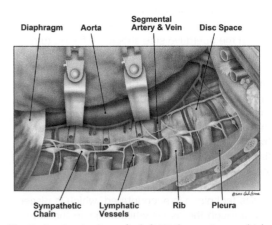

Diaphragm   Aorta   Segmental Artery & Vein   Disc Space

Sympathetic Chain   Lymphatic Vessels   Rib   Pleura

Fig. 6. Anatomic view of a left T7 thoracotomy which is commonly used to address thoracic deformities caused by Scheuermann's disease, fractures, infections, tumors, and other causes of kyphosis by providing an approach to release the anterior column, removal of the discs, facilitate an anterior interbody fusion and implant placement, and corpectomies. For these pathologies the left thoracotomy approach avoids the delicate azygous vein and vena cava, only contending with the more robust aorta during manipulation when exposing the spine. (Image courtesy: John R. Dimar II, MD)

third rib attachments.[39,40] A vertical skin incision in the fashion of a standard Smith–Robinson approach to the cervical spine may be extended distally over the sternum. An L-shaped sternotomy is then made, and the ribs may be elevated and retracted laterally to reveal the upper mediastinum including the major vessels, especially the brachiocephalic vein that crosses the surgical site. These may then be mobilized to access the T1–T4 vertebral levels underneath.

COMPLICATIONS

Safe application of anterior approaches to the spine, especially in complex deformity correction, requires an understanding of the various potential complications, as major organ systems are at risk, with vascular injury being the most dangerous. Although historical reports of complication rates have varied widely, overall complication rates following anterior spine surgery are low, and the literature supports its safety when performed by appropriately trained surgical teams.[19,22] A recent study of 1178 patients showed a 4.8% overall complication rate and a 1.4% vascular injury rate.[21]

Because of the severe sequelae, vascular injuries require special consideration for the surgical team during anterior spine approaches and remain the most commonly reported complications.[19,41,42] Arterial structures at risk include the aorta, common iliac, middle sacral, and renal arteries, and segmental arteries and venous structures include the vena cava, common iliac, iliolumbar, renal, and segmental veins. Lacerations, tearing from inadvertent retraction, or other damage to these vessels can lead to rapid life-threatening exsanguination, and the relatively thin-walled venous vessels are particularly at risk for injury than the more elastic arterial vessels.[19] When a vascular injury occurs immediate pressure and packing should be applied, and here the presence of a surgeon with extensive vascular experience and training is vital. Primary suture repair of the injury should be performed, and patches, grafts, or stents may be considered for larger injuries, with topical hemostatic agents used as a supplement. Ligation of the segmental arteries and veins, as well as smaller branches of the vessels may be accomplished safely, but rarely do the aorta, vena cava, and the common iliac vessels need complete ligation. In such instances, compromise of the vascular inflow and outflow to the affected extremity risks compartment syndrome, amputation, and even death. These possibilities justifiably demand careful preoperative assessment of the vascular anatomy and intervals

and the inclusion of surgeons well trained in vascular repairs. Although vascular injuries from primary anterior approaches are rare, scarring from previous abdominal surgeries can stiffen/obscure the anatomy and vessels, leading to a potentially higher chance of vascular injury with each additional surgery.[32,33,43]

Although rare, injuries to the bowel are also possible from anterior approaches.[31,44,45] Although retroperitoneal approaches are theoretically safer from direct bowel injury than transperitoneal approach, care should always be taken with retractor placement and passage of instrumentation to avoid injury. Lap sponges may be used to help pack bowel away from the operative field in open approaches; in minimally invasive procedures using tubular retractors, blunt dissection with smooth dilators should be used to assist in retractor placement, and retractor blades should be placed and removed with great care under direct visualization to avoid pinching bowel segments. The most common injuries are peritoneal tears that should always be primarily repaired to avoid bowel herniations. When bowel injuries are encountered, primary suture repair is preferred; rarely does the damage necessitate more extensive bowel diversion/ostomy creation. Although adhesions can make revision approaches more challenging, the general favorable mobility of the bowel segments makes these injuries easily avoidable with mindful surgical technique.[45]

Another commonly reported complication in the literature has been abdominal wall hernias/pseudohernias.[26,46] Their incidence has been mitigated by more thoughtful dissection through the musculature with muscle-splitting rather than transecting techniques, preservation of the T11/12 nerves, and avoiding extensile exposures in favor of smaller, targeted incisions.

There are various other reported complications following anterior lumbar approaches, not all of which are exclusive to spine surgery: retroperitoneal hematoma, lymphatic injury, sympathetic chain dysfunction, infection, and ileus.[2] The risks for these can all be controlled with an experienced and well-trained surgical team and proper patient-specific preoperative planning. A rare but particularly reported-upon complication in male patients following anterior surgery has been retrograde ejaculation.[20] Historically, there were concerns that retrograde ejaculation may occur with damage to the superior hypogastric plexus during dissection or due to inflammation with the use of bone morphogenetic protein-2 (rhBMP-2).[2,19,20] Interpretation of these studies, however, is made difficult by differences between patient-self reported data and urologic data with semen

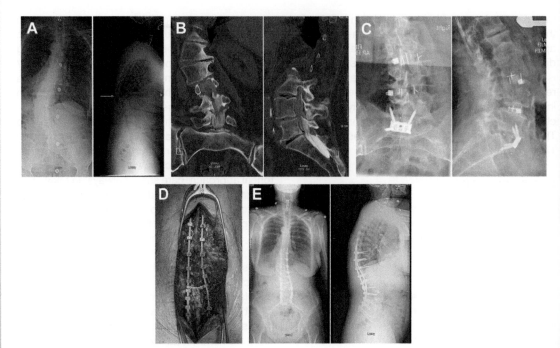

Fig. 7. (*A*) Preoperative 36″ radiographs showing adult lumbar scoliosis presenting with spinal claudication. (*B*) Myelogram/CT showing spinal stenosis. (*C*) Radiograph showing lumbar spine following placement of anterior lordotic cages. (*D*) Intraoperative photograph showing t10 to the pelvis instrumentation, fusion and posterior column osteotomies (PCO) with correction of the deformity. (*E*) Final 36″ standing posterior-anterior and lateral radiographs showing correction.

analyses. A recent meta-analysis has noted that retrograde ejaculation spontaneously resolved in a large proportion of cases, and reported rates have decreased significantly in recent decades with modern techniques of rhBMP-2 dosage and application, suggesting that retrograde ejaculation is an unlikely complication and should not preclude anterior lumbar surgeries when indicated by an experienced and well-trained surgical team.[20]

INSTRUMENTS AND IMPLANTS

With the increased understanding of the benefits of anterior surgery for certain adult spinal deformities, there has been a rise in innovation and development of modern instruments and implants to facilitate anterior spinal realignment. One of the keys to realignment is the direct release of all the anterior soft tissues that are preventing correction, followed by the use of disc space trials and implants that have the ability to restore the disc alignment, height, and rotation, thus correcting global spinal alignment.[47,48] Mobilization of the anterior column is always key before placement of the implants, which are designed to maintain this correction and are now available in a wide variety of shapes, sizes (height, width, and lordosis),

configurations, and materials, in both fixed and expandable iterations.[47] Most implants allow for the use of various bone graft materials including local autograft, allograft, demineralized bone matrix, and bone morphogenic protein (rh-BMP2) in numerous US Food and Drug Administration (FDA) approved cages. Although corrective anterior spinal instrumentation is available, anterior release and realignment for spinal deformity can be universally combined with posterior instrumentation, and thus posterior based correction techniques such as PCOs and pedicular screw/rod instrumentation can enhance deformity correction while facilitating fusion (**Fig. 7**). Ultimately, the goal of anterior instrumentation is to improve sagittal and coronal alignment, fusion rates, and overall global balance of the human spine.

SUMMARY

Anterior approaches offer access to the entire thoracic and lumbar spine, from thoracolumbar to lumbosacral junctions, either as the focal means of deformity correction or to supplement posterior-based reduction and fusion. Regardless of which specific approach is used, a comprehensive and skilled understanding of the anatomy and surgical technique is required by all members of the surgical team. Employed safely in this manner, anterior exposures to the lumbar spine are a powerful tool in correcting spinal deformities.

CLINICS CARE POINTS

- Anterior surgery is useful when the pathology demands direct visualization of the anterior vertebral column.
- Anterior spinal surgery in a flexible, non-ankylosed adult spinal deformity can impart significant anterior column straightening and deformity correction.
- Anterior spinal surgery has low blood loss, less muscle trauma, few complications, and a more extensive visualization of the disc spaces and vertebra.
- Anterior surgery allows for a more complete discectomy, larger endplate footprint for the cage, improved surface area for fusion, and improved stress sharing with the posterior column.
- Anterior surgery allows for a wide variety of cages of different sizes, lordosis, and materials along with the on-label use of bone morphogenic protein in multiple cages.

REFERENCES

1. Matur AV, Mejia-Munne JC, Plummer ZJ, et al. The history of anterior and lateral approaches to the lumbar spine. World Neurosurg 2020;144:213–21.
2. Dimar JR 2nd, Carreon LY. Anterior spine surgery for the treatment of complex spine pathology: a state of-the-art review. Spine Deform 2022;10:973–89.
3. Dimar JR, Carreon LY, Glassman SD, et al. Treatment of pyogenic vertebral osteomyelitis with anterior debridement and fusion followed by delayed posterior spinal fusion. Spine 2004;29:326–32 [discussion: 332].
4. Gjessing MH. Osteoplastic anterior fusion of the lower lumbar spine in spondylolisthesis, localized spondylosis, and tuberculous spondylitis. Acta Orthop Scand 1951;20:200–13.
5. Miyakoshi N, Abe E, Shimada Y, et al. Anterior decompression with single segmental spinal interbody fusion for lumbar burst fracture. Spine 1999; 24:67–73.
6. Tsuchiya K, Bridwell KH, Kuklo TR, et al. Minimum 5-year analysis of L5-S1 fusion using sacropelvic fixation (bilateral S1 and iliac screws) for spinal deformity. Spine 2006;31:303–8.
7. Bridwell KH. Indications and techniques for anterior-only and combined anterior and posterior approaches for thoracic and lumbar spine deformities. Instr Course Lect 2005;54:559–65.
8. Chan AK, Mummaneni PV, Shaffrey CI. Approach selection: multiple anterior lumbar interbody fusion to recreate lumbar lordosis versus pedicle subtraction osteotomy: when, why, how? Neurosurg Clin 2018;29:341–54.
9. Quarto E, Zanirato A, Ursino C. Adult spinal deformity surgery: posterior three-column osteotomies vs anterior lordotic cages with posterior fusion. Complications, clinical and radiological results. A systematic review of the literature. Eur Spine J 2021;30:3150–61.
10. Harmon PH. Anterior excision and vertebral body fusion operation for intervertebral disk syndromes of the lower lumbar spine: three-to five-year results in 244 cases. Clin Orthop Relat Res 1963;26: 107–27.
11. Mobbs RJ, Phan K, Malham G, et al. Lumbar interbody fusion: techniques, indications and comparison of interbody fusion options including PLIF, TLIF, MI-TLIF, OLIF/ATP, LLIF and ALIF. Journal of spine surgery (Hong Kong) 2015;1:2–18.
12. Schwab F, Blondel B, Chay E, et al. The comprehensive anatomical spinal osteotomy classification. Neurosurgery 2014;74:112–20 [discussion: 120].
13. Kim YJ, Bridwell KH, Lenke LG, et al. Pseudarthrosis in primary fusions for adult idiopathic scoliosis: incidence, risk factors, and outcome analysis. Spine 2005;30:468–74.
14. Gumbs AA, Bloom ND, Bitan FD, et al. Open anterior approaches for lumbar spine procedures. Am J Surg 2007;194:98–102.
15. Mayer HM. A new microsurgical technique for minimally invasive anterior lumbar interbody fusion. Spine 1997;22:691–9 [discussion: 700].
16. Ozgur BM, Aryan HE, Pimenta L, et al. Extreme lateral interbody fusion (XLIF): a novel surgical technique for anterior lumbar interbody fusion. Spine J 2006;6:435–43.
17. Silvestre C, Mac-Thiong JM, Hilmi R, et al. Complications and morbidities of mini-open anterior retroperitoneal lumbar interbody fusion: oblique lumbar interbody fusion in 179 patients. Asian Spine J 2012;6:89–97.
18. Pesenti S, Lafage R, Stein D, et al. The amount of proximal lumbar lordosis is related to pelvic incidence. Clin Orthop Relat Res 2018;476:1603–11.
19. Bateman DK, Millhouse PW, Shahi N, et al. Anterior lumbar spine surgery: a systematic review and meta-analysis of associated complications. Spine J 2015; 15:1118–32.
20. Body AM, Plummer ZJ, Krueger BM, et al. Retrograde ejaculation following anterior lumbar surgery: a systematic review and pooled analysis. J Neurosurg Spine 2021;35:427–36.
21. Manunga J, Alcala C, Smith J, et al. Technical approach, outcomes, and exposure-related complications in

patients undergoing anterior lumbar interbody fusion. J Vasc Surg 2021;73:992–8.

22. Mobbs RJ, Phan K, Daly D, et al. Approach-related complications of anterior lumbar interbody fusion: results of a combined spine and vascular surgical team. Global Spine J 2016;6:147–54.

23. Gao L, Wang L, Su B, et al. The vascular supply to the spinal cord and its relationship to anterior spine surgical approaches. Spine J 2013;13:966–73.

24. Davis M, Jenkins S, Bordes S, et al. Iliolumbar vein: anatomy and surgical importance during lateral transpsoas and oblique approaches to lumbar spine. World Neurosurg 2019;128:e768–72.

25. Kim KT, Jo DJ, Lee SH, et al. Oblique retroperitoneal approach for lumbar interbody fusion from L1 to S1 in adult spinal deformity. Neurosurg Rev 2018;41:355–63.

26. Fahim DK, Kim SD, Cho D, et al. Avoiding abdominal flank bulge after anterolateral approaches to the thoracolumbar spine: cadaveric study and electrophysiological investigation. J Neurosurg Spine 2011;15:532–40.

27. Nalbandian MM, Hoashi JS, Errico TJ. Variations in the iliolumbar vein during the anterior approach for spinal procedures. Spine 2013;38:E445–50.

28. Bina RW, Zoccali C, Skoch J, et al. Surgical anatomy of the minimally invasive lateral lumbar approach. J Clin Neurosci 2015;22:456–9.

29. Kwon B, Kim DH. Lateral lumbar interbody fusion: indications, outcomes, and complications. J Am Acad Orthop Surg 2016;24:96–105.

30. Winder MJ, Gambhir S. Comparison of ALIF vs. XLIF for L4/5 interbody fusion: pros, cons, and literature review. Journal of spine surgery (Hong Kong) 2016;2:2–8.

31. Balsano M, Carlucci S, Ose M, et al. A case report of a rare complication of bowel perforation in extreme lateral interbody fusion. Eur Spine J 2015;24(Suppl 3):405–8.

32. Momin AA, Barksdale EM 3rd, Lone Z, et al. Exploring perioperative complications of anterior lumber interbody fusion in patients with a history of prior abdominal surgery: a retrospective cohort study. Spine J 2020;20:1037–43.

33. Osler P, Kim SD, Hess KA, et al. Prior abdominal surgery is associated with an increased risk of postoperative complications after anterior lumbar interbody fusion. Spine 2014;39:E650–6.

34. Kato S. Complications of thoracic spine surgery - their avoidance and management. J Clin Neurosci 2020;81:12–7.

35. Tsirikos AI, Howitt SP, McMaster MJ. Segmental vessel ligation in patients undergoing surgery for anterior spinal deformity. J Bone Joint Surg Br 2008;90:474–9.

36. Wong CA, Cole AA, Watson L, et al. Pulmonary function before and after anterior spinal surgery in adult idiopathic scoliosis. Thorax 1996;51:534–6.

37. Chen C, Wang Z, Hao J, et al. Chylothorax after lung cancer surgery: a key factor influencing prognosis and quality of life. Ann Thorac Cardiovasc Surg 2020;26:303–10.

38. Wang S, Chen Z, Zhang K, et al. Individualized surgical treatment for patients with tumours of the cervicothoracic junction. Interact Cardiovasc Thorac Surg 2022;34:1024–30.

39. Christison-Lagay ER, Darcy DG, Stanelle EJ, et al. "Trap-door" and "clamshell" surgical approaches for the management of pediatric tumors of the cervicothoracic junction and mediastinum. J Pediatr Surg 2014;49:172–6 [discussion: 176-177].

40. Nazzaro JM, Arbit E, Burt M. "Trap door" exposure of the cervicothoracic junction. Technical note. J Neurosurg 1994;80:338–41.

41. Fantini GA, Pappou IP, Girardi FP, et al. Major vascular injury during anterior lumbar spinal surgery: incidence, risk factors, and management. Spine 2007;32:2751–8.

42. Klezl Z, Swamy GN, Vyskocil T, et al. Incidence of vascular complications arising from anterior spinal surgery in the thoraco-lumbar spine. Asian Spine J 2014;8:59–63.

43. Schwender JD, Casnellie MT, Perra JH, et al. Perioperative complications in revision anterior lumbar spine surgery: incidence and risk factors. Spine 2009;34:87–90.

44. Hwang ES, Kim KJ, Lee CS, et al. Bowel injury and insidious pneumoperitoneum after lateral lumbar interbody fusion. Asian Spine J 2022;16:486–92.

45. Siasios I, Vakharia K, Khan A, et al. Bowel injury in lumbar spine surgery: a review of the literature. Journal of spine surgery (Hong Kong) 2018;4:130–7.

46. Jagannathan J, Chankaew E, Urban P, et al. Cosmetic and functional outcomes following paramedian and anterolateral retroperitoneal access in anterior lumbar spine surgery. J Neurosurg Spine 2008;9:454–65.

47. Dimar JR 2nd, Glassman SD, Vemuri VM, et al. Lumbar lordosis restoration following single-level instrumented fusion comparing 4 commonly used techniques. Orthopedics 2011;34:e760–4.

48. Janjua MB, Ozturk AK, Ackshota N, et al. Surgical treatment of flat back syndrome with anterior hyperlordotic cages. Oper Neurosurg (Hagerstown) 2020;18:261–70.

Posterior-based Osteotomies for Deformity Correction

Evan F. Joiner, MD[a], Praveen V. Mummaneni, MD, MBA[b],
Christopher I. Shaffrey, MD[c,d], Andrew K. Chan, MD[e,*]

KEYWORDS

- Adult spinal deformity • Lumbar lordosis • Posterior column osteotomy
- Pedicle subtraction osteotomy • Vertebral column resection

KEY POINTS

- Posterior-based osteotomies are a widely used technique to restore lordosis in adult spinal deformity.
- Posterior-column osteotomies are ideal for patients with an unfused anterior column and non-focal sagittal deformity requiring modest correction in lordosis; multilevel posterior-column osteotomies can provide significant harmonious correction in appropriate patients.
- Pedicle subtraction osteotomies and vertebral column resections, 3-column osteotomies, are appropriate for patients with a fused anterior column and more severe deformity, particularly focal and/or multiplanar deformity.
- Pedicle subtraction osteotomy and vertebral column resection have significantly higher rates of complication than posterior-column osteotomy.

INTRODUCTION

Restoration of physiologic lumbar lordosis is a key principle in adult spinal deformity surgery and an essential strategy in the restoration of sagittal alignment. Extensive literature has established that the restoration of lordosis to within 10° of pelvic incidence is associated with improved postoperative outcomes including lower rates of disability, increased quality of life, and lower incidence of proximal junctional kyphosis.[1-4] More recent studies have focused on the potential need for age-matched pelvic incidence-lumbar lordosis mismatch goals affording less aggressive correction targets in older patients.[5] Likewise, the development of the global alignment and proportion score has sought to capture nuanced impacts of the full pelvic incidence spectrum as well as the distribution of lordosis on overall alignment and surgical success.[6] Relatedly, there is increasing evidence that, throughout the population, proximal lordosis (L1-L4) is significantly influenced by pelvic incidence while distal lordosis (L4-S1) may be relatively fixed across a range pelvic incidence values (ie, less dependent on pelvic incidence).[7] Despite these nuances and ongoing work to optimize

[a] Department of Neurological Surgery, Columbia University-NewYork Presbyterian Hospital, 710 West 168th Street, 4th Floor, New York, NY 10032, USA; [b] Department of Neurological Surgery, University of California San Francisco, 505 Parnassus Avenue M779, San Francisco, CA 94143, USA; [c] Department of Neurosurgery, Duke University, 40 Duke Medicine Circle Clinic 1B/1C, Durham, NC 27710, USA; [d] Department of Orthopaedic Surgery, Duke University, 40 Duke Medicine Circle Clinic 1B/1C, Durham, NC 27710, USA; [e] Department of Neurological Surgery, Columbia University Vagelos College of Physicians and Surgeons, NewYork-Presbyterian Och Spine Hospital, 5141 Broadway, 3FW, New York, NY, USA
* Corresponding author. Department of Neurological Surgery, Columbia University Vagelos College of Physicians and Surgeons, NewYork-Presbyterian Och Spine Hospital, 5141 Broadway, 3FW, New York, NY, USA.
E-mail address: akc2136@columbia.edu
Twitter: @efjoiner (E.F.J.); @andrewchanMD (A.K.C.)

Neurosurg Clin N Am 34 (2023) 555–566
https://doi.org/10.1016/j.nec.2023.06.002

sagittal correction in the individual patient, it is generally accepted that the amount of correction in lordosis required is influenced by the degree of preoperative pelvic incidence-lordosis mismatch.

Posterior-based osteotomies play an important role in the restoration of physiologic lordosis. They are particularly well-suited for patients with contraindications to an anterior or lateral approach to deformity correction (eg, multilevel ALIF, lateral interbody with the release of the anterior longitudinal ligament) and for patients who require direct posterior decompression at the time of deformity correction. This article addresses indications, techniques, and complications of posterior-based osteotomies including posterior-column osteotomy, pedicle subtraction osteotomy, and vertebral column resection.

PREOPERATIVE RADIOGRAPHIC EVALUATION

Candidates for posterior-based osteotomy require standing radiographs from the cranium to the feet. These allow for the assessment of key spinopelvic parameters including sagittal vertical axis, lordosis, pelvic incidence, pelvic tilt, T1 pelvic angle, and sacral slope as well as the visualization of compensatory knee flexion, pelvic obliquity, and leg length discrepancy. Accurate determination of spinopelvic parameters is vital as goals of spinal deformity surgery include the normalization of the sagittal vertical axis and pelvic tilt and restoration of lordosis; the extent of planned correction is thus determined by a patient's preoperative parameters. Flexion and extension radiographs and comparison of upright imaging with supine imaging are helpful for determining rigidity or flexibility of the deformity, which influences the osteotomies required to attain a given degree of correction.[3,8,9] Magnetic resonance imaging and computed tomography are recommended for the assessment of neural elements (eg, central and foraminal compression) and bony structures (eg, bone quality, ankylosis, haloing instrumentation).[10] Patients who have a fused anterior column on computed tomography will require a 3-column osteotomy (ie, pedicle subtraction osteotomy or vertebral column resection) if a gain in lordosis is desired through the anteriorly fused segments.

ANESTHESIA, POSITIONING, AND PERIOPERATIVE MANAGEMENT

Because of the risk of neurologic injury during osteotomy, neuromonitoring with somatosensory evoked potentials and motor evoked potentials is recommended. Electromyography is helpful as well. To optimize neuromonitoring, total intravenous anesthesia and short-acting paralytic should be used.[11] Tranexamic acid safely reduces blood loss by roughly 50% and should be strongly considered in patients without significant contraindications (history of stroke, recent percutaneous cardiac intervention, and so forth).[12,13] An open-bottom Jackson table may optimally induce lordosis, optimize venous return, and reduce blood loss; use of a lower extremity flat board rather than a sling is recommended to provide optimal restoration of lordosis. Alternatively, an open bottom surgical table with a hinged axis— permitting flexion and extension of the lumbar spine during surgery—may be utilized. All patients should receive intraoperative antibiotics.

POSTERIOR COLUMN OSTEOTOMY

Described by Smith-Petersen in 1945 and modified by Ponte in 1984, posterior-column osteotomy has been a mainstay of deformity correction for decades.[14,15] Posterior-column osteotomy, a Schwab grade II osteotomy, involves removal of the posterior elements, including superior and inferior facets and a portion of the spinous process, lamina, and ligamentum flavum at a given level. Smith-Petersen initially described posterior-column osteotomy as a lengthening procedure involving the removal of the posterior elements and disruption of the anterior longitudinal ligament through extension across the disc space. Ponte adapted this approach to characterize what is now considered a standard posterior-column osteotomy, a posterior shortening procedure that involves the removal of the posterior elements and allows for the induction of lordosis across a flexible, unfused disc space without necessarily disrupting the anterior longitudinal ligament. Posterior-column osteotomy provides 5° to 10° of lordotic correction per level. Primary advantages of posterior-column osteotomy include an excellent safety profile and a posterior approach that can readily be combined with pedicle screw placement and posterolateral fusion without the need for a second anterior surgery. The primary disadvantages of posterior-column osteotomy involve its limited correction and inability to address anteriorly fixed deformity.

Indications

Posterior-column osteotomy is ideal for patients with flexible, non-focal sagittal deformity requiring the restoration of lordosis. A single posterior-column osteotomy generates 5° to 10° of lordosis; however, multilevel posterior-column osteotomy affords correction in lordosis similar to that achieved by three-column osteotomy[16] and does so harmoniously across several segments.[17] Patients with moderate to severe sagittal imbalance, global loss of lordosis on standing films, and evidence of some retained flexibility on flexion-extension films or supine radiographs/computed tomography may be good candidates for multi-level posterior-column osteotomies. Because posterior-column osteotomy requires an unfused disc space, it is not an option at levels with evidence of anterior fusion from ankylosis or prior interbody fusion. Multilevel posterior-column osteotomy is also generally less morbid than more aggressive osteotomies and may be suitable for older, frailer patients.[16–22] Posterior-column osteotomy can also be combined with anterior or lateral approaches to help induce lordosis while simultaneously stabilizing the anterior column.

Technique

Level selection

Level selection is influenced by the goals of sagittal correction and restoration of lordosis. As a general rule of thumb, the optimization of sagittal correction targets a postoperative sagittal vertical axis of less than 5 cm.[3,9] Sagittal correction is accomplished primarily through the restoration of lordosis; restoration of 10° allows for roughly 1 cm of sagittal correction.[23] Lordosis should be corrected to bring the pelvic incidence-lumbar lordosis mismatch within 10°. Given that approximately two-thirds of physiologic lordosis occurs between L4 and S1 and 40% at L5-S1, the distal lumbar spine is critical to the restoration of lordosis.[24,25] The level and number of posterior-column osteotomies to be performed should be determined to achieve the restoration of these physiologic parameters assuming that each posterior-column osteotomy will provide 5° to 10° of lordosis.

Surgical technique

Following meticulous midline subperiosteal dissection, pedicle screws are placed. Pedicle screw placement does not interfere with the performance of posterior-column osteotomy at a given level. Screw stimulation and/or intraoperative imaging (eg, x-ray or computed tomography) may be used to confirm screw placement. Next, posterior-column osteotomy—consisting of laminectomy (or extensive caudal and rostral laminotomy), flavectomy, and bilateral facetectomies—is performed using high-speed burr, osteotome, and/or rongeurs (**Fig. 1**).

Posterior-column osteotomy introduces flexibility at a given level that can be utilized to restore lordosis. Lordosis can be optimized through reverse table breaking, bolster manipulation, and compression across posterior instrumentation. The optimal number and arrangement of rods depends upon the extent of surgery. Harmonious rod shape and avoidance of excessive recontouring should be prioritized to optimize rod strength and durability.[26] Cobalt chrome reduces the risk of rod fracture; however, stiffer cobalt chrome may increase the risk of proximal junctional kyphosis.[27,28]

Following compression across the posterior-column osteotomy site(s) and rod placement, it is essential to evaluate for the impingement of the thecal sac and nerve roots, ensuring that compression across each posterior-column osteotomy has not introduced dural buckling or foraminal stenosis. Neuromonitoring and visual/manual inspection are critical in this evaluation. The formal intraoperative x-ray may be helpful to confirm adequate lordotic correction. Alternatively, pre-planned patient-specific rods may also serve as a template to ensure adequate lordotic correction has been achieved. After final tightening, remaining bony surfaces are decorticated;

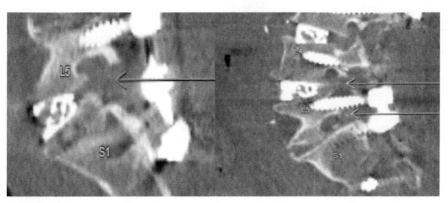

Fig. 1. Postoperative CT scan of a patient who received L4-5 and L5-S1 posterior column osteotomies in addition to L3-S1 ALIF and T2-pelvis posterior spinal instrumented fusion. This demonstrates the complete facetectomies involved in posterior column osteotomies. The arrows note the region where the facets have been removed.

posterolateral fusion may be optimized through the use of autograft, allograft, and demineralized bone matrix.[29,30] Some surgeons choose to supplement their fusion with bone morphogenic protein. Pre- and postoperative radiographic images for a patient who underwent posterior column osteotomies are shown below (**Fig. 2**).

Complications

Posterior-column osteotomies are less morbid than three-column osteotomies, although they are higher risk than inferior facetectomies alone. In a prospective study of 2210 patients undergoing deformity correction, rates of neuromonitoring alerts were higher among patients with posterior-column osteotomy (9.3%) than among those without (4.2%). However, rates of neurologic injury within the posterior-column osteotomy group were relatively low (0.37%) and not significantly higher than those in the non-posterior-column osteotomy group.[18] Posterior-column osteotomy involves greater blood loss than deformity surgery without posterior-column osteotomies.[19] Additional operative and perioperative complications include durotomy, pleural effusion, venous thromboembolic

disease, wound dehiscence, wound infection, urinary tract infection, pneumonia, sepsis, and death. Long-term postoperative complications include hardware failure, pseudarthrosis, and proximal junctional kyphosis.

PEDICLE SUBTRACTION OSTEOTOMY

First described by Thomasen in 1985, pedicle subtraction osteotomy has become integral to the treatment of fixed sagittal deformity.[31] Pedicle subtraction osteotomy involves a wedge-shaped resection of bone from the posterior elements to the anterior cortex of the vertebral body. Pedicle subtraction osteotomy provides significant sagittal correction, obtained through a 25° to 40° correction in lordosis at the index level.[32,33] Advantages of pedicle subtraction osteotomy include the ability to address deformity in the setting of anterior column fusion. The main disadvantage of pedicle subtraction osteotomy is its high complication rate including blood loss, neurologic injury, rod fracture, and pseudoarthrosis.[32,34] Nonetheless, in appropriate patients, pedicle subtraction osteotomy provides durable improvements in radiographic parameters and a wide range of

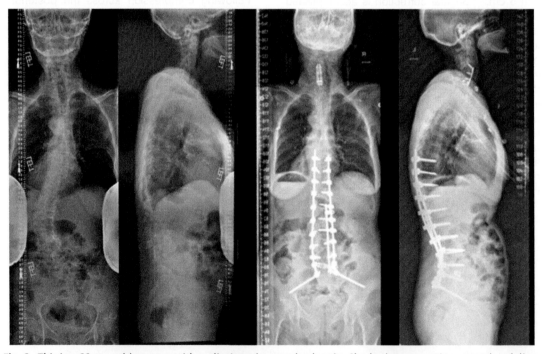

Fig. 2. This is a 66-year-old woman with scoliosis and severe back pain. She had preoperative coronal malalignment with lumbar hypolordosis. Preoperative AP and lateral radiographs (left) demonstrate coronal vertical axis 3.0 cm, sagittal vertical axis 4.2 cm, pelvic incidence-lumbar lordosis mismatch 40 to 5°, and pelvic tilt 20°. She underwent a T9 to pelvis posterior instrumented fusion with L1-S1 posterior column osteotomies, and L5-S1 TLIF. Three-year postoperative AP and lateral radiographs (right) show excellent correction of her coronal alignment while re-establishing her physiologic lumbar lordosis and maintaining her sagittal alignment (cervical vertical axis 0.8 cm, sagittal vertical axis 2.0 cm, pelvic incidence-lumbar lordosis mismatch 40–31°: 9, pelvic tilt 19°).

clinical outcomes including pain, patient satisfaction, disability, and Scoliosis Research Society scores.[35–38]

Indications

Pedicle subtraction osteotomy is indicated for patients with moderate to severe rigid sagittal deformity requiring a minimum of 30° of lordotic correction unlikely to be accomplished through posterior-column osteotomies alone. It is particularly valuable for patients with an anterior column fusion and those requiring focal lordotic correction at a single level as opposed to gradual correction over multiple levels. For patients with concurrent coronal imbalance, asymmetric pedicle subtraction osteotomy may allow for simultaneous coronal and sagittal corrections.[39,40] For patients requiring more aggressive correction, pedicle subtraction osteotomy may be extended to include the entirety of the cephalad disc (Schwab grade IV osteotomy, "extended pedicle subtraction osteotomy").

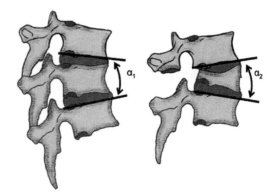

Fig. 3. The pedicle subtraction osteotomy degree of resection is defined as α_2 - α_1. (*From* Smith JS, Bess S, Shaffrey CI, et al. Dynamic changes of the pelvis and spine are key to predicting postoperative sagittal alignment after pedicle subtraction osteotomy: a critical analysis of preoperative planning techniques. *Spine* 2012;37(10):845–53 with permission.).

Technique

Level selection

In patients with focal angular deformity, pedicle subtraction osteotomy should be performed at the apex of deformity. When possible, more caudal levels (L3-S1) should be prioritized for pedicle subtraction osteotomy in order to avoid the conus medullaris and to replicate physiologic lordosis, two-thirds of which arises from L4-S1.[25,41] Furthermore, pedicle subtraction osteotomy performed at lower lumbar levels more effectively corrects pelvic tilt than it does at higher lumbar levels.[42,43]

Osteotomy planning

Pedicle subtraction osteotomy should be tailored to achieve the primary goals of restoration of sagittal balance and physiologic lordosis. While pedicle subtraction osteotomy generally provides between 25° and 40° of correction in lordosis, 30° is a reasonable focal correction goal. Though actual correction may vary between surgeons and may be difficult to determine reliably intraoperatively, the degree of correction, α_2 - α_1 (**Fig. 3**), should nonetheless be planned carefully prior to surgery to avoid inadequate or excessive correction. Dynamic interaction between various spinopelvic parameters and compensatory changes that occur in unfused portions of the spine following deformity surgery add to the complexity of osteotomy planning. Nonetheless, pedicle subtraction osteotomy follows the simple rule that a larger wedge resection achieves greater restoration of lordosis and in turn greater sagittal correction.

Surgical Technique

Following subperiosteal dissection, pedicle screws are placed at least 3 levels above and below the planned pedicle subtraction osteotomy, skipping the index level. Fixation should ideally be extended to the pelvis with iliac or S2-alar-iliac screws.

Pedicle-to-pedicle exposure is subsequently performed in the region of the pedicle subtraction osteotomy: removal of entire posterior elements at the index level, inferior facetectomy at the level above, superior facetectomy at the level below, and removal of the spinous processes, majority of laminae, and ligamentum flavum at the levels above and below. Wide laminectomy and flavectomy above and below the index level—as well as decompression of any scar in revision cases—helps prevent dural buckling and/or nerve impingement at time of osteotomy closure.

At this point, a temporary rod must be placed prior to proceeding because the resection of the anterior column is destabilizing and may result in subluxation or premature closure of the osteotomy. Pedicles of the index level are subsequently removed to the dorsal cortex of the vertebral body; attention must be paid to exiting nerve roots running medially and inferiorly to the pedicles (**Fig. 4**). Psoas is reflected away from the lateral vertebral body using a periosteal elevator or sponge stick. A retractor or temporary sponge may be placed anterior to the body for ventral protection and hemostasis.

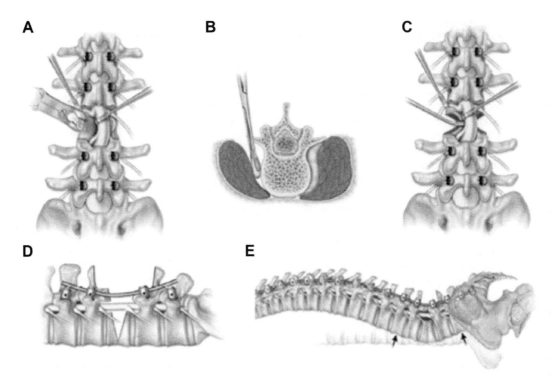

Fig. 4. Key steps of pedicle subtraction osteotomy. (*A*) "Pedicle-to-pedicle" exposure is performed in the region of the pedicle subtraction osteotomy. Pedicles of the index level are removed to the dorsal cortex of the vertebral body. (*B*) Psoas is reflected away from the lateral vertebral body. (*C*) The body is decancellated and the lateral vertebral cortex resected in a wedge-shaped fashion to the anterior cortex. (*D*). Temporary rod placement is necessary during pedicle subtraction osteotomy to stabilize the spinal column. (*E*) Once complete, the osteotomy is closed through extension across the index level. (*From* Mummaneni PV, Dhall SS, Ondra SI, Mummaneni VP, Berven SH. Pedicle Subtraction Osteotomy. *Neurosurgery.* 2008; 63(3 Suppl):171 to 176 with permission.)

The body is then decancellated and the lateral vertebral cortex resected in a wedge-shaped fashion to the anterior cortex using rongeurs and box cutter osteotomes. The anterior cortex should be left intact to serve as a hinge across which correction is performed and to protect anterior visceral and vascular structures. After using a freer-type dissector to establish a plane between ventral dura and posterior cortex, a down-pushing curette is used to mobilize the posterior cortex anteriorly, completing the osteotomy. Failure to establish this plane prior to this maneuver may result in a ventral cerebrospinal fluid leak.

Once complete, the osteotomy is closed through extension across the index level. Reverse table breaking, bolster manipulation, and compression across posterior instrumentation during rod placement may all facilitate closure. Closure of the osteotomy represents a period of heightened risk to neurologic structures. To reduce the risk of ischemia, neural perfusion should be optimized through the maintenance of mean arterial pressures above 90 mm Hg during closure. Following closure, the neural elements must be evaluated through both visual/manual inspection and neuromonitoring. Evidence of dural buckling, neural impingement, or decrement in signals should be addressed through additional removal of bone or soft-tissue structures and/or less aggressive extension.

Several considerations in rod construct selection and promotion of fusion are pertinent given the significant amount of stress across the pedicle subtraction osteotomy. It is important to prevent notching of the rod at the index level; excessive rod recontouring should be avoided. Use of pre-contoured or pre-planned, patient specific-rods and cobalt chrome may reduce rod strain.[27,28,44] Additionally, satellite rods and four-rod constructs reduce pseudarthrosis and rod fracture after pedicle subtraction osteotomy.[45,46] Supplementation of pedicle subtraction osteotomy with anterior column support (eg, ALIF, TLIF, or lateral interbody) may also reduce rod strain and risk of pseudarthrosis.[47,48] In addition to the use of autograft, allograft, bone matrix, and/or bone morphogenic protein,[29,30] fusion can be facilitated through thoracolumbar bracing for the first 3 to 6 month after

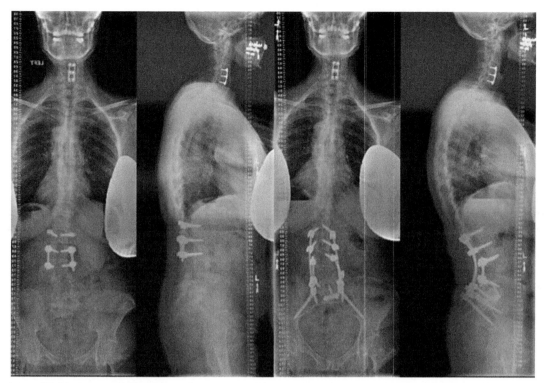

Fig. 5. This is a 66-year-old woman with a prior L1-3 fusion and L3-4 laminectomies who presented with flat back syndrome, sagittal plane imbalance, and inability to stand erect. Preoperative AP and lateral radiographs (left) demonstrate sagittal vertical axis 8.5 cm, pelvic incidence-lumbar lordosis mismatch 60 to 27°, and pelvic tilt 37°. She underwent an L4 pedicle subtraction osteotomy, L1 to pelvis posterior instrumented fusion, and L5-S1 ALIF. Three-month postoperative AP and lateral radiographs (right) show excellent correction in her lumbar lordosis and sagittal alignment (sagittal vertical axis 0 cm, pelvic incidence-lumbar lordosis mismatch 60–60°, and pelvic tilt 24°). Coronal vertical axis remained well aligned pre- and postoperatively.

surgery, which if tolerated, may reduce cyclic loading and rod stress.[43] Pre- and postoperative radiographic images for a patient who underwent pedicle subtraction osteotomy are shown below (**Fig. 5**).

Complications

Complication rates from pedicle subtraction osteotomy are high (~30% to 75%).[16,20,22,36,37,49–51] One prospective study of 71 patients demonstrated nearly twice the blood loss from pedicle subtraction osteotomy (2617 mL) than from multiple pedicle-column osteotomeis (1398 mL).[16] A prospective study with 2-year follow up on 82 patients who underwent three-column osteotomy reported major or minor complications in 78% of patients, including reoperation rate of 33% and neurologic injury rate of 30%. This risk of neurologic injury, reported by many studies to be ~10%,[16,21,22,35,50] should be juxtaposed with the relatively low risk of

neurologic injury from posterior column osteotomy (~0.5%).[18]

Common complications of pedicle subtraction osteotomy include durotomy, pleural effusion, and wound infection. Less common short-term complications include nerve impingement, postoperative ileus, venous thromboembolic disease, urinary tract infection, pneumonia, sepsis, myocardial infarction, and death. Common long-term complications include suboptimal postoperative alignment, which occurs in roughly a third of patients and can cause persistent pain and disability.[33,52] Symptomatic pseudarthrosis after pedicle subtraction osteotomy is reported in roughly 10% of patients.[53] Additional long-term complications include hardware failure (rod fracture, screw fracture) and adjacent segment disease. Indeed, elevated rod stress at the site of the osteotomy and frequently high bending angles result in shorter fatigue life and increased risk of rod fracture after pedicle subtraction osteotomy.[54,55]

VERTEBRAL COLUMN RESECTION

The earliest descriptions of complete vertebrectomy date back to the 1920s; Bradford first reported the use of circumferential vertebral column resection for the treatment of rigid spinal deformities in the 1980s.[56,57] Suk and collaborators subsequently described the modern posterior-based approach to vertebral column resection, which has become one of the most powerful techniques for the treatment of severe fixed deformity.[58,59] Vertebral column resection (Schwab osteotomy grades V/VI), which involves removing an entire vertebra (or vertebrae) as well as adjacent discs, has potential to provide 45° or more of sagittal correction.[60,61] Because vertebral column resection allows for the complete translation of the spinal column, it is a powerful treatment for coronal deformity as well.[62] The power of vertebral column resection comes at the cost of relatively high rates of complication including neurologic injury, blood loss, and proximal junctional kyphosis. Nonetheless, vertebral column resection is a valuable technique for the treatment of severe fixed deformity and yields significant improvements in radiographic and clinical outcomes.[63,64]

Indications

Vertebral column resection is indicated for patients with severe fixed sagittal deformity requiring more correction than can be provided by posterior-column osteotomies and/or pedicle subtraction osteotomy alone. It is particularly valuable for patients with severe focal angular sagittal deformity and for patients with concurrent coronal deformity requiring multiplanar correction.

Technique

Level selection
Unlike pedicle subtraction osteotomy, where level selection may be influenced by a variety of factors, vertebral column resection should typically be performed at the apex of deformity in the sagittal and/or coronal planes.

Osteotomy planning

As with pedicle-column osteotomy and pedicle subtraction osteotomy, osteotomy should provide the angular correction required to achieve the primary goals of restoration of sagittal balance and physiologic lordosis as well as providing coronal correction as needed. The choice between single- and multilevel vertebral column resection should be guided by the principle of resecting the fewest levels required to provide adequate correction.[56]

Surgical technique

Pedicle screw placement at least 3 levels above and 3 levels below the level(s) of the vertebral column resection is recommended; for patients undergoing lumbar vertebral column resection, fixation should be carried through the ilium. Following pedicle screw placement, the entire posterior elements are removed as described for pedicle subtraction osteotomy. For vertebral column resection, it is necessary to remove the bilateral transverse processes at the index level(s) and, for vertebral column resection within the thoracic spine, to remove the articulating rib heads. Removing the posterior elements exposes the exiting nerve roots; in the thoracic spine, these roots may be tied off and ligated if necessary for exposure.

Prior to the resection of the anterior column, temporary rod placement is necessary to stabilize the spinal column. Index level pedicles are then resected to the dorsal cortex of the vertebral body, and psoas is mobilized from the lateral vertebral body as described above for pedicle subtraction osteotomy.

The body is subsequently decancellated and lateral vertebral cortex resected. In contrast to the wedge-shaped osteotomy performed for pedicle subtraction osteotomy, the entire vertebral body and cephalad/caudad discs are resected using high-speed burr, box cutter osteotomes, and/or rongeurs. Care must be taken during the resection of the anterior cortex not to injure the visceral and vascular structures anterior to the spinal column; a thin rim of anterior cortex may be left to promote fusion.[62] As with pedicle subtraction osteotomy, it is necessary to establish a plane between the ventral dural and the posterior cortex of the vertebral body prior to mobilizing the posterior cortex anteriorly.

Once osteotomy is complete, correction is performed. A second temporary rod must be placed at this point if it has not been placed earlier. The deformity is gradually corrected through sequential compression and shortening of the spinal column across temporary rods. Asymmetric compression (eg, convex compression) allows for correction within the coronal plane; distraction should not be performed until sufficient closure of the osteotomy has been performed and adequate slack has been afforded to the concave dura and spinal cord.[62,65] Following gross correction, temporary rods are sequentially replaced by permanent rods; additional correction may be provided by in situ bending, reverse table breaking, and bolster manipulation. Closure of the osteotomy represents a period of heightened risk to neurologic structures which should be mitigated through the maintenance of mean arterial pressures above 90 mm Hg during closure as well as careful evaluation of the neural elements via visual/manual inspection and neuromonitoring.

Finally, interbody placement within the osteotomy site is advised to provide anterior column support and promote fusion.[62] Many of the same considerations regarding rod construct and promotion of fusion apply to both pedicle subtraction osteotomy and vertebral column resection: cobalt chrome, precontoured rods, four-rod constructs, and bone matrix and/or bone morphogenic protein may all help to reduce rates of rod fracture and pseudarthrosis.

Complications

Vertebral column resection is associated with high complication rates (roughly 20% to 75%).[38,59,63–66] As with pedicle subtraction osteotomy, risks include neurologic injury and major medical complications within the perioperative period as well as long-term complications such as pseudarthrosis, proximal junctional kyphosis, and the need for revision surgery.

A systematic review of seven studies with 390 patients who underwent posterior vertebral column resection noted an overall complication rate of 32%.[63] Neurologic injury, the most common complication, occurred in 8% of patients. Average blood loss was 2639 mL, which is comparable to that reported elsewhere for pedicle subtraction osteotomy.[16] Revision surgery was required in 6% of patients.

A retrospective study by Kelly and colleagues suggests vertebral column resection may carry higher risk of major medical complications than pedicle subtraction osteotomy.[21] Among a cohort of 132 patients who underwent pedicle subtraction osteotomy or vertebral column resection, vertebral column resection patients were more likely to experience major medical complications than pedicle subtraction osteotomy patients (73.7% vs 46.9%). However, there was no statistically significant difference in new neurologic deficits between these groups (15.8% vs 8.8%).

In a series of 54 adult and pediatric patients with 5-year follow up after posterior vertebral column resection, Lenke and colleagues have reported a 55.6% complication rate including 9.3% rate of neurologic deficit and 13% rate of revision surgery.[64] Notably, 34.8% of adult patients developed proximal junctional kyphosis; however, none required revision for symptomatic proximal junctional kyphosis. Among adults, common perioperative complications were excessive blood loss, pleural effusion, and postoperative anemia. Common longer-term complications included compression fracture, prominent instrumentation, and pseudarthrosis/rod fracture.

SUMMARY

Posterior-column osteotomy, pedicle subtraction osteotomy, and vertebral column resection represent powerful posterior-based techniques for the treatment of sagittal imbalance through the restoration of physiologic lordosis. While multilevel posterior-column osteotomy is best suited for patients with flexible sagittal deformity, pedicle subtraction osteotomy and vertebral column resection provide greater focal restoration of lordosis and allow for the treatment of both rigid and multiplanar deformity.

CLINICS CARE POINTS

- Posterior-based osteotomies should be considered for the restoration of lordosis in adult spinal deformity.

- Posterior-column osteotomy is well-suited for patients with flexible deformity requiring modest sagittal correction.

- Three column osteotomies, including pedicle subtration osteotomies and vertebral column resection, are powerful techniques for the correction of more severe deformity, particularly focal and multiplanar deformity; however, these techniques carry higher complication rates.

- Regardless of which type of posterior-based osteotomy is implemented, the risk of neurological injury should be mitigated through the use of neuromonitoring and diligent visual/manual inspection following osteotomy closure.

- Techniques to reduce intraoperative blood loss (meticulous subperiosteal dissection, the use of tranexamic acid, utilization of an open table, etc) and methods to optimize fusion (use of bone morphogenic protein, optimal correction of spinopelvic parameters, minimization of rod notching and/or over-contouring, use of satellite rods and four-rod constructs, etc) may help to mitigate key additional short-term complications (acute blood loss and associated medical sequelae) and long-term complications (pseudoarthrosis and adjacent segment disease) associated with posterior-based osteotomies.

DISCLOSURE

Shaffrey: Medtronic (consulting, royalties), NuVasive (consulting, ownership, royalties), Proprio (consulting, ownership), SI Bone (consulting, royalties).

Mummaneni: Depuy Synthes (consultant), Globus (consultant), Nuvasive (consultant), Stryker (consultant), BK Medical (honoraria), Brainlab (honoraria), SI Bone (honoraria), NREF (grant), ISSG (grant), AO Spine (grant), NIH (grant), PCORI (grant), SLIP II (grant), Pacira (grant), Spinicity/ ISD (stock), Springer Publisher (royalties), Thieme Publisher (royalties).

Joiner and Chan: none.

REFERENCES

1. Schwab F, Patel A, Ungar B, et al. Adult spinal deformity-postoperative standing imbalance: how much can you tolerate? An overview of key parameters in assessing alignment and planning corrective surgery. Spine 2010;35(25):2224–31.
2. Smith JS, Singh M, Klineberg E, et al. Surgical treatment of pathological loss of lumbar lordosis (flatback) in patients with normal sagittal vertical axis achieves similar clinical improvement as surgical treatment of elevated sagittal vertical axis: clinical article. J Neurosurg Spine 2014;21(2):160–70.
3. Kuntz C 4th, Shaffrey CI, Ondra SL, et al. Spinal deformity: a new classification derived from neutral upright spinal alignment measurements in asymptomatic juvenile, adolescent, adult, and geriatric individuals. Neurosurgery 2008;63(3 Suppl):25–39.
4. Schwab FJ, Blondel B, Bess S, et al. Radiographical spinopelvic parameters and disability in the setting of adult spinal deformity: a prospective multicenter analysis. Spine 2013;38(13):E803–12.
5. Lafage R, Schwab F, Challier V, et al. Defining Spino-Pelvic Alignment Thresholds: Should Operative Goals in Adult Spinal Deformity Surgery Account for Age? Spine 2016;41(1):62–8.
6. Yilgor C, Sogunmez N, Boissiere L, et al. Global Alignment and Proportion (GAP) Score: Development and Validation of a New Method of Analyzing Spinopelvic Alignment to Predict Mechanical Complications After Adult Spinal Deformity Surgery. J Bone Joint Surg Am 2017;99(19):1661–72.
7. Pesenti S, Lafage R, Stein D, et al. The Amount of Proximal Lumbar Lordosis Is Related to Pelvic Incidence. Clin Orthop 2018;476(8):1603–11.
8. Cheung JPY. The importance of sagittal balance in adult scoliosis surgery. Ann Transl Med 2020;8(2):35.
9. Schwab F, Lafage V, Patel A, et al. Sagittal plane considerations and the pelvis in the adult patient. Spine 2009;34(17):1828–33.
10. Diebo BG, Shah NV, Boachie-Adjei O, et al. Adult spinal deformity. Lancet 2019;394(10193):160–72.
11. Sahinovic MM, Gadella MC, Shils J, et al. Anesthesia and intraoperative neurophysiological spinal cord monitoring. Curr Opin Anesthesiol 2021;34(5):590.
12. Yoo JS, Ahn J, Karmarkar SS, et al. The use of tranexamic acid in spine surgery. Ann Transl Med 2019;7(Suppl 5):S172.
13. Lin JD, Lenke LG, Shillingford JN, et al. Safety of a High-Dose Tranexamic Acid Protocol in Complex Adult Spinal Deformity: Analysis of 100 Consecutive Cases. Spine Deform 2018;6(2):189–94.
14. Smith-Petersen MN, Larson CB, Aufranc OE. Osteotomy of the spine for correction of flexion deformity in rheumatoid arthritis. JBJS 1945;27(1):1.
15. Ponte A, Vero B, Siccardi G. Surgical treatment of Scheuermann's hyperkyphosis. In: Winter R, editor. Progress in spinal pathology: kyphosis. Aulo Gaggi; 1984. p. 75–81.
16. Cho KJ, Bridwell KH, Lenke LG, et al. Comparison of Smith-Petersen versus pedicle subtraction osteotomy for the correction of fixed sagittal imbalance. Spine 2005;30(18):2030–7 [discussion 2038].
17. Wiggins GC, Ondra SL, Shaffrey CI. Management of iatrogenic flat-back syndrome. Neurosurg Focus 2003;15(3):E8.
18. Buckland AJ, Moon JY, Betz RR, et al. Ponte Osteotomies Increase the Risk of Neuromonitoring Alerts in Adolescent Idiopathic Scoliosis Correction Surgery. Spine 2019;44(3):E175–80.
19. Koerner JD, Patel A, Zhao C, et al. Blood loss during posterior spinal fusion for adolescent idiopathic scoliosis. Spine 2014;39(18):1479–87.
20. Smith JS, Shaffrey CI, Klineberg E, et al. Complication rates associated with 3-column osteotomy in 82 adult spinal deformity patients: retrospective review of a prospectively collected multicenter consecutive series with 2-year follow-up. J Neurosurg Spine 2017;27(4):444–57.
21. Kelly MP, Lenke LG, Shaffrey CI, et al. Evaluation of complications and neurological deficits with three-column spine reconstructions for complex spinal deformity: a retrospective Scoli-RISK-1 study. Neurosurg Focus 2014;36(5):E17.
22. Buchowski JM, Bridwell KH, Lenke LG, et al. Neurologic complications of lumbar pedicle subtraction osteotomy: a 10-year assessment. Spine 2007;32(20):2245–52.
23. Noun Z, Lapresle P, Missenard G. Posterior Lumbar Osteotomy for Flat Back in Adults. Clin Spine Surg 2001;14(4):311.
24. Chan AK, Mummaneni PV, Shaffrey CI. Approach Selection: Multiple Anterior Lumbar Interbody Fusion to Recreate Lumbar Lordosis Versus Pedicle Subtraction Osteotomy: When, Why, How? Neurosurg Clin N Am 2018;29(3):341–54.

25. Sparrey CJ, Bailey JF, Safaee M, et al. Etiology of lumbar lordosis and its pathophysiology: a review of the evolution of lumbar lordosis, and the mechanics and biology of lumbar degeneration. Neurosurg Focus 2014;36(5):E1.

26. Slivka MA, Fan YK, Eck JC. The Effect of Contouring on Fatigue Strength of Spinal Rods: Is it Okay to Rebend and Which Materials Are Best? Spine Deform 2013;1(6):395–400.

27. Han S, Hyun SJ, Kim KJ, et al. Rod stiffness as a risk factor of proximal junctional kyphosis after adult spinal deformity surgery: comparative study between cobalt chrome multiple-rod constructs and titanium alloy two-rod constructs. Spine J Off J North Am Spine Soc 2017;17(7):962–8.

28. Shega FD, Zhang H, Manini DR, et al. Comparison of Effectiveness between Cobalt Chromium Rods versus Titanium Rods for Treatment of Patients with Spinal Deformity: A Systematic Review and Meta-Analysis. Adv Orthop 2020;2020:8475910.

29. Tilkeridis K, Touzopoulos P, Ververidis A, et al. Use of demineralized bone matrix in spinal fusion. World J Orthop 2014;5(1):30–7.

30. Lykissas M, Gkiatas I. Use of recombinant human bone morphogenetic protein-2 in spine surgery. World J Orthop 2017;8(7):531–5.

31. Thomasen E. Vertebral osteotomy for correction of kyphosis in ankylosing spondylitis. Clin Orthop 1985;194:142–52.

32. Bridwell KH, Lewis SJ, Lenke LG, et al. Pedicle subtraction osteotomy for the treatment of fixed sagittal imbalance. J Bone Joint Surg Am 2003;85(3):454–63.

33. Rose PS, Bridwell KH, Lenke LG, et al. Role of pelvic incidence, thoracic kyphosis, and patient factors on sagittal plane correction following pedicle subtraction osteotomy. Spine 2009;34(8):785–91.

34. Wang MY, Berven SH. Lumbar pedicle subtraction osteotomy. Neurosurgery 2007;60(2 Suppl 1):ONS140–146 [discussion ONS146].

35. Bridwell KH, Lewis SJ, Edwards C, et al. Complications and outcomes of pedicle subtraction osteotomies for fixed sagittal imbalance. Spine 2003;28(18):2093–101.

36. Barrey C, Perrin G, Michel F, et al. Pedicle subtraction osteotomy in the lumbar spine: indications, technical aspects, results and complications. Eur J Orthop Surg Traumatol Orthop Traumatol 2014;24(Suppl 1):S21–30.

37. Kim YJ, Bridwell KH, Lenke LG, et al. Results of lumbar pedicle subtraction osteotomies for fixed sagittal imbalance: a minimum 5-year follow-up study. Spine 2007;32(20):2189–97.

38. O'Neill KR, Lenke LG, Bridwell KH, et al. Clinical and Radiographic Outcomes After 3-Column Osteotomies With 5-Year Follow-up. Spine 2014;39(5):424.

39. Chan AK, Lau D, Osorio JA, et al. Asymmetric Pedicle Subtraction Osteotomy for Adult Spinal Deformity with Coronal Imbalance: Complications, Radiographic and Surgical Outcomes. Oper Neurosurg (Hagerstown) 2020;18(2):209–16.

40. Bridwell KH. Decision Making Regarding Smith-Petersen vs. Pedicle Subtraction Osteotomy vs. Vertebral Column Resection for Spinal Deformity. Spine 2006;31(19S):S171.

41. Bernhardt M, Bridwell KH. Segmental analysis of the sagittal plane alignment of the normal thoracic and lumbar spines and thoracolumbar junction. Spine 1989;14(7):717–21.

42. Lafage V, Schwab F, Vira S, et al. Does vertebral level of pedicle subtraction osteotomy correlate with degree of spinopelvic parameter correction?: Clinical article. J Neurosurg Spine 2011;14(2):184–91.

43. Berjano P, Aebi M. Pedicle subtraction osteotomies (PSO) in the lumbar spine for sagittal deformities. Eur Spine J Off Publ Eur Spine Soc Eur Spinal Deform Soc Eur Sect Cerv Spine Res Soc 2015;24(Suppl 1):S49–57.

44. Hallager DW, Gehrchen M, Dahl B, et al. Use of Supplemental Short Pre-Contoured Accessory Rods and Cobalt Chrome Alloy Posterior Rods Reduces Primary Rod Strain and Range of Motion Across the Pedicle Subtraction Osteotomy Level: An In Vitro Biomechanical Study. Spine 2016;41(7):E388–95.

45. Gupta S, Eksi MS, Ames CP, et al. A Novel 4-Rod Technique Offers Potential to Reduce Rod Breakage and Pseudarthrosis in Pedicle Subtraction Osteotomies for Adult Spinal Deformity Correction. Oper Neurosurg Hagerstown Md 2018;14(4):449–56.

46. Hyun SJ, Lenke LG, Kim YC, et al. Comparison of standard 2-rod constructs to multiple-rod constructs for fixation across 3-column spinal osteotomies. Spine 2014;39(22):1899–904.

47. Deviren V, Tang JA, Scheer JK, et al. Construct Rigidity after Fatigue Loading in Pedicle Subtraction Osteotomy with or without Adjacent Interbody Structural Cages. Global Spine J 2012;2(4):213–20.

48. Januszewski J, Beckman JM, Harris JE, et al. Biomechanical study of rod stress after pedicle subtraction osteotomy versus anterior column reconstruction: A finite element study. Surg Neurol Int 2017;8:207.

49. Yang BP, Ondra SL, Chen LA, et al. Clinical and radiographic outcomes of thoracic and lumbar pedicle subtraction osteotomy for fixed sagittal imbalance. J Neurosurg Spine 2006;5(1):9–17.

50. Gupta MC, Ferrero E, Mundis G, et al. Pedicle Subtraction Osteotomy in the Revision Versus Primary Adult Spinal Deformity Patient: Is There a Difference in Correction and Complications? Spine 2015;40(22):E1169–75.

51. Schwab FJ, Hawkinson N, Lafage V, et al. Risk factors for major peri-operative complications in adult spinal deformity surgery: a multi-center review of 953 consecutive patients. Eur Spine J Off Publ Eur Spine Soc Eur Spinal Deform Soc Eur Sect Cerv Spine Res Soc 2012;21(12):2603–10.

52. Gottfried ON, Daubs MD, Patel AA, et al. Spinopelvic parameters in postfusion flatback deformity patients. Spine J Off J North Am Spine Soc 2009; 9(8):639–47.

53. Dickson DD, Lenke LG, Bridwell KH, et al. Risk factors for and assessment of symptomatic pseudarthrosis after lumbar pedicle subtraction osteotomy in adult spinal deformity. Spine 2014;39(15):1190–5.

54. Smith JS, Shaffrey E, Klineberg E, et al. Prospective multicenter assessment of risk factors for rod fracture following surgery for adult spinal deformity. J Neurosurg Spine 2014;21(6):994–1003.

55. Tang JA, Leasure JM, Smith JS, et al. Effect of severity of rod contour on posterior rod failure in the setting of lumbar pedicle subtraction osteotomy (PSO): a biomechanical study. Neurosurgery 2013; 72(2):276–82. ; discussion 283.

56. Lenke LG, Sides BA, Koester LA, et al. Vertebral Column Resection for the Treatment of Severe Spinal Deformity. Clin Orthop 2010;468(3):687–99.

57. Bradford D. Vertebral column resection (Printed abstract from the Association of Bone and Joint Surgeons Annual Meeting). Orthop Trans 1987;11:502.

58. Suk SI, Kim JH, Kim WJ, et al. Posterior vertebral column resection for severe spinal deformities. Spine 2002;27(21):2374–82.

59. Suk SI, Chung ER, Lee SM, et al. Posterior vertebral column resection in fixed lumbosacral deformity. Spine 2005;30(23):E703–10.

60. Schwab F, Blondel B, Chay E, et al. The comprehensive anatomical spinal osteotomy classification. Neurosurgery 2014;74(1):112–20 [discussion 120].

61. Kim HJ, Yang JH, Chang DG, et al. Adult Spinal Deformity: A Comprehensive Review of Current Advances and Future Directions. Asian Spine J 2022; 16(5):776–88.

62. Saifi C, Laratta JL, Petridis P, et al. Vertebral Column Resection for Rigid Spinal Deformity. Global Spine J 2017;7(3):280–90.

63. Yang C, Zheng Z, Liu H, et al. Posterior vertebral column resection in spinal deformity: a systematic review. Eur Spine J Off Publ Eur Spine Soc Eur Spinal Deform Soc Eur Sect Cerv Spine Res Soc 2016;25(8):2368–75.

64. Riley MS, Lenke LG, Chapman TMJ, et al. Clinical and Radiographic Outcomes After Posterior Vertebral Column Resection for Severe Spinal Deformity with Five-Year Follow-up. JBJS 2018;100(5):396.

65. Lenke LG, Sides BA, Koester LA, et al. Vertebral column resection for the treatment of severe spinal deformity. Clin Orthop Relat Res 2010;468(3): 687–99.

66. Auerbach JD, Lenke LG, Bridwell KH, et al. Major Complications and Comparison Between 3-Column Osteotomy Techniques in 105 Consecutive Spinal Deformity Procedures. Spine 2012;37(14):1198.

Management of High-Grade Dysplastic Spondylolisthesis

David W. Polly Jr, MD[a,b,]*, Jason J. Haselhuhn, DO[c,]*,
Paul Brian O. Soriano, MD, MBA[d], Kari Odland, DAT, ATC, LAT[d],
Kristen E. Jones, MD[b]

KEYWORDS

- High-grade dysplastic spondylolisthesis • Sagittal alignment • Reduction

KEY POINTS

- Sagittal contour is important for patient outcomes and the risk of slip progression.
- Restoring sagittal contour is more important than reducing slip.
- Benefits of reduction include lower rates of pseudoarthrosis, improved sagittal contour, and improved health-related quality of life for patients.
- There is an increased absolute rate of L5 nerve root injury with reduction versus fusion *in situ*, although this was not statistically significant and most appear to recover.

DEFINITION

Spondylolisthesis is the translation (slip) of a vertebra relative to the adjacent caudal vertebra. The Meyerding classification grades the degree of slippage in the sagittal plane on lateral standing neutral imaging: 0% to 25% Grade I, 25% to 50% Grade II, 50% to 75% Grade III, 75% to 100% Grade IV, and greater than 100% Grade V (Spondyloptosis).[1] Grades I and II are considered low-grade and Grades III-V are considered high-grade.

There are several etiologies of spondylolisthesis. Wiltse and colleagues[2] developed a classification system of the most common causes: Type I – Dysplastic, Type II – Isthmic (including subtypes: A – Lytic, B – Elongation, and C – Acute fracture), Type III – Degenerative, Type IV – Traumatic, Type V – Pathologic, and Type VI – Iatrogenic. Dysplastic spondylolisthesis is a type of spondylolisthesis that occurs at L5-S1 when dysplastic lumbosacral anatomy is present,[3,4] and is associated with high-grade slip and spina bifida occulta.[5–7] It is the senior author's experience that high-grade dysplastic spondylolisthesis (HGDS) is always associated with a significant sacral spina bifida.

Marchetti and Bartolozzi[8] classified spondylolisthesis as developmental or acquired. Developmental can be either low- or high-grade dysplasia depending on the anatomy of L5 and S1 and the risk of progression. HGDS can lead to the lysis or elongation of the pars interarticularis and slip progression, so identifying these patients is particularly important. Lamartina and colleagues[9] developed the severity index, which analyzes pelvic retroversion and is directly proportional to slip severity, to help differentiate low-versus high-grade dysplasia. Previous work by Vidal and Marnay[10] demonstrated that a severity index greater than 20% indicates HGDS, while less than 20% is seen in normal patients and those with low-grade dysplasia.

Funding: The authors received no financial support for the submitted work.
[a] Department of Orthopedic Surgery, University of Minnesota, 2450 Riverside Avenue South, Suite R200, Minneapolis, MN 55454, USA; [b] Department of Neurosurgery, University of Minnesota, Minneapolis, MN, USA;
[c] Department of Orthopedic Surgery, University of Minnesota, 2512 South 7th Street, Suite R200, Minneapolis, MN 55455, USA; [d] Department of Orthopedic Surgery, University of Minnesota, Minneapolis, MN, USA
* Corresponding authors.
E-mail addresses: pollydw@umn.edu (D.W.P.); hasel080@umn.edu (J.J.H.)

Neurosurg Clin N Am 34 (2023) 567–572
https://doi.org/10.1016/j.nec.2023.06.003

THE ROLE OF SAGITTAL ALIGNMENT

HGDS can cause deformity and abnormal sagittal alignment, with kyphosis of L5 relative to S1 and increased pelvic incidence (PI).[2,11] To compensate, lumbar lordosis (LL) and pelvic retroversion increase, causing increased pelvic tilt (PT) and decreased sacral slope (SS).[12] Positive sagittal balance occurs if these compensation mechanisms cannot match the L5-S1 kyphosis. This has been shown to result in worse patient outcomes,[13] most significantly when kyphosis is greatest in the lumbar spine.[14,15] Additionally, Boxall and colleagues[15] found that the angle of slippage, as determined by measuring L5-S1 kyphosis, is as important as the percentage of slip in measuring instability and slip progression in children and adolescents with high-grade L5-S1 spondylolisthesis.

Labelle and colleagues[12] and the Spine Deformity Study Group developed a classification for L5-S1 spondylolisthesis based on grade, PI, and spino-pelvic posture (balanced vs unbalanced) as determined by PT and SS values established by Hresko and colleagues[16] (**Fig. 1**). Types IV-VI are high-grade with a balanced pelvis, retroverted pelvis and balanced spine, and retroverted pelvis and unbalanced spine, respectively. Mac-Thiong et al.[17] found that restoring pelvic balance to normal was associated with improved quality of life as determined by SRS-22 scores, an important consideration in patients with HGDS.

MANAGEMENT

The workup of HGDS should include standing full-length spinal radiographs, which allows the provider to assess the patients' global sagittal alignment. Lateral lumbar films, including flexion and extension views, help assess slip grade and the degree of instability. Magnetic resonance imaging (MRI) or a computed tomography (CT) myelogram can help identify the pathology of the neural elements and intravertebral disks. CT also provides an assessment of bony defects that may not be seen on plan radiographs. Diphosphonate bone scintigraphy or single-photon emission CT (SPECT) can also be used.[18]

Conservative management includes activity modifications, anti-inflammatory medications, physical therapy, and steroid/analgesic injections. However, these treatments do not provide long-term resolution in patients with high-grade spondylolisthesis, and these patients often develop pain and/or neurologic deficits if managed nonoperatively.[19]

The goal of surgical intervention for HGDS is the prevention of slip progression, pain relief, and neural decompression.[18] Current approaches include posterolateral fusion *in situ*, anterior-posterior, or completely posterior with an L5-S1 interbody with or without reduction. However, reduction continues to be debated.

Reducing the spondylolisthesis allows for the improvement of sagittal contour, whereas fusion *in situ* alone does not. If not corrected, patients may present years later with severe sagittal imbalance and pain that is difficult to treat even with surgical intervention. A systematic review by Longo and colleagues[20] found a lower rate of pseudoarthrosis after reduction and fusion compared to fusion *in situ* alone (5.5% vs 17.8%), supporting reduction. While a higher rate of new neurologic injury with reduction versus fusion *in situ* was also reported (8.9% vs 7.8%), this was not statistically significant. A review by the Scoliosis Research Society concluded that the surgical reduction and instrumentation of HGDS lowers the risk of nonunion in pediatric patients.[21] Shear forces at the lumbosacral junction are decreased with either full or partial reduction versus fusion *in situ*,[22] resulting in reduced biomechanical strain which allows fusion to occur. Several reduction techniques have been described with the goal of correcting kyphosis and improving lordosis at L5-S1.

REDUCTION TECHNIQUES

Scaglietti and colleagues[23] described a closed reduction technique with plaster casts that were worn for at least 4 months in 1976. Bradford and

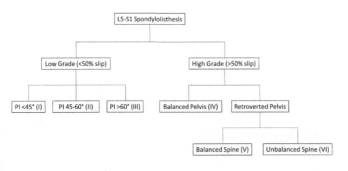

Fig. 1. Labelle and colleagues classification system of L5-S1 spondylolisthesis.

colleagues[24] later developed a three-stage operative technique that began with decompression at L5-S1 and arthrodesis of L4 transverse processes to the sacrum. Traction was then applied (halo-femoral or halo-pelvic) and serial radiographs were taken to assess reduction. Once maximal reduction was achieved (usually 7–10 days), lumbosacral interbody fusion was performed. This was followed by casting for 4 months. Although these techniques resulted in improved sagittal alignment, they are rarely performed today due to the long treatment durations and lengthy bedrest requirements. While these principles are important, these two techniques are primarily of historical interest.

Transpedicular fixation using Schanz pins and an external fixation device was first reported by Magerl.[25] Karampalis and colleagues[26] used this technique to reduce L5-S1 spondylolisthesis and improve sagittal alignment. Edwards[27] achieved a mean total slip correction of 91% and mean slip angle correction of 90% using a progressive reduction technique with similar instrumentation. Prudnikova and colleagues[28] achieved fusion in all patients (5/5) with HGDS using a comparable apparatus followed by transpedicular instrumentation and posterior lumbar interbody fusion. However, 75% (6/8) had pseudoarthrosis at follow-up with external transpedicular fixation alone. Pin site complications, patients being unable to lay supine, and the multiple operations required for this technique limit its use today.

L5 vertebrectomy was described as a two-stage procedure involving the resection of the L5 vertebral body and the L4-5 and L5-S1 discs followed by excision of the posterior elements, articular processes, L5 pedicles, and reduction of L4 onto the sacrum.[29] Gaines[30] reviewed 30 patients who previously underwent L5 vertebrectomy and found a high anterior and posterolateral fusion rate. However, 23 patients (77%) had L5 neuropraxia, of which 21 recovered. This is rarely used today.

Sacral dome osteotomy is used concomitantly with other techniques to facilitate the reduction in patients with S1 endplate rounding, as is often seen in HGDS. This includes wide decompression at L5-S1, an anteriorly directed osteotomy of the S1 vertebral body, and additional osteotomy of the anterior-inferior lip of the L5 vertebral body if needed. Several studies have demonstrated this technique improves LL.[31,32]

Intraoperative posterior distraction (initially popularized by Harms[33,34]) to the spondylolisthesis site facilitates reduction.[35] To begin, bilateral sacral alar hooks are attached to hooks in the mid to upper lumbar spine for temporary distraction, which helps with exposure and reduction.

Sacral dome osteotomy is performed, followed by L5-S1 posterior lumbar interbody fusion (PLIF). L5 and sacral pedicle screws are placed and compressed to provide a posterior force at that level to increase lordosis. The temporary distraction hooks are then removed. Shufflebarger and Geck[35] noted improved sagittal alignment using this technique.

Transpedicular reduction screws can aid with intraoperative reduction and improve sagittal alignment.[6,34,36,37] Pedicle screws are placed into the S1 vertebral body and then reduction screws are inserted into L5 using a transpedicular technique. Two rods are locked in place on the sacral screws, and then the reduction screws are used to perform the reduction by the utilization of the double thread, which is held against the immobile rod. A similar technique described by Schlösser and colleagues[38] to treat HGDS provided significant improvements in all local, regional, and global sagittal alignment parameters except LL. While LL did improve from a mean of 66° to 62°, this was not statistically significant. Additionally, patients with a balanced pelvis (L5 incidence <60°)[39] had significantly higher SRS-22 total and self-image scores at follow-up.

Ilharreborde and colleagues[40] described the use of a cantilever maneuver in HGDS. First, a sacral dome osteotomy is performed, followed by the placement of pedicle screws at L4, L5, and S1. Bilateral transsacral rods are placed caudal to the S1 pedicle screws, extending intraosseously to S2 or S3. This creates an "iliac buttress" to resist distal cut-out during reduction. The sacrum is then anteverted in the sagittal plane and reduced to the inferior endplate of L5 by locking the rods into the L4 and L5 pedicle screw heads. Bouyer and colleagues[41] reported a 100% L4-S1 fusion rate and improved sagittal parameters with this reduction maneuver. A similar technique using S2AI screws instead of transsacral rods can be done as well.

AUTHORS' PREFERRED SURGICAL TECHNIQUE

Our preferred technique has been described previously.[3] This is a single-stage, posterior-only approach with circumferential fusion using a transforaminal lumbar interbody fusion (TLIF), pelvic fixation, and a cantilever reduction maneuver.

1. Position the patient prone with the hips flexed in a leg sling
2. Perform a posterior midline incision and subperiosteal exposure
3. Posted threaded reduction screws are placed through the L5 pedicles

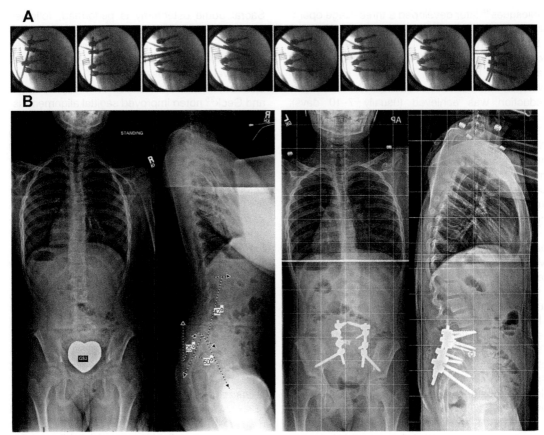

Fig. 2. (*A*) Fluoroscopic progression of the Author's described reduction maneuver. (*B*). Pre- and postoperative standing full-length spine films.

4. Pedicle screws placed in S1 (and L4 if necessary)
   - Place S1 screws low in the pedicle to allow for sacral dome osteotomy
5. Placement of bilateral S2 alar-iliac screws
6. L5-S1 gill laminectomy
7. L4 caudal hemilaminectomy performed to identify the L5 nerve roots, which are followed out to the neuroforamina bilaterally
8. Discectomy at L5-S1
9. Sacral dome osteotomy
10. L5-S1 TLIF
    - Insert and rotate distractors used to elevate L5 for interbody cage placement
11. Reduction maneuver (**Fig. 2**)
    - Rods are locked to the sacral screws
    - The pelvis is anteverted by extending the hips, reducing the pelvis to the lumbar spine
    - A cantilever maneuver is used to further reduce the pelvis to the lumbar spine, bringing the rods into contact with the L4 & L5 screw heads
    - Reduction screws in the L5 vertebral body are used to persuade L5 posteriorly
    - Assess reduction with fluoroscopy - The primary goal is to restore lumbosacral lordosis
12. Posterolateral fusion - Maximize decortication to achieve the greatest fusion surface area, given the known hypoplastic transverse processes
13. Surgical site irrigation and closure
14. Postoperatively the patient is positioned on their side or supine with hips extended and knees bent to minimize L5 nerve root tension

The goal of reduction is the restoration of lumbosacral lordosis, and a full translational reduction is not necessary. Reducing the lumbar spine to the pelvis could increase anterior thecal sac pressure and lead to cauda equina syndrome. To potentially lower this risk, the pelvis should be reduced to the lumbar spine.

SUMMARY

Based on current evidence we know that most patients with HGDS will benefit from surgical intervention to prevent disease progression, pain, and neurologic symptoms. Restoration of sagittal alignment should be prioritized in order to maximize patient outcomes. This may require the reduction of the slip, which has been shown to lower pseudoarthrosis rates without significantly higher new neurologic deficits compared to fusion *in situ*. Improvement of kyphosis and restoration of lordosis at the lumbosacral junction should be the goal of any reduction maneuver.

CLINICS CARE POINTS

- High grade dysplastic spondylolisthesis should have full spine films obtained to assess sagittal balance
- Preventing progression in young patients is important
- Correcting lumbosacral kyphosis is more important than slip reduction
- Slip reduction does improve fusion rates at some L5 nerve root risk

DECLARATIONS

D.W. Polly - declares consulting fees from Globus Medical and Alexion; institutional grant/research support from Medtronic and MizuhoOSI; consulting fees, royalties, and honoraria from SI-Bone; and royalties/other financial or material support from Springer. K.E. Jones - declares consulting fees and institutional grant/research support from Medtronic and SI-Bone. J.J. Haselhuhn, P.B.O. Soriano, and K. Odland - have nothing to declare.

REFERENCES

1. Meyerding HW. Spondylolisthesis. Surg Gynecol Obstet 1932;54:371–7.
2. Wiltse LL, Newman PH, Macnab I. Classification of spondylolysis and spondylolisthesis. Clin Orthop 1976;117:23–9.
3. Hoel RJ, Brenner RM, Polly DW Jr. The Challenge of Creating Lordosis in High-Grade Dysplastic Spondylolisthesis. Neurosurg Clin N Am 2018;29(3): 375–87.
4. Vialle R, Dauzac C, Khouri N, et al. Sacral and lumbar-pelvic morphology in high-grade spondylolisthesis. Orthopedics 2007;30(8):642–9.
5. Wynne-Davies R, Scott JH. Inheritance and spondylolisthesis: a radiographic family survey. J Bone Joint Surg Br 1979;61-B(3):301–5.
6. Fredrickson BE, Baker D, McHolick WJ, et al. The natural history of spondylolysis and spondylolisthesis. J Bone Joint Surg Am 1984;66(5):699–707.
7. Pfeil J, Niethard FU, Cotta H. Die Pathogenese kindlicher Spondylolisthesen [Pathogenesis of pediatric spondylolisthesis]. Z Orthop Ihre Grenzgeb 1987; 125(5):526–33. German.
8. Marchetti PG, Bartolozzi P. Spondylolisthesis: classification of spondylolisthesis as a guideline for treatment. In: The Textbook of spinal Surgery. 2nd edition. Philadelphia: Lippincott-Raven; 1997. p. 1211–54.
9. Lamartina C, Zavatsky JM, Petruzzi M, et al. Novel concepts in the evaluation and treatment of high-dysplastic spondylolisthesis. Eur Spine J 2009; 18(Suppl 1):133–42.
10. Vidal J, Marnay T. Morphology and anteroposterior body equilibrium in spondylolisthesis L5/S1. Rev Chir Orthop 1983;69(1):17–28.
11. Labelle H, Roussouly P, Berthonnaud E, et al. Spondylolisthesis, pelvic incidence, and spinopelvic balance: a correlation study. Spine 2004;29(18): 2049–54.
12. Labelle H, Mac-Thiong JM, Roussouly P. Spino-pelvic sagittal balance of spondylolisthesis: a review and classification. Eur Spine J 2011;(Suppl 5): 641–6.
13. Glassman SD, Bridwell K, Dimar JR, et al. The impact of positive sagittal balance in adult spinal deformity. Spine 2005;30(18):2024–9.
14. Harroud A, Labelle H, Joncas J, et al. Global sagittal alignment and health-related quality of life in lumbosacral spondylolisthesis. Eur Spine J 2013;22(4): 849–56.
15. Boxall D, Bradford DS, Winter RB, et al. Management of severe spondylolisthesis in children and adolescents. J Bone Joint Surg Am 1979;61(4):479–95.
16. Hresko MT, Labelle H, Roussouly P, et al. Classification of high-grade spondylolistheses based on pelvic version and spine balance: possible rationale for reduction. Spine 2007;32(20):2208–13.
17. Mac-Thiong JM, Hresko MT, Alzakri A, et al. Criteria for surgical reduction in high-grade lumbosacral spondylolisthesis based on quality of life measures. Eur Spine J 2019;28(9):2060–9.
18. Wu HH, Brown K, Flores M, et al. Diagnosis and Management of Spondylolysis and Spondylolisthesis in Children. JBJS Rev 2022;10(3). https://doi. org/10.2106/JBJS.RVW.21.00176.
19. Harris IE, Weinstein SL. Long-term follow-up of patients with grade-III and IV spondylolisthesis. Treatment with and without posterior fusion. J Bone Joint Surg Am 1987;69(7):960–9.
20. Longo UG, Loppini M, Romeo G, et al. Evidence-based surgical management of spondylolisthesis: reduction or arthrodesis in situ. J Bone Joint Surg Am 2014;96(1):53–8.
21. Crawford CH 3rd, Larson AN, Gates M, et al. Current Evidence Regarding the Treatment of Pediatric Lumbar Spondylolisthesis: A Report From the Scoliosis

Research Society Evidence Based Medicine Committee. Spine Deform 2017;5(5):284–302.

22. Agabegi SS, Fischgrund JS. Contemporary management of isthmic spondylolisthesis: pediatric and adult. Spine J 2010;10(6):530–43.

23. Scaglietti O, Frontino G, Bartolozzi P. Technique of anatomical reduction of lumbar spondylolisthesis and its surgical stabilization. Clin Orthop Relat Res 1976;117:165–75.

24. Bradford DS, Boachie-Adjei O. Treatment of severe spondylolisthesis by anterior and posterior reduction and stabilization. A long-term follow-up study. J Bone Joint Surg Am 1990;72(7):1060–6.

25. Magerl FP. Stabilization of the lower thoracic and lumbar spine with external skeletal fixation. Clin Orthop Relat Res 1984;189:125–41.

26. Karampalis C, Grevitt M, Shafafy M, et al. High-grade spondylolisthesis: gradual reduction using Magerl's external fixator followed by circumferential fusion technique and long-term results. Eur Spine J 2012;21(Suppl 2):S200–6.

27. Edwards CC, Bradford DS. Instrumented reduction of spondylolisthesis. Spine 1994;19(13):1535–7.

28. Prudnikova OG, Shchurova EN. Operative management of high-grade dysplastic L5 spondylolisthesis with the use of external transpedicular fixation: advantages and drawbacks. Int Orthop 2016;40(6):1127–33.

29. Gaines RW, Nichols WK. Treatment of spondyloptosis by two stage L5 vertebrectomy and reduction of L4 onto S1. Spine 1985;10(7):680–6.

30. Gaines RW. L5 vertebrectomy for the surgical treatment of spondyloptosis: thirty cases in 25 years. Spine 2005;30(6 Suppl):S66–70.

31. Min K, Liebscher T, Rothenfluh D. Sacral dome resection and single-stage posterior reduction in the treatment of high-grade high dysplastic spondylolisthesis in adolescents and young adults. Eur Spine J 2012;(Suppl 6):S785–91.

32. Tian W, Han X-G, Liu B, et al. Posterior reduction and monosegmental fusion with intraoperative three-dimensional navigation system in the treatment of high-grade developmental spondylolisthesis. Chin Med J (Engl) 2015;128(7):865–70.

33. Harms J. True spondylolisthesis reduction and monosegmental fusion in spondylolisthesis. In: Bridwell K, DeWald R, editors. The Textbook of spinal Surgery. 2nd edition. Philadelphia: Lippincott-Raven; 1997. p. 1337–47.

34. Ruf M, Koch H, Melcher RP, et al. Anatomic reduction and monosegmental fusion in high-grade developmental spondylolisthesis. Spine 2006;31(3):269–74.

35. Shufflebarger HL, Geck MJ. High-grade isthmic dysplastic spondylolisthesis: monosegmental surgical treatment. Spine 2005;30(6 Suppl):S42–8.

36. Martiniani M, Lamartina C, Specchia N. "In situ" fusion or reduction in high-grade high dysplastic developmental spondylolisthesis (HDSS). Eur Spine J 2012;21(Suppl 1):S134–40.

37. Thomas D, Bachy M, Courvoisier A, et al. Progressive restoration of spinal sagittal balance after surgical correction of lumbosacral spondylolisthesis before skeletal maturity. J Neurosurg Spine 2015;22(3):294–300.

38. Schlösser TPC, Garrido E, Tsirikos AI, et al. Health-related quality of life and sagittal balance at two to 25 years after posterior transfixation for high-grade dysplastic spondylolisthesis. Bone Jt Open 2021;2(3):163–73.

39. Sebaaly A, El Rachkidi R, Grobost P, et al. L5 incidence: an important parameter for spinopelvic balance evaluation in high-grade spondylolisthesis. Spine J 2018;18(8):1417–23.

40. Ilharreborde B, Fitoussi F, Morel E, et al. Jackson's intrasacral fixation in the management of high-grade isthmic spondylolisthesis. J Pediatr Orthop B 2007;16(1):16–8.

41. Bouyer B, Bachy M, Courvoisier A, et al. High-grade lumbosacral spondylolisthesis reduction and fusion in children using transsacral rod fixation. Childs Nerv Syst 2014;30:505–13.

Proximal Junctional Kyphosis and Failure: Strategies for Prevention

Ayush Arora, BSE[a], Zachary T. Sharfman, MD[a], Aaron J. Clark, MD, PhD[b], Alekos A. Theologis, MD[a],*

KEYWORDS

- Adult spinal deformity • Proximal junctional kyphosis • Prevention • Kyphoplasty • Vertebroplasty
- Tethers • Ligamentoplasty

KEY POINTS

- Proximal junctional kyphosis (PJK) and proximal junctional failure (PJF) are common complications following long-segment posterior instrumented fusions for adult spinal deformity (ASD).
- Failures at the thoracolumbar junction are generally secondary to fractures, whereas those in the upper thoracic spine are typically caused by ligamentous failure.
- Ligamentous banding and use of transition rods may present cost-effective options that have potential to reduce PJF secondary to ligamentous failure.
- Two-level cement augmentation of the upper instrumented vertebra (UIV) and supra-adjacent vertebra to the UIV (UIV+1) may also benefit patients by reducing the incidence of PJF.
- Regional implant-focused strategies combined with careful planning and correction of the sagittal profile are important for minimizing the development of PJK and PJF and ensuring financial viability of ASD surgery.

INTRODUCTION

Balanced and patient-specific harmonious spinal alignment is important for upright posture maintenance, biomechanical stability, and to decrease energy used to stand and ambulate.[1,2] Deviations in alignment can be secondary to idiopathic, congenital neuromuscular, degenerative changes, and iatrogenic causes, which may manifest as sagittal malalignment, scoliosis, kyphosis, rotatory subluxation, and spondylolisthesis.[1,3] Such pathologies are categorized under the umbrella term, "Adult Spinal Deformity" (ASD).[3,4] These deformities are common and current prevalence data likely underestimate the true burden of disease due to mixed diagnoses and multiple subclassifications.[5] The prevalence of adult scoliosis has been estimated to be as high as 68% in elderly individuals.[6–10] As the global population ages, it is likely that the incidence of ASD will continue to increase, as will the economic burden associated with its surgical and nonsurgical management.

In an evolving value driven health care economy, there is increasing focus on defining the benefits of complex spine surgery.[11] Clinical outcome assessment via health-related quality of life (HRQOL) outcome scores is critical in defining the value and role for surgery in treating ASD. These outcome measures should incorporate measures of overall quality of life, functional measurements, pain levels, and disability.[12] Given the high prevalence and severity of complications following operations for

[a] Department of Orthopaedic Surgery, UCSF, 500 Parnassus Avenue, MUW 3Road Floor, San Francisco, CA 94143, USA; [b] Department of Neurological Surgery, UCSF, 521 Parnassus Avenue, 6307, San Francisco, CA 94117, USA
* Corresponding author.
E-mail address: alekos.theologis@ucsf.edu

Neurosurg Clin N Am 34 (2023) 573–584
https://doi.org/10.1016/j.nec.2023.06.004
1042-3680/23/© 2023 Elsevier Inc. All rights reserved.

ASD (ie, >70%), quantifying the benefits of surgery in this patient population is important in justifying its value proposition.[13] Importantly, multiple investigations have demonstrated the utility of operative intervention for ASD. Specifically, in a study of 427 ASD patients with 4-year mean follow-up, patients reported significant improvements in terms of pain, activity, appearance, mental status and SF-36.[14] In addition to improved patient-reported outcomes, the benefits of surgery are tangible in terms of increased productivity and decreased absenteeism from school and work, as demonstrated in a cohort of 1188 patients who underwent operative intervention to address ASD.[15] Even in patients who undergo the most complex ASD surgeries, including three column osteotomies, clinically relevant improvement in Scoliosis Research Society-22r (SRS-22r) HRQOL scores are achievable.[11] High postoperative satisfaction is reported in patients undergoing ASD surgery regardless of the approach used.[16]

Despite good outcomes, high satisfaction, and increased productivity after ASD surgery, complications can jeopardize outcomes and negatively affect quality of life. Included in these complications are surgical complications of which proximal junctional kyphosis (PJK) and proximal junctional failure (PJF) often require revision procedures. As PJK and PJF can be devastating complications for patients and vexing problems for surgeons, the authors present a detailed outline of PJK and PJF with a focus on surgical strategies aimed at preventing their occurrence.

DEFINITION, PREVALENCE, AND CLASSIFICATION OF PROXIMAL JUNCTIONAL KYPHOSIS AND PROXIMAL JUNCTIONAL FAILURE

PJK is defined by a postoperative proximal junction sagittal cobb angle $\geq$ 10° between the lower end plate of the upper instrumented vertebra (UIV) and the upper end plate of the two supra-adjacent vertebrae (UIV+2).[17] The prevalence of PJK following posterior fusion for ASD has been reported to range between 17% and 46%, with two-thirds of cases occurring within the 3-month postoperative period.[18–20] Many patients with PJK do not require revisions and may have equivalent functional outcomes when compared with those without PJK.[17,21–23] However, the progression of PJK to failure that necessitates revision is termed PJF and is clinically important (Fig. 1), as it can result in catastrophic neural compromise, severe disability, and challenging and costly revision operations.[24] Hostin and colleagues and the International Spine Study Group specifically

defined PJF as occurring due to $\geq$ 15° postoperative increase in PJK, vertebral fracture of UIV or UIV+1, failure of UIV fixation, new onset of myelopathy, and/or other causes that require revision surgery (see Fig. 1; Fig. 2).[25] Revision operations for PJF typically consist of proximal extension of instrumented fusion with or without neural decompression and deformity correction via osteotomies, as they are commonly indicated for clinical symptoms of pain, spinal instability, neurologic deficits, significant kyphosis, ambulatory difficulties, and/or inability to maintain a horizontal gaze.[21,23,26–28]

The occurrence of PJK and PJF following surgery varies in time. In a cohort of 150 patients, Wang and colleagues reported that 80% of PJK cases are diagnosed within 18 months postoperatively, whereas Yagi and colleagues found that 66% of PJK cases were present at the 3-month mark in a study of 76 patients with 5-year follow-up.[23,29] In a series of 1218 posterior segmental instrumented fusions for ASD, Hostin and colleagues noted 5.6% of patients had PJF, with a mean time to failure occurring at 11.4 weeks.[25] The study reported that fractures were significantly more common for thoracolumbar PJF, whereas whole soft-tissue failures were more common in constructs that terminated in the upper thoracic spine.[25] Risk factors associated with PJF included older age, fewer fusion levels, worse postoperative sagittal vertical axis, fusion to the sacrum, and posterior spine fusion.[25] Even in cases where clinically irrelevant PJK is present at the 3-month mark, PJK may continuously progress and result in more extensive kyphosis within the 5-year postoperative period.[23]

Two categories of PJK/PJF include ligamentous failure and osseous fracture (see Figs. 1 and 2; Figs. 3 and 4).[23] Ligamentous failure comprises greater than 70% of PJK cases and is hypothesized to occur due to surgical interventions that alter the integrity of the posterior supraspinous and interspinous ligaments, spinous process, and paraspinal musculature (see Fig. 4).[23] The insufficiency of the posterior ligamentous complex secondary to surgery may not be reversible.[23] Alternatively, PJK/PJF due to fractures present a differing presentation, of which there are two modalities (see Figs. 1, 3, and 4).[23] One type is where the supra-adjacent vertebrae above the UIV (UIV+1) undergoes a compression fracture with kyphosis (see Figs. 1 and 3), whereas the second is UIV collapse and subluxation of UIV+1 (see Fig. 4). Although the former may not be symptomatic, the latter is often clinically significant and produces myelopathy that necessitates a revision.

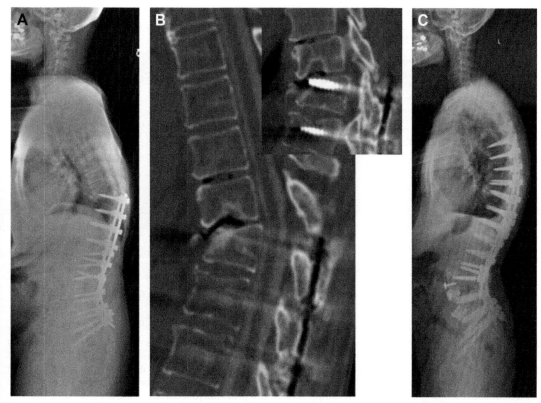

Fig. 1. A 73-year-old woman with osteoporosis underwent a T10 to pelvis posterior instrumented fusion (PSIF) with L4–S1 transforaminal lumbar interbody fusions (TLIF). Two years after operation, she reported worsening mid-thoracic back pain, progressively more difficulty standing upright, and subjective weakness of the lower extremities. Radiographs and CT scan demonstrated proximal junctional kyphosis (PJK) and a compression fracture at T10 (*A*, *B*). Note the risk for developing PJK and PJF was the undercorrection of her lumbar lordosis resulting in persistent lumbopelvic mismatch (*A*). No preventative strategies were used at the proximal junction. After undergoing an L3–S1 anterior lumbar interbody fusion (ALIF) and revision of T4 to pelvis PSIF, her back pain and posture were greatly improved (*C*).

COSTS OF PROXIMAL JUNCTIONAL KYPHOSIS AND PROXIMAL JUNCTIONAL FAILURE

The high costs associated with revision surgeries for PJF may undermine the ultimate utility of ASD surgery. The average direct costs associated with readmissions for PJF are among the largest and only second to pseudoarthrosis.[30] In a study of deformity patients, Yeramaneni and colleagues reported the average direct costs associated with readmission for PJF to be $55,516 while the average direct costs for revisions for any other cause to be $38,754.[30] Although available literature indicates direct costs associated with PJF revision operations to range from $20,000 to $120,000, estimations are likely underapproximations due to the lack of accounting for indirect costs. As for reasons PJF accounts for high expenditures, Theologis and colleagues noted that PJF revisions are of high complexity and require intensive postoperative care.[31,32] In the study, patients required the following average metrics: 6.3 posterior levels of instrumented fusion, blood loss of 1.2 L, operative time of 5.3 hours, and length of stay of 7.2 days.[32] Although surgical intervention for ASD may confer quality of life improvement for patients, overall utility depends on the associated costs and potential for revision surgery. As PJF presents a highly prevalent occurrence after posterior thoracolumbar instrumented spinal fusions with costs that are unsustainable for health care systems, preventative strategies to minimize the occurrence of PJF are of tremendous importance.

TECHNIQUES FOR PREVENTION OF LIGAMENTOUS FAILURE

Ligamentous failures afflict long posterior instrumented fusions that end cranially at the thoracolumbar junction and at the upper thoracic spine,

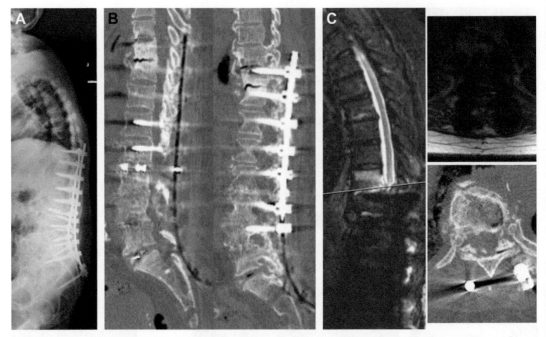

Fig. 2. A 79-year-old woman with osteoporosis presented with worsening back pain, gait instability, and lower extremity weakness after multiple prior spine operations, the last of which included a T10 to pelvis posterior instrumented fusion (PSIF) (*A*). Radiographs and CT scan demonstrated advanced disc degeneration and collapse at the proximal junction associated with loosening of the upper instrumented vertebral level's screws (*B*). An MRI also demonstrated high-grade spinal cord compression at this proximal junction (*C*). Note the risk for developing PJK and PJF was the undercorrection of her lumbar lordosis resulting in persistent lumbopelvic mismatch (*A*). No preventative strategies were used at the proximal junction.

although the latter constitutes a larger percentage. Techniques aimed at preventing ligamentous failure include implant focused solutions that dampen proximal forces. Such techniques use an approach known as "topping-off," implementing semi-rigid fixation at the proximal end of a rigid construct and thereby mitigating focal peak stresses at junctional levels.[33] Techniques to be discussed include the following: transverse process hooks (TPHs), ligamentous banding, multi-level stabilization screws (MLSSs), and flexible transition rods.

Transverse Process Hooks

TPHs may be used for constructs terminating in the upper thoracic spine, especially because failure at such levels is commonly due to ligamentous fatigue (**Fig. 5**). The benefits of hook fixation stem from the fact that it requires less dissection of surrounding muscle and facet and does not require subperiosteal exposure.[34] Although the use of TPHs at the proximal end of constructs has been suggested, their demonstrated clinical utility in reducing PJK/PJF risk in adults is limited. Although Kim and colleagues found no significant difference in incidences of PJK in ASD patients undergoing

posterior spinal fusion using TPHs, pedicle screws, or hybrid constructs, the TPH group did have lower average proximal level kyphosis.[35,36] In terms of PJF incidence, Line and colleagues and Matsumura and colleagues also found no significant reduction with the use of TPH.[37,38] Only one study by Hassanzadeh and colleagues with 47 ASD patients found that PJK/PJF rates were lower when compared with a pedicle screw control group, though the TPH group had a shorter mean follow-up time compared with the pedicle screw group (2.8 vs 5.7 years).[39] Although TPH has shown clinical benefit in adolescents with scoliosis, limited evidence exists for adult deformity patients.[35,36,40]

Ligamentous Banding

Ligamentous banding at the UIV-1, UIV, and/or UIV+1 may provide a cornerstone method of reducing PJK rates that is superior to TPH. Implantation involves drill holes in the center of the spinous processes and weaving of a cable composed of allograft tendon or Mersilene tape through the holes in a variety of configurations. The cable is placed under tension so that the spinous processes are loaded into slight extension

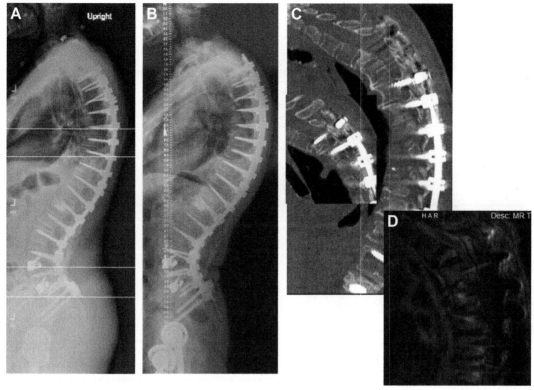

Fig. 3. A 68-year-old woman with osteoporosis with a degenerative lumbar scoliosis and adult Scheuermann's kyphosis underwent an L4–S1 ALIF and T3 to pelvis PSIF (*A*). Within 3 months of the index operation, she reported progressive difficulty maintaining horizontal gaze and decompensation of her neck posture. Radiographs and CT scan demonstrated PJK secondary to a UIV compression fracture and translation of the UIV+1 on the UIV (*B, C*) despite having ligament banding with mersilene tape at the UIV+1, UIV, and UIV-1. Although there was ventral spinal cord compression at the level of the UIV, she was neurologically intact (*D*).

and resist flexion at the UIV.[34] Each configuration (see **Fig. 5**) is associated with its own respective efficacy in preventing PJK/PJF.

Tether Connector Configuration

The tether connector configuration (see **Fig. 5**) was studied by Alluri and colleagues and Safaee and colleagues, who both found PJF to be significantly less common in tether connector groups than in patients with no posterior ligamentous augmentation.[41,42] Of note, the former study used a semitendinosus allograft,[41] whereas the latter used polyethylene tape.[42] No studies have compared whether one material is better than the other but the semitendinosus allograft may be a more cost-effective option. The tether connector configuration presents moderate efficacy in preventing progression of PKJ to failure.

Tether-Only and Tether-Crosslink

The tether-only (see **Fig. 5**) and tether-crosslink (see **Fig. 5**) configurations show less promise than

the tether connector configuration. The tether-only configuration involves hand-tightening the band through the spinous processes of UIV+1 and UIV-1, whereas the tether-crosslink configuration involves the tape threaded through the spinous process of UIV-1 and tensioned by a cross-link between UIV-1 and UIV-2. No difference in PJF incidences was found by Buell and colleagues and Line and colleagues for either configuration when compared with pedicle screws without these ligamentous augmentation techniques.[37,43]

Tether-Pedicle Loop Configuration

The tether-pedicle loop configuration involves threading the band through the spinous process of UIV+1 and then tensioned and looped underneath the UIV pedicle screws, with the same process applied to the UIV and UIV-1 (see **Fig. 5**). There is limited scientific evidence to support this technique, as only one retrospective series has investigated this tether-pedicle loop configuration.[44] In this study of 108 patients, Iyer and

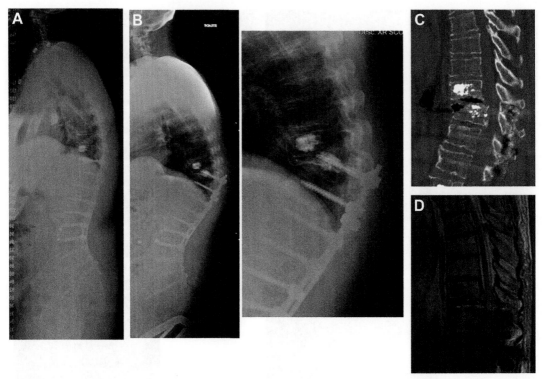

Fig. 4. A 56-year-old man underwent a T10 to pelvis posterior instrumented fusion including two-level cement augmentation of the UIV+1 and UIV (*A*). Six weeks postoperatively, he presented with progressive motor weakness of the lower extremities following a fall at home. Radiographs demonstrated an unstable three-column fracture with bilateral perched facets between the UIV and UIV+1 secondary to a ligamentous failure at the UIV and UIV+1 (*B*). A CT scan demonstrated a fracture of the anterior-superior endplate of the UIV and partial reducibility of the fracture-dislocation (*C*). At the proximal junction, MRI demonstrated severe central stenosis with cord signal change from a thoracic disc herniation and a dorsal epidural hematoma (*D*).

colleagues found no impact on PJK/PJF rates in patients with or without banding after controlling for sagittal correction.[44]

Figure-of-8 Tether

The figure-of 8 tether configuration consists of passing the band through the spinous process of UIV+1 and looping the band in a figure-of-8 pattern around the spinous process of UIV (see **Fig. 5**). In a study of 80 patients, Rodriguez-Fontan and colleagues found mersilene tape in the figure-of-8 configuration significantly decreased the risk of PJK following posterior instrumented fusions for ASD when matched to patients with this augmentation technique for sagittal cobb angle, lumbar lordosis, pelvic tilt, sacral slope, and pelvic incidence.[45]

Multilevel Stabilization Screws

MLSSs present a promising approach for reducing PJK and PJF incidence (see **Fig. 5**). In a cohort analysis, Kaufmann and colleagues demonstrated

a significant independent association between MLSS and PJF rates, with an odds ratio of 0.11 when compared with patients with no MLSS.[46] In a separate case series of 15 patients, Sandquist and colleagues confirmed the possible clinical utility of LSS, finding that no patients with MLSS developed PJK/PJF.[47]

Flexible Transition Rods

Flexible transition rods over the UIV have shown promise in biomechanical studies but remain to be evaluated clinically (see **Fig. 5**). In a finite-element analysis, Cahill and colleagues found that the use of titanium transition rods may reduce disc nucleus pressure by 23% and angular displacement by 18% to 19% at the UIV.[48] Although Lee and colleagues found that the use of flexible titanium rods allowed 15° flexion and 10° extension at the proximal junction and produced a significantly lower PJK incidence when compared with pedicle screws (15% vs 38%), the follow-up duration of the pedicle screw group was longer.[49] The rod material favored in the

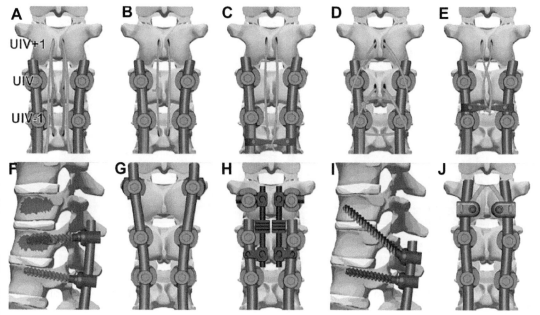

Fig. 5. Surgical prophylactic techniques for proximal junctional kyphosis and proximal junctional failure (*A*) tether-connectors, (*B*) tether-only, (*C*) tether-crosslink, (*D*) tether-pedicle loop, (*E*) tether in a figure-8 configuration, (*F*) prophylactic two-level vertebroplasty, (*G*) transverse process hooks, (*H*) flexible rods, (*I*) multilevel stabilization screw (MLSS) 44, and (*J*) sublaminar tapes. Adapted with permission from Vercoulen and colleagues.[33]

literature is titanium, with Han and colleagues reporting that PJK occurred much later for patients with titanium rods compared with cobalt rods (mean of 26.3 months postop vs 3.6 months postop, respectively).[50] However, the same study found that titanium transition rods had a significantly higher rate of rod fracture compared with cobalt-chrome rods (32.4% vs 0%).[50]

TECHNIQUES FOR PREVENTION OF FRACTURES

PJFs due to fractures most commonly occur at the thoracolumbar junction but may also occur in constructs that extend to the upper thoracic spine (see **Figs. 1**, **3** and **4**). The primary method for prevention of fractures is cement augmentation (**Fig. 6**).

Cement Augmentation

Cement augmentation may be performed when the UIV is at any thoracic and lumbar spinal level (see **Fig. 6**). There are numerous ways by which cement augmentation can be accomplished in regard to exposure technique, cement delivery method, and number of levels augmented.[34] For example, cement augmentation may be performed via an open exposure, through an all-percutaneous method, or through a hybrid open and percutaneous method. In addition, there

can be variation in cement deliver, including performing a vertebroplasty or a kyphoplasty, or both if two levels are involved.

Regarding level selection for cement augmentation, prior *in vitro* and clinical studies have demonstrated that cement augmentation of both the UIV and UIV+1 provides a stronger construct more apt at the prevention of fractures than no cement or only one-level cement augmentation of the UIV or UIV+1 (see **Fig. 6**). In a biomechanical study, Kebaish and colleagues found that 67% of specimens treated with one-level vertebroplasty and 100% of specimens without cement augmentation had a PJF, whereas only one of six cadavers with two-level cement augmentation (UIV and UIV+1) sustained a PJF.[51] Certain studies have found significant reduction in PJK/PJF rates when two-level cement is applied, whereas others have found that the two-level cement plays a role in delaying progression to PJK/PJF.[50,52–54] For example, in a retrospective study with minimum 6-month follow-up, Theologis and colleagues demonstrated that two-level cement augmentation resulted in significantly fewer revision operations for PJF compared with patients with no augmentation or augmentation at only one level.[54] In a separate prospective study of 39 ASD surgical patients with two-level cement, Raman and colleagues determined that cement augmentation minimized

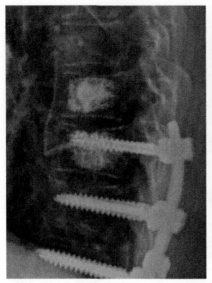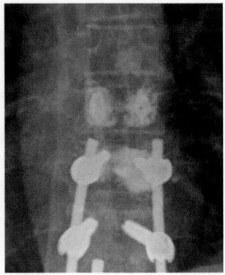

Fig. 6. Example of prophylactic two-level cement augmentation at the UIV and UIV+1 for prevention of proximal junctional fracture.

risk of PJF in the early postoperative period but had no decrease in incidence at 5-years.[55] Most patients in the study who developed PJK did so at 2 to 5 years, a follow-up duration that few other studies adhere toward. Hence, although PJF and PJF are typically early findings, two-level cement augmentation may delay the time course of the condition. Although rates reported in the literature for PJF in patients with cement augmentation are likely underestimated due to follow-up less than 2 years, patients may still functionally benefit from cement augmentation, with Martin and colleagues and Theologis and colleagues noting that patients receiving two-level cement augmentation had less disability, as assessed by the Oswestry Disability Index.[54,56]

Cement augmentation may also be cost-effective when compared with costs of revision operations for PJF. In a study of 28 ASD patients, Hart and colleagues noted that none of the 15 patients with two-level cement augmentation at the UIV and UIV+1 incurred PJF, whereas PJF occurred in the remaining 2/13 patients with constructs extending to the thoracolumbar junction.[24] The study determined that the cost of revision instrumented fusion (average $77,432) outweighed the costs of prophylactic two-level cement augmentation (average of $47,240).[24]

Potential negative effects of cement augmentation include cement embolization to the lungs, cement leakage to the adjacent surround tissues, including the spinal canal, acceleration of degenerative disc disease at the UIV, UIV+1, and UIV+2, and increased adjacent vertebral level

fracture risk, which all may lead to future disability and costs.[24,57,58]

THE IMPORTANCE OF ALIGNMENT IN PREVENTING PROXIMAL JUNCTIONAL KYPHOSIS/PROXIMAL JUNCTIONAL FAILURE

Although the aforementioned text has focused on focal surgical strategies aimed at preventing PJK/PJF by augmenting the anterior column with cement and/or reinforcing the posterior ligamentous structures at the proximal junction of long thoracolumbar constructs, it is also important to take into consideration spinal alignment as a tool for minimizing the occurrence of PJK/PJF. Striking a balance between ideal correction of spinal alignment and avoiding overcorrection and undercorrection of the sagittal plane is important in preventing PJK/PJF (see **Figs. 1** and **2**; **Fig. 7**).[59–61] Although the "ideal" sagittal alignment parameters remain debatable and under continued investigation, the degree of sagittal plane correction is also important, as alignment measurements even within ideal postoperative ranges have been implicated with increased rates of PJK/PJF in older patients. In a retrospective review, Mauro and colleagues reported that changes in lumbar lordosis greater than 30° and thoracic kyphosis greater than 30° were significant risk factors for PJK.[59] On a similar note, Kim and colleagues determined that patients with PJF requiring revisions were older and had larger sagittal balance corrections in a case-control study of 206 ASD.[62] Specifically, older patients with "ideal alignment" (ie, postoperative

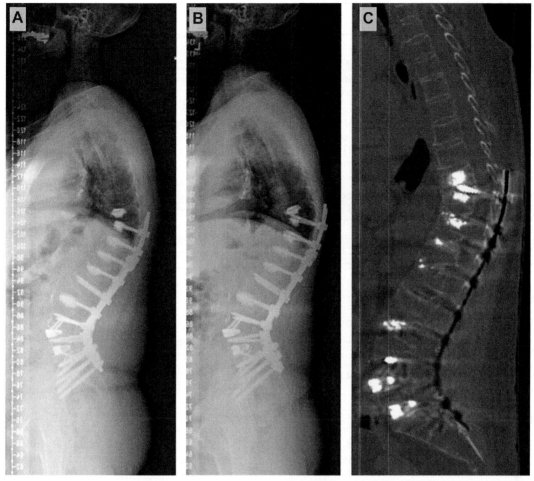

Fig. 7. A 56-year-old obese woman with osteoporosis underwent an L4–S1 ALIF and T10 to pelvis PSIF with two-level cement augmentation at the UIV and UIV+1 (*A*). At the 6-month postoperative visit, radiographs and CT scan demonstrated PJK from a compression fracture the UIV and cut out of the proximal screws into the disc space between the UIV and UIV+1 (*B*, *C*). Note the risk factors for development of PJK/PJF were obesity, osteoporosis, and likely overcorrection of the deformity with a posteriorly displaced L1 relative to the gravity line (*A*).

sagittal vertical axis [SVA] near 0 mm and lumbar lordosis [LL] approximating the pelvic incidence [PI]) were at an elevated risk of PJF compared with those patients with "non-ideal alignment" (ie, SVA nearer to 40 mm and LL closer to PI-10°).[62] Additional reports have verified corrections in SVA beyond 50 mm to be associated with PJK.[16,28,63] As such, a combination of implant-based solutions and avoidance of overcorrection and undercorrection of sagittal alignment represents the best path forward in mitigating PJK risk.

SUMMARY

PJK and PJF are common complications following long-segment posterior instrumented fusions for ASD. Progression to PJF involves clinical consequences for patients and requires costly revisions that may undermine the utility of surgery. Failures at the thoracolumbar junction are generally due to fractures, whereas those in the upper thoracic spine are typically caused by ligamentous failure. Ligamentous banding and use of transition rods may present cost-effective options that have potential to reduce PJF secondary to ligamentous failure. Two-level cement augmentation of the UIV and UIV+1 may also benefit patients by reducing the incidence of PJF and/or offering a delayed progression of PJK to PJF. These regional implant-focused strategies combined with careful planning and correction of the sagittal profile are important for minimizing the development of PJK and PJF and ensuring financial viability of ASD surgery.

CLINICS CARE POINTS

- Ligamentous banding and use of transition rods may present cost-effective options that have potential to reduce PJF secondary to ligamentous failure.

- Two-level cement augmentation of the upper instrumented vertebra (UIV) and supra-adjacent vertebra to the UIV (UIV+1) may also benefit patients by reducing the incidence of PJF.

- Regional implant-focused strategies combined with careful planning and correction of the sagittal profile are important for minimizing the development of PJK andPJF and ensuring financial viability of ASD surgery.

FUNDING

No funding was obtained for the submitted work.

DISCLOSURE

None of the authors have any relevant disclosures related to the submitted work.

REFERENCES

1. Ames CP, Scheer JK, Lafage V, et al. Adult spinal deformity: epidemiology, health impact, evaluation, and management. Spine Deform 2016;4(4):310–22.

2. Scheer JK, Smith JS, Clark AJ, et al. Comprehensive study of back and leg pain improvements after adult spinal deformity surgery: analysis of 421 patients with 2-year follow-up and of the impact of the surgery on treatment satisfaction. J Neurosurg Spine 2015;22(5):540–53.

3. Grubb SA, Lipscomb HJ, Coonrad RW. Degenerative adult onset scoliosis. Spine 1988;13(3):241–5.

4. BERNHARDT M, BRIDWELL KH. Segmental analysis of the sagittal plane alignment of the normal thoracic and lumbar spines and thoracolumbar junction. Spine 1989;14(7):717–21.

5. Gum JL, Carreon LY, Glassman SD. State-of-the-art: outcome assessment in adult spinal deformity. Spine Deform 2021;9(1):1–11.

6. Carter OD, Haynes SG. Prevalence rates for scoliosis in US adults: results from the first National Health and Nutrition Examination Survey. Int J Epidemiol 1987;16(4):537–44.

7. Francis RS. Scoliosis screening of 3,000 college-aged women. The Utah Study–phase 2. Phys Ther 1988;68(10):1513–6.

8. Kostuik JP, Bentivoglio J. The incidence of low-back pain in adult scoliosis. Spine 1981;6(3):268–73.

9. Perennou D, Marcelli C, Herisson C, et al. Adult lumbar scoliosis. Epidemiologic aspects in a low-back pain population. Spine 1994;19(2):123–8.

10. Schwab F, Dubey A, Gamez L, et al. Adult scoliosis: prevalence, SF-36, and nutritional parameters in an elderly volunteer population. Spine 2005;30(9):1082–5.

11. Riley MS, Bridwell KH, Lenke LG, et al. Health-related quality of life outcomes in complex adult spinal deformity surgery. J Neurosurg Spine 2018;28(2):194–200.

12. Faraj SSA, van Hooff ML, Holewijn RM, et al. Measuring outcomes in adult spinal deformity surgery: a systematic review to identify current strengths, weaknesses and gaps in patient-reported outcome measures. Eur Spine J 2017;26(8):2084–93.

13. Smith MW, Annis P, Lawrence BD, et al. Early proximal junctional failure in patients with preoperative sagittal imbalance. Evid Based Spine Care J 2013;4(2):163–4.

14. Elias E, Bess S, Line B, et al. Outcomes of operative treatment for adult spinal deformity: a prospective multicenter assessment with mean 4-year follow-up. J Neurosurg Spine 2022;1–10. https://doi.org/10.3171/2022.3.SPINE2295.

15. Durand WM, Babu JM, Hamilton DK, et al. Adult spinal deformity surgery is associated with increased productivity and decreased absenteeism from work and school. Spine 2022;47(4):287–94.

16. Ryu WHA, Cheong M, Platt A, et al. Patient satisfaction following minimally invasive and open surgeries for adult spinal deformity. World Neurosurg 2021;155:e301–14.

17. Glattes RC, Bridwell KH, Lenke LG, et al. Proximal junctional kyphosis in adult spinal deformity following long instrumented posterior spinal fusion: incidence, outcomes, and risk factor analysis. Spine 2005;30(14):1643–9.

18. Kim HJ, Iyer S. Proximal junctional kyphosis. J Am Acad Orthop Surg 2016;24(5):318–26.

19. Kim HJ, Lenke LG, Shaffrey CI, et al. Proximal junctional kyphosis as a distinct form of adjacent segment pathology after spinal deformity surgery: a systematic review. Spine 2012;37(22 Suppl):S144–64.

20. Lau D, Clark AJ, Scheer JK, et al. Proximal junctional kyphosis and failure after spinal deformity surgery: a systematic review of the literature as a background to classification development. Spine 2014;39(25):2093–102.

21. Kim YJ, Bridwell KH, Lenke LG, et al. Proximal junctional kyphosis in adult spinal deformity after segmental posterior spinal instrumentation and fusion: minimum five-year follow-up. Spine 2008;33(20):2179–84.

22. Kim YJ, Bridwell KH, Lenke LG, et al. Is the T9, T11, or L1 the more reliable proximal level after adult

lumbar or lumbosacral instrumented fusion to L5 or S1? Spine 2007;32(24):2653–61.

23. Yagi M, King AB, Boachie-Adjei O. Incidence, risk factors, and natural course of proximal junctional kyphosis: surgical outcomes review of adult idiopathic scoliosis. Minimum 5 years of follow-up. Spine 2012;37(17):1479–89.

24. Hart RA, Prendergast MA, Roberts WG, et al. Proximal junctional acute collapse cranial to multi-level lumbar fusion: a cost analysis of prophylactic vertebral augmentation. Spine J 2008;8(6):875–81.

25. Hostin R, McCarthy I, O'Brien M, et al. Incidence, mode, and location of acute proximal junctional failures after surgical treatment of adult spinal deformity. Spine 2013;38(12):1008–15.

26. Kim HJ, Bridwell KH, Lenke LG, et al. Proximal junctional kyphosis results in inferior SRS pain subscores in adult deformity patients. Spine 2013;38(11): 896–901.

27. McClendon J Jr, O'Shaughnessy BA, Sugrue PA, et al. Techniques for operative correction of proximal junctional kyphosis of the upper thoracic spine. Spine 2012;37(4):292–303.

28. Sardar ZM, Kim Y, Lafage V, et al. State of the art: proximal junctional kyphosis-diagnosis, management and prevention. Spine Deform 2021;9(3): 635–44.

29. Wang J, Zhao Y, Shen B, et al. Risk factor analysis of proximal junctional kyphosis after posterior fusion in patients with idiopathic scoliosis. Injury 2010;41(4): 415–20.

30. Yeramaneni S, Gum JL, Carreon LY, et al. Impact of readmissions in episodic care of adult spinal deformity: event-based cost analysis of 695 consecutive cases. J Bone Joint Surg Am 2018;100(6):487–95.

31. Theologis AA, Gussous YM, Berven SH. Economic impact of proximal junctional kyphosis. Tech Orthop 2021;36(1):12–7.

32. Theologis AA, Miller L, Callahan M, et al. Economic impact of revision surgery for proximal junctional failure after adult spinal deformity surgery: a cost analysis of 57 operations in a 10-year experience at a major deformity center. Spine 2016;41(16): E964–72.

33. Vercoulen TFG, Doodkorte RJP, Roth A, et al. Instrumentation techniques to prevent proximal junctional kyphosis and proximal junctional failure in adult spinal deformity correction: a systematic review of clinical studies. Global Spine J 2022;12(6):1282–96.

34. Safaee MM, Osorio JA, Verma K, et al. Proximal junctional kyphosis prevention strategies: a video technique guide. Oper Neurosurg (Hagerstown) 2017;13(5):581–5.

35. Helgeson MD, Shah SA, Newton PO, et al. Evaluation of proximal junctional kyphosis in adolescent idiopathic scoliosis following pedicle screw, hook, or hybrid instrumentation. Spine 2010;35(2):177–81.

36. Kim YJ, Lenke LG, Bridwell KH, et al. Proximal junctional kyphosis in adolescent idiopathic scoliosis after 3 different types of posterior segmental spinal instrumentation and fusions: incidence and risk factor analysis of 410 cases. Spine 2007;32(24): 2731–8.

37. Line BG, Bess S, Lafage R, et al. Effective prevention of proximal junctional failure in adult spinal deformity surgery requires a combination of surgical implant prophylaxis and avoidance of sagittal alignment overcorrection. Spine 2020;45(4):258–67.

38. Matsumura A, Namikawa T, Kato M, et al. Effect of different types of upper instrumented vertebrae instruments on proximal junctional kyphosis following adult spinal deformity surgery: pedicle screw versus transverse process hook. Asian Spine J 2018;12(4): 622–31.

39. Hassanzadeh H, Gupta S, Jain A, et al. Type of anchor at the proximal fusion level has a significant effect on the incidence of proximal junctional kyphosis and outcome in adults after long posterior spinal fusion. Spine Deform 2013;1(4):299–305.

40. O'Leary PT, Bridwell KH, Lenke LG, et al. Risk factors and outcomes for catastrophic failures at the top of long pedicle screw constructs: a matched cohort analysis performed at a single center. Spine 2009;34(20):2134–9.

41. Alluri R, Kim A, Ton A, et al. Semitendinosus tendon augmentation for prevention of proximal junctional failure. Spine 2021;46(4):241–8.

42. Safaee MM, Deviren V, Dalle Ore C, et al. Ligament augmentation for prevention of proximal junctional kyphosis and proximal junctional failure in adult spinal deformity. J Neurosurg Spine 2018;28(5):512–9.

43. Buell TJ, Chen CJ, Quinn JC, et al. Alignment risk factors for proximal junctional kyphosis and the effect of lower thoracic junctional tethers for adult spinal deformity. World Neurosurg 2019;121:e96–103.

44. Iyer S, Lovecchio F, Elysee JC, et al. Posterior ligamentous reinforcement of the upper instrumented vertebrae +1 does not decrease proximal junctional kyphosis in adult spinal deformity. Global Spine J 2020;10(6):692–9.

45. Rodriguez-Fontan F, Reeves BJ, Noshchenko A, et al. Strap stabilization for proximal junctional kyphosis prevention in instrumented posterior spinal fusion. Eur Spine J 2020;29(6):1287–96.

46. Kaufmann A, Claus C, Tong D, et al. Multilevel stabilization screws prevent proximal junctional failure and kyphosis in adult spinal deformity surgery: a comparative cohort study. Oper Neurosurg (Hagerstown) 2022;22(3):150–7.

47. Sandquist L, Carr D, Tong D, et al. Preventing proximal junctional failure in long segmental instrumented cases of adult degenerative scoliosis using a multilevel stabilization screw technique. Surg Neurol Int 2015;6:112.

48. Cahill PJ, Wang W, Asghar J, et al. The use of a transition rod may prevent proximal junctional kyphosis in the thoracic spine after scoliosis surgery: a finite element analysis. Spine 2012;37(12):E687–95.

49. Lee KY, Lee JH, Kang KC, et al. Preliminary report on the flexible rod technique for prevention of proximal junctional kyphosis following long-segment fusion to the sacrum in adult spinal deformity. J Neurosurg Spine 2019;12:1–8.

50. Han S, Hyun SJ, Kim KJ, et al. Rod stiffness as a risk factor of proximal junctional kyphosis after adult spinal deformity surgery: comparative study between cobalt chrome multiple-rod constructs and titanium alloy two-rod constructs. Spine J 2017;17(7):962–8.

51. Kebaish KM, Martin CT, O'Brien JR, et al. Use of vertebroplasty to prevent proximal junctional fractures in adult deformity surgery: a biomechanical cadaveric study. Spine J 2013;13(12):1897–903.

52. Ghobrial GM, Eichberg DG, Kolcun JPG, et al. Prophylactic vertebral cement augmentation at the uppermost instrumented vertebra and rostral adjacent vertebra for the prevention of proximal junctional kyphosis and failure following long-segment fusion for adult spinal deformity. Spine J 2017;17(10): 1499–505.

53. Han S, Hyun SJ, Kim KJ, et al. Effect of vertebroplasty at the upper instrumented vertebra and upper instrumented vertebra +1 for prevention of proximal junctional failure in adult spinal deformity surgery: a comparative matched-cohort study. World Neurosurg 2019. https://doi.org/10.1016/j.wneu.2018.12. 113.

54. Theologis AA, Burch S. Prevention of acute proximal junctional fractures after long thoracolumbar posterior fusions for adult spinal deformity using 2-level cement augmentation at the upper instrumented vertebra and the vertebra 1 level proximal to the upper instrumented vertebra. Spine 2015;40(19): 1516–26.

55. Raman T, Miller E, Martin CT, et al. The effect of prophylactic vertebroplasty on the incidence of proximal junctional kyphosis and proximal junctional failure following posterior spinal fusion in adult spinal deformity: a 5-year follow-up study. Spine J 2017; 17(10):1489–98.

56. Martin CT, Skolasky RL, Mohamed AS, et al. Preliminary results of the effect of prophylactic vertebroplasty on the incidence of proximal junctional complications after posterior spinal fusion to the low thoracic spine. Spine Deform 2013;1(2):132–8.

57. Trout AT, Kallmes DF, Kaufmann TJ. New fractures after vertebroplasty: adjacent fractures occur significantly sooner. AJNR Am J Neuroradiol 2006;27(1): 217–23.

58. Watanabe K, Lenke LG, Bridwell KH, et al. Proximal junctional vertebral fracture in adults after spinal deformity surgery using pedicle screw constructs: analysis of morphological features. Spine 2010; 35(2):138–45.

59. Maruo K, Ha Y, Inoue S, et al. Predictive factors for proximal junctional kyphosis in long fusions to the sacrum in adult spinal deformity. Spine 2013; 38(23):E1469–76.

60. Reames DL, Kasliwal MK, Smith JS, et al. Time to development, clinical and radiographic characteristics, and management of proximal junctional kyphosis following adult thoracolumbar instrumented fusion for spinal deformity. J Spinal Disord Tech 2015;28(2):E106–14.

61. Xi Z, Duan PG, Mummaneni PV, et al. Posterior displacement of L1 may be a risk factor for proximal junctional kyphosis after adult spinal deformity correction. Global Spine J 2021. https://doi.org/10. 1177/21925682211015651. 21925682211015651.

62. Kim HJ, Bridwell KH, Lenke LG, et al. Patients with proximal junctional kyphosis requiring revision surgery have higher postoperative lumbar lordosis and larger sagittal balance corrections. Spine 2014;39(9):E576–80.

63. Park SJ, Lee CS, Chung SS, et al. Different risk factors of proximal junctional kyphosis and proximal junctional failure following long instrumented fusion to the sacrum for adult spinal deformity: survivorship analysis of 160 patients. Neurosurgery 2017;80(2): 279–86.

Strategies to Avoid Distal Junctional Pathology

Gerard F. Marciano, MD[a],*, Matthew E. Simhon, MD[a], Ronald A. Lehman, MD[b], Lawrence G. Lenke, MD[c]

KEYWORDS

- Distal junctional kyphosis • Distal junctional failure • Lumbosacral junctional pathology

KEY POINTS

- Distal junctional pathology remains an unsolved problem in spine surgery and a less well-studied issue than proximal junctional pathology
- Depending on the etiology of the spine deformity there are techniques to reduce distal junctional pathology with the basic strategy of appropriate lowest instrumented vertebra (LIV) selection and fixation methods.
- When distal junctional pathology requiring intervention occurs, the basic principles require strengthening the area of failure and usually extending the construct to a more caudal LIV.

INTRODUCTION AND HISTORY, DEFINITIONS, BACKGROUND

The advent of modern segmental spinal instrumentation has allowed for greater control of spinal deformity correction over previous techniques such as Harrington rods. However, postoperative decompensation was soon recognized as an entity and the sagittal plane subsequently gained significant attention in the literature. The first report of kyphosis at the distal junction of the instrumented and non-instrumented spine following segmental spinal instrumentation came when Richards and colleagues[1] demonstrated that in their series of 53 patients with adolescent idiopathic scoliosis (AIS) treated with Cotrel-Dubousset instrumentation, one-third developed postoperative radiographic junctional kyphosis.

The definition of distal junctional kyphosis (DJK) as the development of kyphotic angulation $\geq 10°$ at the distal segment of a fusion construct was first introduced by Lowe and colleagues[2] in 2006 in their retrospective series of 375 patients with AIS. They reported the postoperative incidence of DJK in this population to be 7.1% for those undergoing anterior fusion and 14.6% in those undergoing posterior fusion.[2]

While DJK is a radiographic definition, distal junctional failure (DJF) is understood to be clinical or radiographic signs of failure at the caudal end of the construct for a variety of reasons (Fig. 1). These include but are not limited to symptomatic DJK, construct failure including rod fracture and/or screw plowing/pull out, pseudarthrosis, fracture, and adjacent segment disease.

Unlike the proximal junction, pathology at the distal junction has been less studied overall. Perhaps due to its lower incidence. It remains an unsolved problem in multiple surgical settings such as AIS, Scheuermann's Kyphosis, and adult spinal deformity (ASD) surgery.

NATURE OF THE PROBLEM/DIAGNOSIS
Diagnosis

Distal junctional pathology (DJP) is typically diagnosed by radiographic imaging postoperatively with or without patient symptoms. Patients may be asymptomatic with only a radiographic diagnosis of DJK. Others may report more acute

a Department of Orthopedics, Columbia University Medical Center, 622 West 168th Street, PH 11- Center, New York, NY 10032, USA; b The Daniel and Jane Och Spine Hospital at New York-Presbyterian/Allen, 5141 Broadway, New York, NY 10034, USA; c The Daniel and Jane Och Spine Hospital at New York-Presbyterian/ Allen, Och Spine/Allen NYP Hospital, 5141 Broadway, New York, NY 10034, USA
* Corresponding author.
E-mail address: gfm2113@cumc.columbia.edu

Neurosurg Clin N Am 34 (2023) 585–597
https://doi.org/10.1016/j.nec.2023.06.006

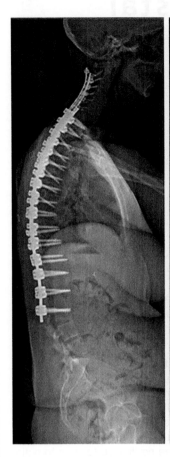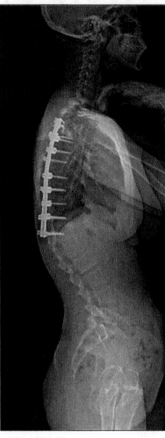

Fig. 1. The radiograph on the left illustrates radiographic DJK. The radiograph on the right demonstrates DJF in a short thoracic fusion with screw pullout at the LIV.

events and report a sound or sensation related to construct failure such as rod fracture or screw failure. It may present more insidiously with continued pain postoperatively and observed pseudarthrosis, or adjacent segment disease diagnosed on advanced imaging.

The obvious goal is to eliminate or decrease DJP as a reduction in postoperative complications of spine surgery is beneficial for outcomes. While DJK can be observed radiographically without deterioration of clinical outcomes it could be considered a first step toward a pathway leading toward DJF which can be clinically problematic.

The burden of disease for DJP can be variable depending on the clinical setting. In ASD, DJF has been reported with an incidence between 1.8% and 15.6%.[3] DJP has been reported as high as 15%, 50%, and 24% in AIS,[2] Scheuermann's Kyphosis,[4] and cervical spine surgery[5] respectively with modern instrumentation.

While the problem has been long identified, it remains unsolved. However, risk factors have been elucidated in the literature that fall into one of two categories, technical and patient specific.

Technical risk factors that have been addressed include the selection of the lowest instrumented vertebra and methods of fixation at the distal end of the construct. With the discovery of technical risk factors, DJP avoidant strategies have been developed although are still not entirely agreed upon by the surgical community. Patient-specific risk factors described broadly fall under preoperative radiographic alignment parameters, anatomy, and other medical conditions.

Current evidence

The lowest instrumented vertebra Much of the literature investigating DJP has been focused on the lowest instrumented vertebra (LIV) because of surgeons' desire to obtain the most rigid, stable construct and limit the risk of distal failure while maintaining as much flexibility in the spine as possible.

Adult spinal deformity Many ASD patients with posterior fusions require fusion to the sacrum or ilium in the index procedure due to apriori distal lumbar degeneration which will ultimately serve to protect the construct against DJP. Yasuda and colleagues found that lumbosacral failure decreased when using iliac screws in a study of 25 patients.[6] The authors advocated for spinopelvic fixation using an iliac screw as the lower fusion level in contrast to L5 or S1 due to a 76% incidence of complications in the cohort fused to L5 or S1 versus a 12.0% rate in the iliac fusion group. In a recent meta-analysis by Cavagnaro and colleagues, it was similarly reported that pelvic fixation had a protective effect against junctional failure as measured by pseudarthrosis at the lumbosacral junction.[7] The enhanced stiffness and strength of the construct with pelvic fixation was likely the reason behind this clinical finding and is supported by biomechanical reports that iliac fixation produces higher load to failure than only sacral fixation regardless of configuration.[8]

Similar recommendations for pelvic fixation were made by Ushio and colleagues based on patient-specific pre-operative radiographic parameters. Ushio and colleagues reported a cohort of 52 patients undergoing fusion to L5 with LIV failure in 20 patients and revision surgery in 6 patients. The authors noted a significantly higher pelvic incidence (PI) in the failure group.[9] Consequently, sacropelvic fixation should be considered in patients with a high preoperative PI and long fusion stopping at L5 should be avoided in this patient group.[10]

In addition to level selection for primary constructs, when using accessory rods the LIV should be carefully considered. Lee and colleagues found that when utilizing sacro-pelvic fixation the level of the accessory rods at S2/ilium was protective in a study of 253 ASD patients. The authors reported that pelvic fixation failure was significantly reduced when the accessory rod LIV was S2/ilium versus S1.[11]

While many surgeons advocate for index fusion to the pelvis there are select patients that can have the fusion short of the pelvis where the correct level is widely debated. In particular, it has yet to be determined if patients with a healthy L5-S1 segment should have fusion stopped at L5 or extend to the sacrum. Results reported have been equivocal and each level has been shown to come with its own corresponding complications such as higher pseudarthrosis rate in fusions ending in the sacrum and increased adjacent segment disease and loss of sagittal balance in fusions stopping at L5.[12,13]

While fusion to the sacrum/pelvis seems a reliable standard for long constructs it should be noted when selecting to fuse into the sacrum or ilium there is an increased risk for proximal junctional kyphosis.[10] Additionally exposing the sacrum adds to the length and morbidity of surgery and has a higher pseudarthrosis rate. Fusing L5-S1 may also alter the mechanics of patient gait. As such, the decision to fuse to the sacrum must be balanced by the deformity correction required, length of the fusion, status of the L5-S1 disc space, and risk of pseudarthrosis and revision surgery.

Scheuermann's kyphosis In the setting of thoracic hyperkyphosis or Scheuermann kyphosis, historically it had been advocated all patients should have constructs from T3-L2[14] or that the distal level should include the end vertebra and first lordotic disc (FLD).[15,16] However, FLD selection can be challenging as the true FLD can be difficult to determine as patients often have compensatory hyperlordosis below the hyperkyphotic segment leading to inappropriately short fusions. Due to this challenge and the continued rate of DJK, the stable sagittal vertebra (SSV) concept was proposed to select the LIV (**Fig. 2**). The SSV is defined as the most proximal vertebra touched by a vertical line from the posterior superior corner of the sacrum on lateral imaging. Cho and colleagues reported a significant decrease in DJK (4% vs 71%) when fusion extended to a more distal SSV than the first lordotic vertebra (FLV).[17] In another direct comparison of FLV to SSV methodology using all posterior all pedicle screw instrumentation, Kim and colleagues found a lower rate of revision surgery explicitly for DJK (5.0% vs 36.3%) when the SSV was selected.[18] Luzzi and colleagues further investigated appropriate LIV selection/fusion and found fusion to the second vertebrae below the first lordotic disc decreased the development of DJK.[19]

While evidence supports fusion to or beyond the SSV, other authors suggest longer fusion than the FLV is unnecessary because they found similar rates of DJK and revision surgery in patients fused to the SSV and FLV. Xu and colleagues stratified Scheuermann's Kyphosis into different curve patterns based on the kyphotic apex, as thoracic kyphosis versus thoracolumbar kyphosis and found that shorter fusions stopping at the FLV, which coincided with the vertebra above SSV, achieved comparable outcomes to SSV fusion and did not increase DJK incidence in either curve patterns.[20] Authors contend fusing to the FLV preserves levels and aids in avoiding adjacent segment degenerative disc disease in the lumbar spine, which may be caused by posterior fusions to L4 and L5 (**Fig. 3**).[21] However, this adjacent segment degeneration in the lumbar spine may not be clinically relevant as suggested by MRI and patient-reported outcomes.[22]

Adolescent idiopathic scoliosis Optimal level selection is essential in AIS to prevent

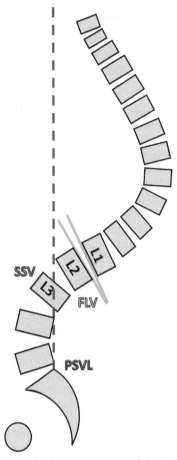

Fig. 2. Graphical representation of the lateral spine in Scheuermann's kyphosis. The posterior sacral vertical line (PSVL) is represented by the dashed red line. The most proximal vertebra touched by the PSVL is the SSV. The FLD is represented by the green lines and is the distal first lordotic disc space. The FLV is the first vertebra immediately caudal to the FLD. In this example, L2 is the FLV and L3 is the SSV.

decompensation and avoid the adding-on phenomenon and DJK. Similar to other deformity etiologies, preventing complications by utilizing longer fusions have to be weighed against the loss of mobile segments.[23,24] Various methods have been proposed for level selection in AIS with a historical focus on the coronal plane and the prevention of the adding on. Goldstein described fusing 1 to 3 levels below the primary curve in 1964.[25] Harrington introduced the concept of the stable zone to select the LIV[26] which was further expounded on by King and colleagues into the concept of the stable vertebra, the vertebra most bisected by the central stable vertical line.[27] Suk and colleagues[28] demonstrated the relationship between the end vertebra and the neutral vertebra in main thoracic curves, showing satisfactory outcomes with fusion

to the neutral vertebra when the preoperative neutral vertebra was the same level as or one level distal to the end vertebra. When the neutral vertebra was two or more levels distal to the end vertebra, fusion to one level shorter than the neutral vertebra resulted in satisfactory outcomes.[28] The last touched vertebra (LTV), initially promoted by Lenke and colleagues, defined as the most cephalad thoracolumbar/lumbar vertebra "touched" by the CSVL has been proposed as the LIV with good outcomes from multiple authors.[29,30] Cho and colleagues[31] introduced the concept of the last substantially touched vertebra, defined as the most cephalad lumbar vertebra in which the CSVL intersects the pedicle or is medial to it. Multiple authors have demonstrated a higher risk of adding on when the LTV is selected as the LIV versus the LSTV.[32,33]

Fischer and colleagues[34] synthesized the concepts of the stable vertebra, neutral vertebra, and LTV in a large retrospective study of 544 patients with thoracic AIS and found higher rates of adding on or DJK in patients with LIV proximal to the LTV and three or more vertebra proximal to the neutral vertebra as well as in those with open triradiate cartilage. In order to prevent adding on or DJK they recommended the selection of an LIV that is touched by the CSVL and within 2 vertebra proximal to the neutral vertebra in patients following closure of the triradiate cartilage.[34]

More recent literature has begun to focus on the sagittal plane in level selection in AIS, especially as awareness has grown for its implications in the development of DJK. As previously discussed, Lowe and colleagues[2] found that in their series of 375 patients with AIS, DJK was twice as common (14.6% compared to 7.1%) in patients undergoing posterior fusion as opposed to anterior fusion. Development of DJK in the posterior group was associated with a lowest instrumented vertebra (LIV) at the end vertebra rather than 1 or 2 levels beyond. They also demonstrated that failure to restore or maintain normal sagittal alignment in the thoracic and thoracolumbar region were risk factors for the development of DJK. They hypothesized that this was less of a problem in the anterior group through the use of interbody structural support.

Yang and colleagues[35] first applied the concept of the SSV to AIS in 2018 to identify the effectiveness of using the SSV for selecting the LIV to prevent DJK in selective thoracic fusions. In their series of 113 patients, 17% of those with an LIV above the SSV developed DJK whereas 0% of those with an LIV at or distal to the SSV developed DJK. Segal and colleagues[36] demonstrated that at 5 years postoperatively, 15.6% of patients with LIV

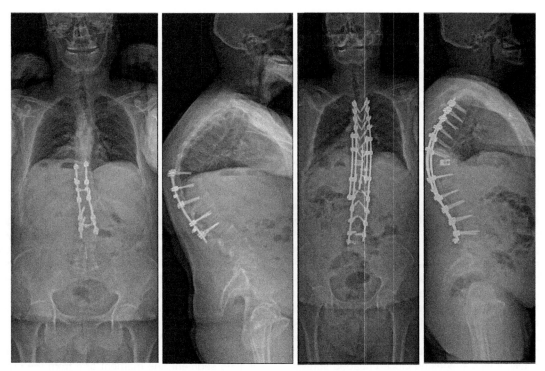

Fig. 3. Example Scheuermann's kyphosis pre- and post-operatively. The patient underwent the removal of hardware from T9-L2 followed by PSF T3-L4. Anterior fusion was performed at T8-T11. Posterior column osteotomies were performed at T6-T8 and L2-L3. Additional VCR performed at T9-T10.

above the SSV developed DJK versus 2.2% in those with fusions below the LIV. In a large retrospective study of 856 patients, Marciano and colleagues[37] found that 13.3% of patients had an LTV and an SSV that were not at the same level. Of these patients with a discordant LTV and SSV, 7.7% of those with fusions including the SSV developed DJK whereas 45.5% of patients with fusions short of the SSV developed DJK. Patients with shorter fusions demonstrated improvements in pain scores measured by SRS-22, but only when they did not develop DJK.[37] Segal and colleagues[38] expanded on these findings with a multicenter study demonstrating that 18.5% of patients with an SSV below the LTV who were fused to the LTV developed DJK while no patients with an SSV above the LTV developed DJK, regardless of fusion to the LTV, SSV, or between. Notably, they found that 95% of DJK occurred in patients with fusions ending at T11, T12, and more rarely L1.[38] In their study, preoperative thoracolumbar hyperkyphosis was identified as a risk factor for the development of DJK, as was a postoperative distal junctional angle greater than 5°, with the latter resulting in a greater than 16 times risk of DJK.[38]

Methods of fixation in the distal segment After LIV selection, optimal methods of fixation should be considered.

There can be a great deal of variety in pelvic fixation constructs including screw size, number of screws, number of rods, and level of fixation which was previously discussed. A standardized approach that limits distal junctional pathology has yet to be devised. However, the literature does have some significant recommendations. Lee and colleagues suggest that the number of rods crossing the lumbopelvic junction likely increase construct stiffness without creating a stress riser at the junction and found that higher number of rods and an accessory rod to LIV of S2 or ilium was protective against pelvic fixation failure.[11]

Interbody fusion in the junctional segment can also be utilized to provide greater lordotic correction while simultaneously enhancing the stiffness of the construct allowing the segment to withstand mechanical stresses after fusion and providing indirect neural decompression. While the use of interbody devices has proliferated in deformity surgery as means of correction the evidence remains equivocal. In a meta-analysis, Cavagnaro and colleagues conclude that the widely adopted use of interbody fusion at L5/S1 in long fusion is unsupported in a review of 12 retrospective studies containing 1216 patients. The primary outcome defined as pseudarthrosis rate was reported as having no difference between those receiving and not receiving interbody fusion.[7] Similarly, McDonnell et al reviewed risk factors for DJF in ASD and found no difference in the rate of DJF in those receiving interbody fusion and those not concluding it is not a risk factor for DJF, however, there was heterogeneity of levels and technique included in analysis.[3] More high-quality investigations are necessary to understand the effect of interbody fusion on DJF. The authors of this article regularly use interbody devices and support their use in the lumbar spine for deformity correction and indirect neural decompression.

When index surgery requires fixation to the pelvis there are a variety of factors that can be addressed to avoid pelvic fixation failure. Historical pelvic fixation failure rates have been reported as high as 36%.[39] Recently Lee and colleagues published 2 year results of pelvic fixation in 253 patients with a failure rate of only 4.3%. The authors investigated protective strategies against pelvic fixation failure and found significant support for multiple rods across the lumbosacral junction and accessory rod LIV to ilium/S2 (**Fig. 4**). Additionally, it was suggested closed headed screws, larger diameter pelvic screws, longer length pelvic screws, and cobalt chrome rods may be protective when evaluating the much lower fixation rate

against historical outcomes.[11] In prior investigations, Guler and colleagues found higher rates of failure in S2AI fixation versus iliac fixation, however, it should be noted the authors used titanium rods and open head pelvic screws which may account for the screw disengagement and rod breakages that were seen in the study.[39]

ANATOMY

While numerous risk factors have been identified for DJK, it is biomechanically the breakdown of the transition point from the rigid fused segment to the unfused mobile spine. This transition point becomes an axis of rotation on which flexing deforming forces can ultimately exceed the ability of the instrumentation-bone interface or adjacent disc to resist. When the spine is well-balanced and an appropriate fusion level is chosen, the distance from the LIV (the axis of rotation) to the force applied by the weight of the fused body segment is small (**Fig. 5**). Therefore, there is a small amount of torque across the LIV and a decreased risk of DJK. When the spine is fused to a more proximal kyphotic segment, the moment arm from the LIV to the force applied by the weight of the body segment is increased, leading to increased torque across the LIV and a higher risk of DJK. This may

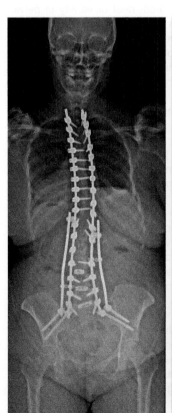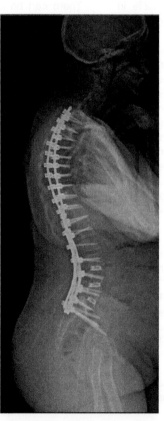

Fig. 4. The author's preferred fixation is shown when fusing to the sacrum.

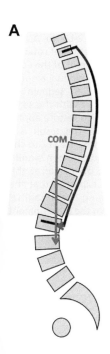

A

COM

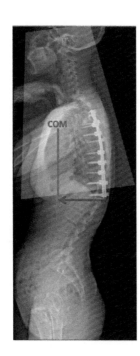

B

COM

Fig. 5. A shows a balanced spine with a fusion construct from T2-L2 and B shows a fusion construct from T4-T12 with radiographic DJK. The gray trapezoid represents the body mass above the LIV. "COM" represents the center of mass of the body above the LIV, with the blue arrow representing the force vector of the center of mass. The red arrow represents the lever arm of the LIV. In A, the moment arm from the center of rotation of the LIV to the force vector of the COM is small, resulting in a small amount of torque across the L2-L3 segment. In B, there is a much larger moment arm from the center of rotation of the LIV, resulting in a large amount of torque across the T12-L1 segment. This torque ultimately caused rotation around the LIV resulting in DJK.

explain why increased rates of DJK are seen when an LIV is chosen that is proximal to the SSV in AIS and Scheurmann's Kyphosis.[17,19,35–37,40]

It has also been shown that longer fusion constructs, especially those with an LIV at L5 or S1 without pelvic fixation increase the risk for developing DJK.[3,41,42] It is well known that long fusions in ASD to L5 significantly increase the risk of L5-S1 degeneration.[43] The increased weight of the body segments above the LIV as well as fewer mobile segments to compensate for changes in posture contribute to increased junctional stress. This is especially true with sagittal malalignment. When sagittal malalignment is not restored in a long fusion resulting in positive sagittal imbalance, a larger moment arm results in significantly more force transmitted through the LIV from the entire weight of the rigid fusion segments above **(Fig. 6)**. The resulting junctional stress results in subsequent disc degeneration, further exacerbation of positive sagittal imbalance, and the ultimate development of DJK.[43,44]

Patient-specific factors such as anatomic variation in the L5 vertebra are also speculated to play a role in the development of DJK. Edwards and colleagues[44] examined a series of patients with ASD fused to L5 and found that the depth of L5 within the pelvis was a significant risk factor for loss of L5 fixation, where an L5 depth of 12 mm or more led to an implant failure rate of 55%. The authors hypothesized that a deep-seated L5 provided stability to the L5-S1 motion segment with fusions ending at L5, thus concentrating stress at the L5 bone-implant interface.[44]

PREOPERATIVE/PRE-PROCEDURE PLANNING

A surgical plan should be defined prior to entrance in the operating room to facilitate efficiency and safety. Obviously, this plan must account for the unique characteristics of each patient including etiology of deformity and goals of correction.

With regard to distal junctional pathology the major preoperative/planning steps involve deciding the distal level of fusion and the method of fixation. As previously described, there is literature to help make these decisions. In certain cases, classification systems have been developed to help guide the decision, such as the Lenke Classification for Adolescent Idiopathic Scoliosis.[45,46] In other areas such as ASD, as many patients are fused to the sacrum the decision is more focused on the method of fixation. In isolated thoracic hyperkyphosis, the literature is less consistent on level selection; however, the authors' preference is to fuse to at least the SSV.

A few consistent rules for the distal LIV selection can be applied regardless of the etiology and surrounding patient characteristics:

- It is necessary to understand the deformity and magnitude of correction required
- The planned distal fusion level should not have substantial degeneration, instability, or kyphosis
- Preservation of the posterior ligament complex at the distal segment is necessary
- In the setting of a preoperative fusion mass, the fused area should be restored to normal

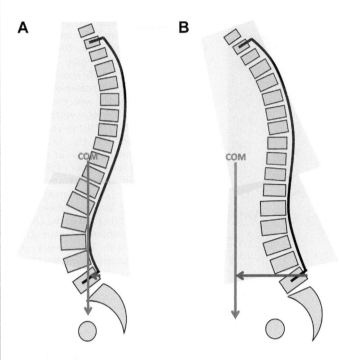

Fig. 6. A shows a balanced spine with a fusion construct from T2-L5. In A, the moment arm from the center of rotation of the LIV to the force vector of the COM is minute, resulting in a minimal amount of torque across the L5-S1 segment. B demonstrates a construct with the same levels as A with failure to restore appropriate lumbar lordosis. The result is a larger moment arm from the LIV to the COM force vector, indicating a significantly larger amount of torque at this level. Over time it is expected that the higher torque resulting from sagittal imbalance will result in the development of DJK with subsequent increases in torque across the LIV as the deformity worsens.

alignment if possible. This may be achieved with planned osteotomies.

PREP AND PATIENT POSITIONING

The authors preferred skin prep includes a 4% chlorhexidine gluconate mechanical scrub that is removed with a clean towel followed by a 70% alcohol solution that is allowed to dry on the skin followed finally by a chlorhexidine gluconate and isopropyl alcohol skin prep applicator prior to draping. After draping an additional chlorhexidine gluconate and isopropyl alcohol skin prep applicator is used again followed by an iodine impregnated adhesive over the entire surgical area. Standard patient positioning is demonstrated in the included images. Special attention is paid to padding all bony prominences. Regarding room set up, all surgical electronics are run to power sources at the foot of the patient. The surgical instrument table is set up behind the primary surgeon with the surgical technician and mayo stand on the same side at the foot of the patient. The first assistant is on the opposite side. If robotics or intraoperative imaging are to be used they are brought in from the first assistants' side.

PROCEDURAL APPROACH
Adult spinal deformity

- Long fusion should be extended to the sacrum or pelvis in the following cases:[47]
  - Poor bone quality
  - Spondylolisthesis or degenerative disease at L5-S1
  - Sagittal imbalance
  - Lumbar hypolordosis
  - Concomitant coronal plane deformity
  - High pelvic incidence[9]
  - Prior laminectomy at L5-S1[48]
  - Oblique take-off at L5-S1[48]
- When fusing to the sacrum or pelvis
  - Consider interbody structural support at L5-S1 and other lower lumbar levels on a case by case basis[7]
  - Consider accessory rods and if utilizing, S2/ilium is the preferred LIV[11]
  - Consider the use of multiple pelvic screws to enhance pelvic fixation[49]
  - Use wider diameter and length pelvic screws. At least 8.5-mm and 85-mm is suggested
  - Aim for minimal residual coronal malalignment to avoid pelvic fixation failure[11]
  - It is highly recommended that S1 pedicle screws be tricortical, especially in elderly patients, and should be directed medially in the sacral promontory for both greater insertional torque and safe application[48,50]
  - Preserve the posterior ligament complex of the distal junction segment if fusing short of the sacrum

Adolescent Idiopathic Scoliosis
- Consider utilizing the LTV rather than LSTV to preserve an additional motion segment in mature patients

- When there is discordance between the SSV and the LTV, fuse to the more distal segment to decrease risk of junctional pathology
- Consider determining LTV and SSV on supine radiographs to assess curve flexibility and spontaneous curve correction

Thoracic Hyperkyphosis/Scheuermann's Kyphosis

- Fusion to the SSV, FLV+1, or FLV+2 should be considered to maximize avoidance of clinically significant DJK/DJF[17–19]
- Patients with thoracic type Scheuermann's Kyphosis, consideration of fusion above the SSV to the FLV can be considered[20]
- Preserve the posterior ligament complex of the distal junction segment

RECOVERY AND REHABILITATION (INCLUDING POST-PROCEDURE CARE)

While much has been published on postoperative measures after spine surgery such as enhanced recovery protocols and surgical site infection avoidance, little to no literature has been published on recovery and rehab protocols to aid the avoidance of distal junctional pathology. As such no standardized protocol has been implemented; however, there are commonsense principles that can be applied to any patient undergoing spine surgery where DJK/DJF is a concern.

- Initiation of physical therapy to aid cuing the patient to adopt an erect sitting position and activation of extension muscles as soon as permitted
- Avoidance of passive flexion in the junctional segment
- Patient education on safe ergonomic practices such as avoiding lifting weights at a distance from the body, and knee flexion instead of back flexion when picking an item off the floor
- Consideration of walker use to decrease the flexion moment in patients with an unbalanced trunk
- Consideration of a brace to protect the distal junction from flexion for a limited time period post operatively[51]

MANAGEMENT

When distal junctional pathology occurs it may or may not need to be addressed depending on the etiology. Asymptomatic distal junctional kyphosis may not always need intervention, but it can be considered if it is thought to be the initial finding in a trend toward distal junctional failure. Other pathologic etiologies that are less equivocal which should be intervened upon include junctional failure from fracture or implant-related issues.

In general, distal junctional failure should be addressed on an individual basis, but the following principles can guide treatment:

1. Restore alignment
2. Decompress any stenotic areas
3. Improve mechanical support at the failed junction
4. Extend the construct distally (if able, as many long constructs end in the ilium during the index procedure)
5. Select a new distal sagittal stable level in patients initially fused short of the sacrum. Ensure the level is stable coronally and rotationally as well.

Improved mechanical support can be achieved by multiple methods. This can include adding additional rods in accessory, kick-stand, or delta rod configuration. Additionally, anterior interbody devices can be added to off load posterior constructs of the junction segment. Upsizing distal screws can also be considered.

OUTCOMES
Outcomes for distal junctional pathology avoidant strategies

Distal junctional pathology avoidant strategies often select for longer constructs and more significant fixation distally such as iliac fixation. The argument against such constructs is that it fuses a greater number of segments decreasing spine mobility and increases operative morbidity.

In ASD, outcomes reported on DJP avoidant strategies suggest patients need to be evaluated on a case-by-case basis as there are unique advantages and disadvantages of lumbar fusion versus sacro-iliac fusion with regard to complication avoidance.[3,52,53] Additionally, the evidence is not always consistent. In a meta-analysis of 12 studies assessing risk factors for DJF in ASD, it was found that fusion stopping at L5 compared to the sacrum was at increased risk of DJF (11.6% vs 3.7%).[3] A higher DJF rate would imply a higher revision rate. However, in another meta-analysis of 11 studies, no significant difference in overall complication rate and revision surgery rate was noted between fusing to the sacrum or L5.[52]

After deciding to fuse to the sacrum in ASD patient, outcomes are more clear that iliac fixation is most beneficial in avoiding distal junctional pathology with improved sagittal balance and no detriment to patient-reported outcomes.[11,54,55]

Outcomes reported on thoracic hyperkyphosis and AIS appear to be more consistent. Most reports agree that fusing to at least the SSV provide a significant advantage in reducing DJP.[17,18,40] In AIS, recent outcome literature focused on the sagittal plane suggests fusion to the SSV is most protective against DJP.[35-38]

Outcomes after distal junctional pathology revision surgery

Clinical and radiographic outcomes related to revision surgery for DJK are currently lacking in the literature. Further research is necessary to determine the optimal management of patients in whom DJK develops.

While emerging literature is identifying risk factors for DJK as well as strategies to avoid it, the outcomes of these strategies are a necessary area of further study. This is especially true as these strategies may demonstrate further consequences. For example, in long fusions in the setting of ASD, fusion to the sacrum vs L5 in patients without L5-S1 degeneration results in a higher reoperation rate, particularly for pseudarthrosis, and an increased rate of medical morbidities such as pulmonary embolism.[13] Therefore, the risk of subsequent DJK must be weighed against the risks of extending the fusion to the sacrum in this population. However, among these patients, patient-reported outcome scores are similar.[13] It has also been shown that the addition of iliac fixation to long fusions does not have a negative influence on patient-reported quality of life.[55] Further high-quality studies are required to analyze the effects of these and other DJK avoidant strategies on patient outcomes.

SUMMARY

Distal junctional pathology remains an unsolved problem in spine surgery. There is no definitive answer regardless of deformity etiology, however, there is a growing literature which suggest strategies to avoid it. When DJP is encountered, it can be on a spectrum from asymptomatic radiographic finding or marked distal construct failure necessitating early revision. Asymptomatic radiographic findings, however, may be the first step toward total failure. Utilizing the literature focused on avoiding distal junctional pathology along with basic principles of deformity correction will improve outcomes. Distal junctional pathology requiring revision surgery should focus on restoration of alignment and improved mechanical support at the level of pathology and distal extension as is usually required.

CLINICS CARE POINTS

- Avoiding Distal Junctional Pathology
  - In all scenarios, preserve the posterior ligament complex of the distal junction segment.
- Adult spinal deformity
  - Extend fusion to the sacrum in the setting of any lumbar pathology that may predispose to failure such as osteopenia or disc space degeneration
  - Consider accessory rods across the distal junction and if utilizing, S2/ilium is the preferred LIV[11]
  - When fusing into the sacrum, consider using sacro-iliac fixation to reduce the risk of distal junctional pathology
  - Cobalt rods, closed head screws, larger diameter screws, and longer screws for pelvic fixation may be protective against failure
- Adolescent Idiopathic Scoliosis
  - When there is discordance between the SSV and the LTV, fuse to the more distal segment to decrease the risk of distal junctional pathology
- Scheuermann's Kyphosis
  - Fusion to the SSV, FLV+1, or FLV+2 should be considered to maximize avoidance of clinically significant DJK/DJF[17-19]

DISCLOSURE

G.F. Marciano and M.E. Simhon have nothing to disclose. R.A. Lehman, MD has the following disclosures: Medtronic: 1) Consulting; 2) Royalties; Stryker: 1) Royalties; Pacira: 1) Consulting; Department of Defense: 1) Principal Investigator: Grants for Research Support; National Institutes of Health: 1) Co-Investigator: Grants for Research Support. L.G. Lenke, MD has the following disclosures: 1. Broadwater- 1) Reimbursement For Airfare/Hotel; 2. Medtronic- 1) Paid Consultant - Monies Donated To A Charitable Foundation; 2) Royalties; 3. Scoliosis Research Society- 1) Reimbursement For Airfare/Hotel; 2) Grant Support - Monies To Institution; 4. Setting Scoliosis Straight Foundation- 1) Grant Support - Monies To Institution; 5. Evans Family Donation-1) Philanthropic Research Funding From Grateful Patient/Family; 6. Fox Family Foundation-1) Philanthropic Research Funding From Grateful Patient; 7.

AOSpine-1) Reimbursement For Airfare/Hotel; 2) Grant Support - Monies To Institution; 3) Fellowship Support To Institution; 8. Acuity Surgical- 1) Paid Consultant- Monies Donated To Charitable Foundation; 2. Royalties; 9. Abryx −1) Paid Consultant- Monies Donated To Charitable Foundation; 10. EOS Technology - 1) Grant Support - Monies To Institution.

REFERENCES

1. Richards BS, Birch JG, Herring JA, et al. Frontal Plane and Sagittal Plane Balance following Cotrel-Dubousset Instrumentation for Idiopathic Scoliosis. Spine 1989;14(7):733.

2. Lowe TG, Lenke L, Betz R, et al. Distal Junctional Kyphosis of Adolescent Idiopathic Thoracic Curves Following Anterior or Posterior Instrumented Fusion: Incidence, Risk Factors, and Prevention. Spine 2006;31(3):299.

3. McDonnell JM, Ahern DP, Wagner SC, et al. A Systematic Review of Risk Factors Associated With Distal Junctional Failure in Adult Spinal Deformity Surgery. Clin Spine Surg 2021;34(9):347.

4. Lundine K, Turner P, Johnson M. Thoracic hyperkyphosis: assessment of the distal fusion level. Glob Spine J 2012;2(2):65–70.

5. Passias PG, Vasquez-Montes D, Poorman GW, et al. Predictive model for distal junctional kyphosis after cervical deformity surgery. Spine J 2018;18(12):2187–94.

6. Yasuda T, Hasegawa T, Yamato Y, et al. Lumbosacral Junctional Failures After Long Spinal Fusion for Adult Spinal Deformity-Which Vertebra Is the Preferred Distal Instrumented Vertebra? Spine Deform 2016;4(5):378–84.

7. Cavagnaro MJ, Orenday-Barraza JM, Khan N, et al. Is L5/S1 interbody fusion necessary in long-segment surgery for adult degenerative scoliosis? A systematic review and meta-analysis. J Neurosurg Spine 2021;36(6):997–1004.

8. Tis JE, Helgeson M, Lehman RA, et al. A Biomechanical Comparison of Different Types of Lumbopelvic Fixation. Spine 2009;34(24):E866.

9. Ushio S, Yoshii T, Otani K, et al. Pelvic incidence is a risk factor for lower instrumented vertebra failure in adult spinal deformity patients who underwent corrective fusion terminating at the L5 vertebra. J Orthop Sci 2021. https://doi.org/10.1016/j.jos.2021.11.008. S0949-2658(21)00373-0.

10. Yao YC, Kim HJ, Bannwarth M, et al. Lowest Instrumented Vertebra Selection to S1 or Ilium Versus L4 or L5 in Adult Spinal Deformity: Factors for Consideration in 349 Patients With a Mean 46-Month Follow-Up. Glob Spine J 2021. https://doi.org/10.1177/21925682211009178. 21925682211009176.

11. Lee NJ, Marciano G, Puvanesarajah V, et al. Incidence, mechanism, and protective strategies for 2-year pelvic fixation failure after adult spinal deformity surgery with a minimum six-level fusion. J Neurosurg Spine 2022;1(aop):1–9.

12. Cho KJ, Suk SI, Park SR, et al. Arthrodesis to L5 versus S1 in long instrumentation and fusion for degenerative lumbar scoliosis. Eur Spine J 2009;18(4):531–7.

13. Edwards CCI, Bridwell KH, Patel A, et al. Long Adult Deformity Fusions to L5 and the Sacrum A Matched Cohort Analysis. Spine 2004;29(18):1996.

14. Wenger DR, Frick SL. Scheuermann Kyphosis. Spine 1999;24(24):2630.

15. Tg L, Md K. An analysis of sagittal curves and balance after Cotrel-Dubousset instrumentation for kyphosis secondary to Scheuermann's disease. A review of 32 patients. Spine 1994;19(15). https://doi.org/10.1097/00007632-199408000-00005.

16. Otsuka NY, Hall JE, Mah JY. Posterior fusion for Scheuermann's kyphosis. Clin Orthop 1990;(251):134–9.

17. Cho KJ, Lenke LG, Bridwell KH, et al. Selection of the Optimal Distal Fusion Level in Posterior Instrumentation and Fusion for Thoracic Hyperkyphosis: The Sagittal Stable Vertebra Concept. Spine 2009;34(8):765.

18. Kim HJ, Nemani V, Boachie-Adjei O, et al. Distal Fusion Level Selection in Scheuermann's Kyphosis: A Comparison of Lordotic Disc Segment Versus the Sagittal Stable Vertebrae. Glob Spine J 2017;7(3):254–9.

19. Luzzi A, Sardar Z, Cerpa M, et al. Risk of distal junctional kyphosis in scheuermann's kyphosis is decreased by selecting the LIV as two vertebrae distal to the first lordotic disc. Spine Deform 2022;10(6):1437–42.

20. Xu Y, Hu Z, Zhang L, et al. Selection of the optimal distal fusion level for Scheuermann kyphosis with different curve patterns: when can we stop above the sagittal stable vertebra? Eur Spine J 2022;31(7):1710–8.

21. Harding IJ, Charosky S, Vialle R, et al. Lumbar disc degeneration below a long arthrodesis (performed for scoliosis in adults) to L4 or L5. Eur Spine J 2008;17(2):250–4.

22. Green DW, Lawhorne TWI, Widmann RF, et al. Long-Term Magnetic Resonance Imaging Follow-up Demonstrates Minimal Transitional Level Lumbar Disc Degeneration After Posterior Spine Fusion for Adolescent Idiopathic Scoliosis. Spine 2011;36(23):1948.

23. Wilk B, Karol LA, Johnston CE, et al. The effect of scoliosis fusion on spinal motion: a comparison of fused and nonfused patients with idiopathic scoliosis. Spine 2006;31(3):309–14.

24. Takahashi J, Newton PO, Ugrinow VL, et al. Selective thoracic fusion in adolescent idiopathic scoliosis: factors influencing the selection of the optimal

lowest instrumented vertebra. Spine 2011;36(14): 1131–41.

25. Goldstein LA. The surgical management of scoliosis. Clin Orthop 1964;35:95–115.

26. Harrington PR. Treatment of scoliosis. Correction and internal fixation by spine instrumentation. J Bone Joint Surg Am 1962;44-A:591–610.

27. King HA, Moe JH, Bradford DS, et al. The selection of fusion levels in thoracic idiopathic scoliosis. J Bone Joint Surg Am 1983;65(9):1302–13.

28. Suk SI, Lee SM, Chung ER, et al. Determination of distal fusion level with segmental pedicle screw fixation in single thoracic idiopathic scoliosis. Spine 2003;28(5):484–91.

29. Matsumoto M, Watanabe K, Hosogane N, et al. Postoperative distal adding-on and related factors in Lenke type 1A curve. Spine 2013;38(9): 737–44.

30. Lenke L, Newton P, Lehman R, et al. Adolescent Scoliosis 1A001: Radiographic Results of Selecting the Touched Vertebra as the Lowest Instrumented Vertebra in Lenke Type 1 (Main Thoracic) & Type 2 (Double Thoracic) Curves at a Minimum 5-year Follow-up. Glob Spine J 2017;7(2 Suppl):2S–189S.

31. Cho RH, Yaszay B, Bartley CE, et al. Which Lenke 1A Curves Are at the Greatest Risk for Adding-On... and Why? Spine 2012;37(16):1384.

32. Murphy JS, Upasani VV, Yaszay B, et al. Predictors of Distal Adding-on in Thoracic Major Curves With AR Lumbar Modifiers. Spine 2017;42(4):E211–8.

33. Qin X, Sun W, Xu L, et al. Effectiveness of Selective Thoracic Fusion in the Surgical Treatment of Syringomyelia-associated Scoliosis: A Case-control Study With Long-term Follow-up. Spine 2016; 41(14):E887–92.

34. Fischer CR, Lenke LG, Bridwell KH, et al. Optimal Lowest Instrumented Vertebra for Thoracic Adolescent Idiopathic Scoliosis. Spine Deform 2018;6(3): 250–6.

35. Yang J, Andras LM, Broom AM, et al. Preventing Distal Junctional Kyphosis by Applying the Stable Sagittal Vertebra Concept to Selective Thoracic Fusion in Adolescent Idiopathic Scoliosis. Spine Deform 2018;6(1):38–42.

36. Segal DN, Orland KJ, Yoon E, et al, Harms Study Group. Fusions ending above the sagittal stable vertebrae in adolescent idiopathic scoliosis: does it matter? Spine Deform 2020;8(5):983–9.

37. Marciano G, Ball J, Matsumoto H, et al. Including the stable sagittal vertebra in the fusion for adolescent idiopathic scoliosis reduces the risk of distal junctional kyphosis in Lenke 1-3 B and C curves. Spine Deform 2021;9(3):733–41.

38. Segal DN, Ball J, Fletcher ND, et al. Risk factors for the development of DJK in AIS patients undergoing posterior spinal instrumentation and fusion. Spine Deform 2022;10(2):377–85.

39. Guler UO, Cetin E, Yaman O, et al. Sacropelvic fixation in adult spinal deformity (ASD); a very high rate of mechanical failure. Eur Spine J 2015;24(5):1085–91.

40. Gong Y, Yuan L, He M, et al. Comparison Between Stable Sagittal Vertebra and First Lordotic Vertebra Instrumentation for Prevention of Distal Junctional Kyphosis in Scheuermann Disease: Systematic Review and Meta-analysis. Clin Spine Surg 2019; 32(8):330.

41. Passias PG, Naessig S, Kummer N, et al. Predicting development of severe clinically relevant distal junctional kyphosis following adult cervical deformity surgery, with further distinction from mild asymptomatic episodes. J Neurosurg Spine 2021; 36(6):960–7.

42. Bouloussa H, Ghailane S. P101. Distal junctional failure: a feared complication of adult spinal deformity surgery. Spine J 2020;20(9, Supplement):S194–5.

43. Kuhns CA, Bridwell KH, Lenke LG, et al. Thoracolumbar Deformity Arthrodesis Stopping at L5: Fate of the L5-S1 Disc, Minimum 5-Year Follow-up. Spine 2007;32(24):2771.

44. Edwards CCI, Bridwell KH, Patel A, et al. Thoracolumbar Deformity Arthrodesis to L5 in Adults: The Fate of the L5-S1 Disc. Spine 2003;28(18):2122.

45. Lenke LG, Betz RR, Harms J, et al. Adolescent Idiopathic Scoliosis : A New Classification to Determine Extent of Spinal Arthrodesis. JBJS 2001;83(8): 1169.

46. Lenke LG. The Lenke Classification System of Operative Adolescent Idiopathic Scoliosis. Neurosurg Clin N Am 2007;18(2):199–206.

47. Bridwell KH. Selection of instrumentation and fusion levels for scoliosis: where to start and where to stop: Invited submission from the Joint Section Meeting on Disorders of the Spine and Peripheral Nerves, March 2004. J Neurosurg Spine 2004;1(1):1–8.

48. Bridwell KH, Edwards CCI, Lenke LG. The Pros and Cons to Saving the L5–S1 Motion Segment in a Long Scoliosis Fusion Construct. Spine 2003;28(20S): S234.

49. Park PJ, Lin JD, Makhni MC, et al. Dual S2 Alar-Iliac Screw Technique With a Multirod Construct Across the Lumbosacral Junction: Obtaining Adequate Stability at the Lumbosacral Junction in Spinal Deformity Surgery. Neurospine 2020;17(2):466–70.

50. Lehman RAJ, Kuklo TR, Belmont PJJ, et al. Advantage of Pedicle Screw Fixation Directed Into the Apex of the Sacral Promontory Over Bicortical Fixation: A Biomechanical Analysis. Spine 2002;27(8):806.

51. Berjano P, Damilano M, Pejrona M, et al. Revision surgery in distal junctional kyphosis. Eur Spine J 2020;29(1):86–102.

52. Jia F, Wang G, Liu X, et al. Comparison of long fusion terminating at L5 versus the sacrum in treating adult spinal deformity: a meta-analysis. Eur Spine J 2020; 29(1):24–35.

53. Taneichi H, Inami S, Moridaira H, et al. Can we stop the long fusion at L5 for selected adult spinal deformity patients with less severe disability and less complex deformity? Clin Neurol Neurosurg 2020;194:105917.

54. Tsuchiya K, Bridwell KH, Kuklo TR, et al. Minimum 5-Year Analysis of L5–S1 Fusion Using Sacropelvic Fixation (Bilateral S1 and Iliac Screws) for Spinal Deformity. Spine 2006;31(3):303.

55. Martín-Buitrago MP, Pizones J, Sánchez Pérez-Grueso FJ, et al. Impact of Iliac Instrumentation on the Quality of Life of Patients With Adult Spine Deformity. Spine 2018;43(13):913–8.

Section III: MIS Approaches for Deformity

Algorithmic Patient Selection for Minimally Invasive Versus Open Lumbar Interbody Fusion Surgery

Jacob L. Goldberg, MD, Ibrahim Hussain, MD, Kai-Ming Fu, MD, PhD,
Michael S. Virk, MD, PhD*

KEYWORDS

- Minimally invasive spine surgery • Spine deformity • Selection algorithm

KEY POINTS

- MISDEF2 algorithm guides approach selection for adult spinal deformity.
- Minimally invasive interbody selection algorithm (MIISA) guides technique selection.
- Data driven algorithms help guide patient selection for minimally invasive lumbar interbody fusion

INTRODUCTION

Symptomatic adult spinal deformity (ASD) encompasses a range of spinal alignment disorders that can significantly influence quality of life, with both sagittal and coronal plane deformities recognized as determinants of health status.[1] In extreme cases, the health impact of cervical or thoracolumbar spinal deformity is on par with chronic diseases and disabilities such as low-vision/blindness, emphysema, renal failure, and stroke.[2,3] ASD results from degeneration of structural support elements of the spinal column but can also develop from untreated pediatric or adolescent idiopathic scoliosis, trauma, infection, neoplasm, or earlier spine surgery. ASD can become symptomatic when (1) muscle pain and fatigue result from increased biomechanical work required to maintain upright posture in the setting of spinal malalignment, (2) nociceptive pain resulting from spondylotic disc or zygohypophyseal joint disease accumulates, or (3) when compression of neural elements leads to radicular pain and/or myelopathy. Symptoms also develop from compensatory maneuvers and increased spino-pelvic rigidity negatively affecting activities of daily living.[4] ASD is found at a prevalence of up to 32% in the general adult population and up to 68% among the elderly.[5] The elderly population meeting surgical criteria based on symptomatic burden is expected to increase in direct proportion to the aging population structure, which must be considered from a health-care policy and demographic standpoint.[6] Additionally, the elderly are increasingly healthier at older ages, have increased life expectancy,[7] and are acceptable candidates for surgical treatment across multiple specialties at higher rates due to these factors.[8]

In appropriately selected patients, traditional open operative treatment of symptomatic ASD provides improvements in patient reported quality of life compared with conservative (nonoperative) treatment.[9] However, not all patients are candidates for open surgical correction. Earlier studies evaluating open techniques demonstrate significant morbidity due to extensive muscle dissection, blood loss, infection risk, and postoperative narcotic requirement, with many patients requiring discharge to rehabilitation centers rather than home. Further, the most powerful alignment correction techniques are associated with high-complication rates. For example, minor and major complication rates after 3-column osteotomy have been reported to be as high as 78% and 61%,

Department of Nerosurgery, Weill Cornell Medical Center, New York Presbyterian Hospital, 525 E 68th Street, Box 99, New York, NY 10065, USA
* Corresponding author.
E-mail address: virkm1@gmail.com

Neurosurg Clin N Am 34 (2023) 599–607
https://doi.org/10.1016/j.nec.2023.06.007
1042-3680/23/© 2023 Elsevier Inc. All rights reserved.

respectively.[10] In addition, the cumulative revision rate during 4 years is 18%. Although technical advances in open deformity surgery have mitigated complication rates, it is commonly recognized that perioperative complications have been associated with worse outcomes.[11]

The techniques and technology that have enabled minimally invasive approaches in degenerative spine pathologic condition have been adapted to treat ASD. MIS approaches can offer several potential advantages and noninferior outcomes in appropriately selected patients.[12–14] The MIS approach in this context generally refers to interbody implants used to achieve alignment goal through anterior column reconstruction and facilitation of arthrodesis. Posterior percutaneous pedicle screw instrumentation is also a part of the MIS philosophy resulting in additional correction and stabilization. Variations of posterior MIS techniques may incorporate miniopen approaches for selective osteotomies or facet fusion. Advantages of such strategies include less intraoperative blood loss, decreased transfusion rates, decreased postoperative narcotic use, shorter length of hospital stay, faster rates of postoperative mobilization, and fewer patients discharged to inpatient rehab.[15–17] Additionally, patients presenting with increased preoperative risk stratification may be more suitable candidates for MIS approaches.

Several potential drawbacks are inherent in the MIS approach to spine deformity.[18–20] MIS techniques are evolving rapidly and associated with a significant initial learning curve. Until recently, many surgeons did not receive formal training in these approaches that require selective surgical corridors devoid of traditional anatomic landmarks resulting in orientation loss. Additionally, the smaller MIS corridors targeting the interbody disc space for primary correction may impose limits on the extent of correction given lack of osteotomies that require hybrid approaches. Although providing a more harmonious segmental correction, MIS techniques are limited in ankylosed segments or earlier fusion surgery. Furthermore, given less posterior element exposure, there is decreased surface area for arthrodesis, which can contribute to higher rates of pseudoarthrosis in some cases.[21] Cost is a further barrier as the fundamental instruments and technology require significant upfront investment, such as with intraoperative CT scanners, computer navigation systems, robotics, and sophisticated implants. Finally, optimal patient selection requires proper pairing of the patient-specific spinal alignment goals to the proper MIS technique, as well as recognizing when hybrid or traditional open techniques are optimal.[18–20]

Postoperative outcomes as determined by patient reported symptoms and radiographic parameters are contingent on achieving realistic surgical goals and this begins with appropriate patient selection. There is a lack of consensus among spine surgeons regarding optimal surgical approach and extent of treatment of ASD.[22] To standardize care, multicenter study groups have pooled resources to develop algorithms that provide guidance for determining whether MIS techniques may be able to achieve the desired surgical goals. Patient selection algorithms have evolved considerably during the past decade because intraoperative techniques and technologies have expanded the armamentarium of MIS surgeons and because the goals of deformity surgery have changed. The purpose of this article is to review the algorithms available to surgeons to help guide decision-making regarding MIS versus open surgical approaches for ASD.

Lenke-Silva Levels of Treatment Classification

The Lenke-Silva algorithm describes 6 increasingly invasive levels of treatment of adult degenerative scoliosis based on severity of patient reported symptoms, clinical history, and radiographic findings.[23] Nonoperative management is reserved for patients with radiographic findings including scoliotic curves less than 30° and less than 2 mm subluxation with anterior osteophytes, and a lack of significant clinical symptoms including stenotic, radicular, or back pain. Among operative candidates, the 6 distinct treatment options include the following: (1) decompression of neural elements, (2) decompression + posterior instrumented fusion limited to the levels decompressed, (3) decompression + posterior instrumented fusion of the entire lumbar curve, (4) decompression with both anterior and posterior instrumented fusion of the entire lumbar curve, (5) extension of level 4 treatment into the thoracic spine, and (6) targeted osteotomies.

MiSLAT

In 2013, Mummaneni and colleagues published an MIS adaptation of the Lenke-Silva treatment levels establishing the MiSLAT algorithm.[24] MiSLAT similarly incorporated both clinical symptoms and radiographic findings to establish 6 levels of increasing complexity. Because this algorithm considered the technical capabilities of MIS techniques at the time, it suggests the 2 most complex levels of deformity (5 and 6) are best treated with open surgical correction to extend fusions through the thoracic spine and when osteotomies are required.

The Minimally Invasive Spinal Deformity Surgery Algorithm

The minimally invasive spinal deformity surgery algorithm (MISDEF) algorithm is a further refinement of MiSLAT designed to increase intraobserver reliability by focusing the decision-making algorithm solely on radiographic findings.[25] MISDEF simplified decision-making by creating 3 radiographically based treatment classes. Patients with class I and II deformities could be treated with MIS surgery involving decompression ± limited fusion or decompression with longer segment fusion with or without interbody grafts. Class III deformities, involving a nonflexible curve or more severe deformity defined by PT greater than 25°, LL-PI mismatch greater than 30°, lateral listhesis greater than 6 mm, or thoracic kyphosis lesser than 60°, were best treated with open surgery for osteotomies and/or fusion extension into the thoracic spine.

MISDEF2

The MISDEF algorithm accounted for the limited capability of MIS to achieve sagittal deformity correction. As MIS techniques continued to be validated, tools and technology to support sagittal correction had emerged and gained acceptance including anterior column release, hyperlordotic interbody cages, and miniopen pedicle subtraction osteotomy.[26–30] With the consideration of these techniques, the MISDEF-2 algorithm was developed.[31] MISDEF2 has 4 treatment levels with class 3 modified to include MIS treatment options for severe and/or rigid deformities using anterior column release (ACR), expandable cages, miniopen pedicle subtraction osteotomy (PSO), and hybrid MIS/open techniques. Class 4 describes deformities best addressed via open techniques due to the requirement of long constructs or revision of previous multilevel fusions (**Fig. 1**).

Minimally Invasive Interbody Selection Algorithm

Arthrodesis and correction through the interbody space via cage implants and bone grafting is an essential MIS technique. Depending on the surgical goals, interbody grafts can be used to aid in sagittal or coronal deformity correction, anterior column realignment, and both indirect central canal and foraminal decompressions. The most common MIS interbody graft techniques in the lumbar spine include transforaminal lumbar interbody fusion (TLIF), anterior lumbar interbody fusion (ALIF), and lateral lumbar interbody fusion (LLIF) via retroperitoneal transpsoas or prepsoas approaches and with or without anterior longitudinal ligament (ALL) release. The choice of technique requires consideration of the surgical goals, patient anatomy, spinal level, and surgeon comfort.

To aid in technique selection, the minimally invasive interbody selection algorithm (MIISA) was

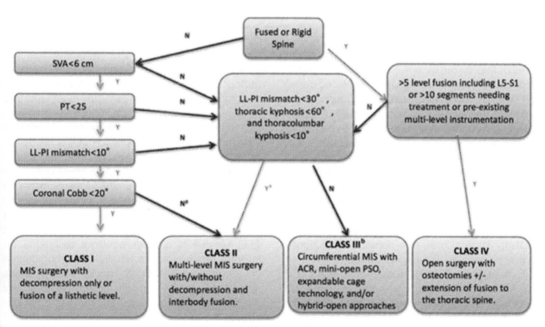

Fig. 1. MISDEF2 decision tree. The MISDEF2 deformity algorithm uses purely radiographic parameters to guide surgical decision-making to 1 of 4 general classes of treatment options. The treatment classes increased in complexity and invasiveness with class 4 being open surgery.

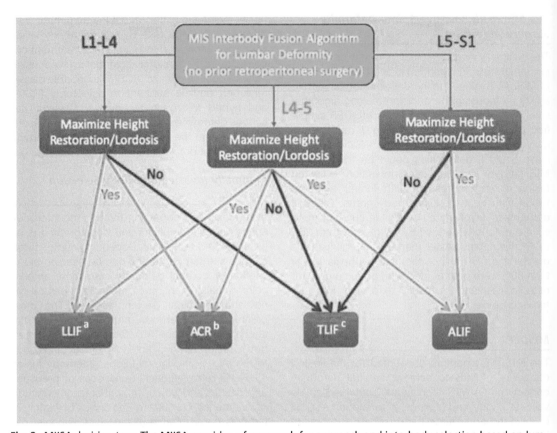

Fig. 2. MIISA decision tree. The MIISA provides a framework for approach and interbody selection based on lumbar spinal level and surgical goal. [a]LLIF: Prepsoas or transpsoas lateral interbody fusion; use when up to 5° of segmental lordosis is desired. Lordosis between L1-L4 is inconsistent while height restoration is consistent. [b]ACR: Use when ≥10° of segmental lordosis is desired. [c]TLF: Allows direct decompression of foraminal/lateral recess stenosis.

created.[32] This algorithm was created by an expert panel of MIS deformity spine surgeons who evaluated greater than 300 interbody grafts placed during 100 MIS ASD surgeries at multiple institutions maintained via the MIS International Spine Study Group database. Both clinical and long-term (2-year) radiographic outcomes were analyzed in the context of the surgical goals. Four interbody graft techniques were considered: ALIF, TLIF, LLIF without ACR, and LLIF with ACR. Among the statistically significant cohort, beneficial impacts were observed in lumbar lordosis, PI-LL mismatch, and coronal cobb angle. Assessment of the overall Oswestry Disability Index scores also demonstrated significant improvement. The expert surgeons preferred LLIF at L1-2, L2-3, L3-4, and L4-5. Overall, LLIF with ACR was performed in 5% of cases and most commonly at L3-4 (8%) and L2-3 (6%). At L5-S1, TLIF and ALIF were most performed at rates of 61% and 39%, respectively.

MIISA provides a framework for MIS lumbar interbody grafting between L1 and S1 spinal levels among patients without prior retroperitoneal surgery (**Fig. 2**). At L1-4, the surgical goals of maximizing interbody height restoration and restoration of lordosis can be most robustly accomplished via LLIF alone (if desired segmental lordosis is 5° or less) and combine with ALL release if more than 10° of segmental lordosis is needed. If maximal interbody height restoration and/or lordosis is not needed, TLIF is a good option for direct lateral recess or foraminal decompression at L1-L4. At the L4-5 level, all 4 techniques can be used. ALIF was found to be the most powerful for restoration of lordosis. LLIF (with or without ALL release) is another powerful technique for lordosis restoration but requires a higher degree of surgeon expertise to avoid complications related to psoas muscle and/or lumbosacral plexus nerve trauma. At L5-S1, the iliac crest obstructs the lateral approach; maximal disc height and lordosis restoration is accomplished via ALIF. If the primary goal is not maximal disc height and lordosis restoration, TLIF is a good option.

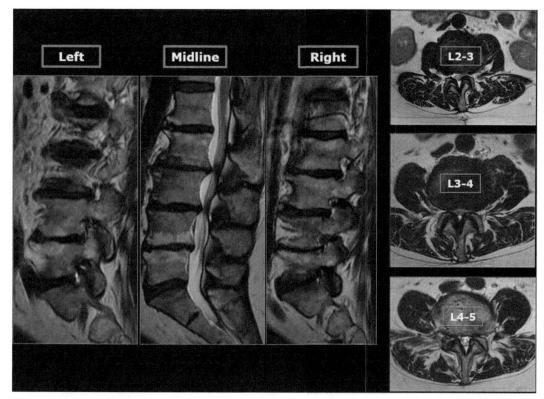

Fig. 3. Preoperative MRI.

TLIF, when combined with posterior column osteotomies, however, can both restore interbody height to accomplish foraminal decompression as well as achieve significant segmental lordosis (see **Fig. 2**).

Global Alignment Proportion Score

The global alignment proportion (GAP) score is a radiographic tool comparing measured pelvic-incidence proportional parameters to ideal spinopelvic parameters to predict mechanical complications.[33] Unlike traditional parameters for sagittal balance, such as correlation between sagittal vertical axis (SVA) and patient reported outcome measure (PROMs), the GAP score focuses on hardware complications rather than quality of life measures.[34] The principle underlying the GAP score is the focus on obtaining correction at ideal physiologic levels. For example, ACRs are generally reserved for L4-5-S1 (predominantly with ALIFs) rather than L2-3-4 (predominantly with LLIFs) to avoid placing the maximum degree of lordosis in a nonphysiological location. Several studies including traditional open deformity techniques have demonstrated a significant correlation between a moderately or severely disproportioned spinopelvic state after surgery for malalignment

and higher rates of mechanical complications including proximal and distal junctional kyphosis and hardware failure.[33,35,36] However, 2 recent studies examining patients after open deformity correction found no correlation between GAP score and rates of hardware failure.[37,38] The predictive value of the GAP score in the MIS setting is under active investigation. In a retrospective study of 182 patients who underwent cMIS ASD correction, Gendelberg and colleagues found no correlation between GAP score and mechanical complications.[39] Last, a study of asymptomatic, nonoperative volunteers revealed 26% with a moderately or severely disproportioned GAP score suggesting further refinement of GAP targets is possible.[40] The GAP score remains a potentially powerful tool to aid in decision-making with additional target refinement and study in the MIS setting is ongoing.

Case 1

A 70-year-old woman with past medical history significant only for hypertension and hyperlipidemia presented with 1 year of subjectively worsening right leg weakness, bilateral radicular pain in the posterolateral distribution, neurogenic claudication including bilateral calf and foot

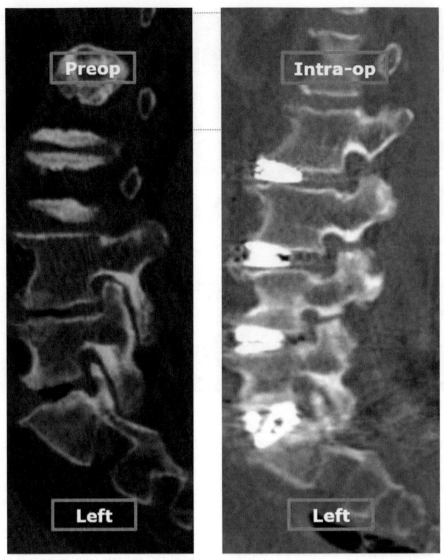

Fig. 4. Indirect decompression achieved via interbody placement.

paresthesias, and severe back pain. She had failed 1 year of oral pain medication, physical therapy, and epidural steroid injections. Her neurologic examination did not reveal any motor deficits. Her MRI demonstrated significant degenerative changes include spondylosis at L2-3, L3-4, and L4-5 with severe central and bilateral foraminal stenosis and severe left L5-S1 foraminal stenosis. Standing plain films revealed a lumbar flat back morphology with a lumbar lordosis of 11°, no significant coronal deformity, and no ankylosis. The primary pathology was thus localized to L2-S1 based on spondylosis, foraminal, and central stenosis (**Fig. 3**).

She is a MISDEF class 2 and was planned for a multilevel MIS procedure. She was positioned,

prepped, and draped in lateral decubitus position. C-arm fluoroscopy was used for this portion of the procedure. A vascular approach surgeon gained access to the L5-S1 disc space via a mini-open, lateral-anterior approach (lateral ALIF). A 15° titanium interbody cage was placed at this level. A lateral, retroperitoneal, transpsoas approach was taken to place 10° titanium interbody cages at L2-3, L3-4, and L4-5 (LLIFs) **Fig. 4**. The patient was then flipped prone onto a modified Jackson table compatible with intraoperative CT navigation and posterior percutaneous pedicle screws were placed L2-S1. The patient was discharged home on postoperative day 2. At 12 months follow-up, she reports an average pain score of 0 without the use of pain

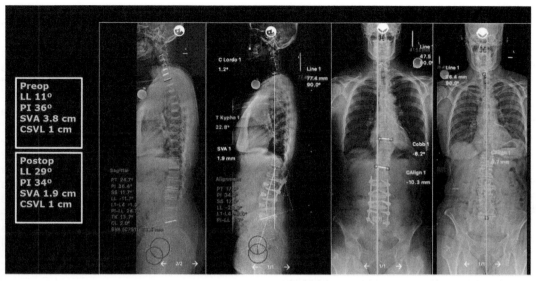

Fig. 5. Preoperative and postoperative standing radiographs for example, case 1 demonstrating a MISDEF class 2.

medication and has no ongoing limitations to her activities of daily living (ODI preop 24, postop 10). Preoperative and 1-year postoperative standing films (**Fig. 5**).

Case 2

A 69-year-old woman with 1.5 years of worsening severe axial back pain with radicular pain radiating into the right leg presented for surgical evaluation after failing conservative management. Her preoperative standing long cassette x-rays were notable

for: SVA 3 cm, LL 18°, PI 49°, Coronal cobb 41°, and CSVL 3 cm. She was found to be a MISDEF class 3 and underwent a staged anterior posterior procedure. Stage 1 Anterior: L3-4, 4 to 5, 5 to 1 ALIF. Stage 2 posterior: midline incision with percutaneous pedicle screw placement through thoracolumbar fascia L1-pelvis (L1 and L2 cement augmentation via fenestrated screws), L3-4, 4 to 5 tubular posterior column osteotomies, and L1-2, 2 to 3 facet joint fusion through tubular retractors (**Fig. 6**).

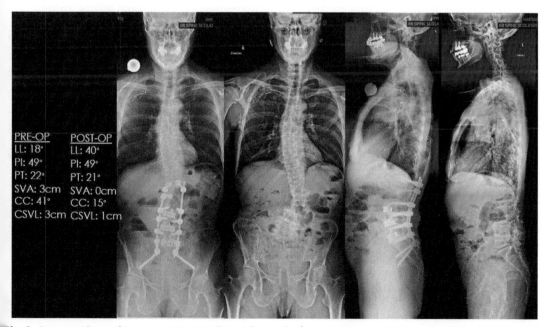

Fig. 6. Preoperative and postoperative standing radiographs for example, case 2 demonstrating a MISDEF class 3.

SUMMARY

ASD can be associated with significant morbidity and has been found to be comparable with other systemic chronic diseases. Appropriately selected patients can benefit from surgery aimed at decompression of neural elements and restoration of spinal alignment. Traditional open surgery, although often effective, is associated with high rates of certain complications. In select patients with flexible deformities of less severe magnitude, MIS techniques allow for correction with decreased surgical morbidity. Early attempts at MIS deformity correction were hampered by high rates of pseudarthrosis and inadequate deformity correction. The capabilities of MIS deformity surgery have since evolved supported by significant advances in MIS surgical tools, techniques, and intraoperative navigation technology. Decision-making algorithms to guide patient and approach selection have been formed based on data from multi-institution working groups. As patient outcomes data continue to emerge and new technology becomes part of surgical practice, the selection algorithms will continue to evolve. Furthermore, the emergence of artificial intelligence to analyze big data cohorts and variables will continue to drive refinement including predictive metrics, of these algorithms.

REFERENCES

1. Ames CP, Scheer JK, Lafage V, et al. Adult spinal deformity: epidemiology, health impact, evaluation, and management. Spine Deform 2016;4(4):310–22.
2. Smith JS, Line B, Bess S, et al. The Health Impact of Adult Cervical Deformity in Patients Presenting for Surgical Treatment: Comparison to United States Population Norms and Chronic Disease States Based on the EuroQuol-5 Dimensions Questionnaire. Neurosurgery 2017;80(5):716–25.
3. Bess S, Line B, Fu K-M, et al. The health impact of symptomatic adult spinal deformity: comparison of deformity types to united states population norms and chronic diseases. Spine 2016;41(3):224–33.
4. Daniels AH, Smith JS, Hiratzka J, et al. Functional limitations due to lumbar stiffness in adults with and without spinal deformity. Spine 2015;40(20): 1599–604.
5. Schwab F, Dubey A, Gamez L, et al. Adult scoliosis: prevalence, SF-36, and nutritional parameters in an elderly volunteer population. Spine 2005;30(9):1082–5.
6. Spencer G. Projections of the Population of the United States, by Age, Sex, and Race: 1983 to 2080. Curr Popul Rep 1984.
7. Statistical Abstract of the United States, Volume 128, Part 2009. U.S. Government Printing Office; 2009.
8. Blanche C, Matloff JM, Denton TA, et al. Cardiac operations in patients 90 years of age and older. Ann Thorac Surg 1997;63(6):1685–90.
9. Bridwell KH, Glassman S, Horton W, et al. Does treatment (nonoperative and operative) improve the two-year quality of life in patients with adult symptomatic lumbar scoliosis: a prospective multicenter evidence-based medicine study. Spine 2009;34(20):2171–8.
10. Smith JS, Shaffrey CI, Klineberg E, et al. Complication rates associated with 3-column osteotomy in 82 adult spinal deformity patients: retrospective review of a prospectively collected multicenter consecutive series with 2-year follow-up. J Neurosurg Spine 2017;27(4):444–57.
11. Glassman SD, Hamill CL, Bridwell KH, et al. The impact of perioperative complications on clinical outcome in adult deformity surgery. Spine 2007; 32(24):2764–70.
12. Anand N, Chung A, Kong C, et al. Prevalence and modes of posterior hardware failure with a staged protocol for circumferential minimally invasive surgical correction of adult spinal deformity: a 13-year experience. Int J Spine Surg 2022;16(3):481–9.
13. Anand N, Alayan A, Kong C, et al. Management of severe adult spinal deformity with circumferential minimally invasive surgical strategies without posterior column osteotomies: a 13-year experience. Spine Deform 2022;10(5):1157–68.
14. Chou D, Lafage V, Chan AY, et al. Patient outcomes after circumferential minimally invasive surgery compared with those of open correction for adult spinal deformity: initial analysis of prospectively collected data. J Neurosurg Spine 2021;1–12. https://doi.org/10.3171/2021.3.SPINE201825.
15. Vora D, Kinnard M, Falk D, et al. A comparison of narcotic usage and length of post-operative hospital stay in open versus minimally invasive lumbar interbody fusion with percutaneous pedicle screws. J Spine Surg 2018;4(3):516–21.
16. Patel AA, Zfass-Mendez M, Lebwohl NH, et al. Minimally invasive versus open lumbar fusion: a comparison of blood loss, surgical complications, and hospital course. Iowa Orthop J 2015;35:130–4.
17. Lu VM, Kerezoudis P, Gilder HE. Minimally invasive surgery versus open surgery spinal fusion for spondylolisthesis: a systematic review and meta-analysis. Spine 2017;42(3):E177–85.
18. Goldberg JL, Härtl R, Elowitz E. Minimally invasive spine surgery: an overview. World Neurosurg 2022; 163:214–27.
19. Goldberg JL, Härtl R, Elowitz E. Challenges hindering widespread adoption of minimally invasive spine surgery. World Neurosurg 2022.
20. Goldberg JL, Hussain I, Sommer F, et al. The future of minimally invasive spinal surgery. World Neurosurg 2022.

21. Mummaneni PV, Park P, Fu K-M, et al. Does minimally invasive percutaneous posterior instrumentation reduce risk of proximal junctional kyphosis in adult spinal deformity surgery? a propensity-matched cohort analysis. Neurosurgery 2016;78(1): 101–8.

22. Uribe JS, Koffie RM, Wang MY, et al. Are Minimally Invasive Spine Surgeons or Classical Open Spine Surgeons More Consistent with Their Treatment of Adult Spinal Deformity? World Neurosurg 2022; 165:e51–8.

23. Silva FE, Lenke LG. Adult degenerative scoliosis: evaluation and management. Neurosurg Focus 2010;28(3):E1.

24. Mummaneni PV, Tu T-H, Ziewacz JE. The role of minimally invasive techniques in the treatment of adult spinal deformity. Neurosurg Clin N Am 2013;24(2): 231–48.

25. Mummaneni PV, Shaffrey CI, Lenke LG, et al. The minimally invasive spinal deformity surgery algorithm: a reproducible rational framework for decision making in minimally invasive spinal deformity surgery. Neurosurg Focus 2014;36(5):E6.

26. Chou D, Lau D. The Mini-Open Pedicle Subtraction Osteotomy for Flat-Back Syndrome and Kyphosis Correction: Operative Technique. Oper Neurosurg (Hagerstown) 2016;12(4):309–16.

27. Wang MY, Madhavan K. Mini-open pedicle subtraction osteotomy: surgical technique. World Neurosurg 2014;81(5–6):843.e11–4.

28. Wang MY, Bordon G. Mini-open pedicle subtraction osteotomy as a treatment for severe adult spinal deformities: case series with initial clinical and radiographic outcomes. J Neurosurg Spine 2016;24(5): 769–76.

29. Turner JD, Akbarnia BA, Eastlack RK, et al. Radiographic outcomes of anterior column realignment for adult sagittal plane deformity: a multicenter analysis. Eur Spine J 2015;24(Suppl 3):427–32.

30. Akbarnia BA, Mundis GM, Moazzaz P, et al. Anterior column realignment (ACR) for focal kyphotic spinal deformity using a lateral transpsoas approach and ALL release. J Spinal Disord Tech 2014;27(1):29–39.

31. Mummaneni PV, Park P, Shaffrey CI, et al. The MIS-DEF2 algorithm: an updated algorithm for patient selection in minimally invasive deformity surgery. J Neurosurg Spine 2019;32(2):221–8.

32. Mummaneni PV, Hussain I, Shaffrey CI, et al. The minimally invasive interbody selection algorithm for spinal deformity. J Neurosurg Spine 2021;1–8. https://doi.org/10.3171/2020.9.SPINE20230.

33. Yilgor C, Sogunmez N, Boissiere L, et al. Global alignment and proportion (GAP) score: development and validation of a new method of analyzing spino-pelvic alignment to predict mechanical complications after adult spinal deformity surgery. J Bone Joint Surg Am 2017;99(19):1661–72.

34. Schwab F, Ungar B, Blondel B, et al. Scoliosis Research Society-Schwab adult spinal deformity classification: a validation study. Spine 2012; 37(12):1077–82.

35. Noh SH, Ha Y, Obeid I, et al. Modified global alignment and proportion scoring with body mass index and bone mineral density (GAPB) for improving predictions of mechanical complications after adult spinal deformity surgery. Spine J 2020;20(5):776–84.

36. Jacobs E, van Royen BJ, van Kuijk SMJ, et al. Prediction of mechanical complications in adult spinal deformity surgery-the GAP score versus the Schwab classification. Spine J 2019;19(5):781–8.

37. Bari TJ, Ohrt-Nissen S, Hansen LV. Ability of the global alignment and proportion score to predict mechanical failure following adult spinal deformity surgery-validation in 149 patients with two-year follow-up. Spine Deform 2019;7(2):331–7.

38. Kawabata A, Yoshii T, Sakai K, et al. Identification of predictive factors for mechanical complications after adult spinal deformity surgery: a multi-institutional retrospective study. Spine 2020;45(17):1185–92.

39. Gendelberg D, Rao A, Chung A, et al. Does the global alignment and Proportion score predict mechanical complications in circumferential minimally invasive surgery for adult spinal deformity? Neurosurg Focus 2023;54(1):E11.

40. Wegner AM, Iyer S, Lenke LG. Global alignment and proportion (GAP) scores in an asymptomatic, nonoperative cohort: a divergence of age-adjusted and pelvic incidence-based alignment targets. Eur Spine J 2020;29(9):2362–7.

Transpsoas Approaches to the Lumbar Spine
Lateral and Prone

Michael D. White, MD, Nima Alan, MD, Juan S. Uribe, MD*

KEYWORDS

- Lateral lumbar fusion • Lateral lumbar interbody fusion • LLIF • Prone lateral
- Transpsoas approach

KEY POINTS

- The lateral transpsoas approach requires thoughtful patient selection and careful preoperative assessment and planning to be performed safely and effectively.
- Performing the lateral transpsoas approach in the prone position can circumvent the need for repositioning during surgery and reduce operative time for patients who also require posterior fixation.
- Although the steps to this approach in the prone and lateral decubitus positions are similar, some nuances make performing LLIF in the prone position difficult to master.

INTRODUCTION

The lateral lumbar interbody fusion (LLIF) approach is a minimally invasive approach to the lateral lumbar spine, which is accessed via a working corridor through the psoas muscle. The technique was first described by McAfee and colleagues[1] and further developed into the modern LLIF procedure by Ozgur and colleagues.[2] This transpsoas approach allows surgeons to place large interbody cages that span the length of the vertebral body, which takes advantage of the strong epiphyseal ring of cortical bone around the endplate.[3] Studies have established the effectiveness of LLIF in treating degenerative spinal pathologic conditions, including degenerative disc disease and spondylolisthesis.[4–6] The addition of hyperlordotic cages and anterior column release to this approach has improved our ability to correct severe sagittal imbalance and better achieve preoperative alignment goals for patients with spinal deformity.[7,8]

It should be mentioned that LLIF can be either antepsoas or transpsoas, with this article focusing on the transpsoas approach. However, both approaches have demonstrated high rates of fusion and good postoperative outcomes.[9] Performing LLIF through the transpsoas approach has a few notable advantages compared with the antepsoas approach, with the first being the ability to perform a single-position lateral interbody fusion with posterior pedicle screw fixation in the prone-lateral position. Additionally, the transpsoas approach facilitates placement of a longer and wider interbody cage that spans from the ipsilateral to the contralateral diaphysis, taking advantage of the strongest areas of the endplate. The interbody cage placement with the antepsoas approach is at an oblique angle, which limits the length of the interbody cage, so that it does not necessarily extend from diaphysis to diaphysis. Finally, the transpsoas approach is associated with significantly lower risk of major vascular injury or sympathetic nerve injury compared with the transpsoas approach.[10]

Lateral interbody fusion can be performed as a stand-alone construct or supplemented with

Department of Neurosurgery, Barrow Neurological Institute, St. Joseph's Hospital and Medical Center, Phoenix, AZ, USA
* Corresponding author. c/o Neuroscience Publications, Barrow Neurological Institute, St. Joseph's Hospital and Medical Center, 350 W. Thomas Road, Phoenix, AZ 85013.
E-mail address: Neuropub@barrowneuro.org

Neurosurg Clin N Am 34 (2023) 609–617
https://doi.org/10.1016/j.nec.2023.06.008
1042-3680/23/© 2023 Elsevier Inc. All rights reserved.

posterior pedicle screw fixation for cases involving instability or malalignment, such as cases of spondylolisthesis. In the traditional lateral transpsoas technique, lateral interbody placement is performed with the patient in the lateral decubitus position, and the patient is then repositioned prone for the placement of percutaneous pedicle screws. Recent technological advances have led to the development of the single-position prone, lateral approach, which allows LLIF and posterior pedicle screw fixation to be performed without patient repositioning. In addition to enabling easier placement of posterior pedicle screws and requiring less time in the operating room, the prone lateral transpsoas approach allows the abdomen to hang down on the Jackson table in a more lordotic position, which improves the segmental lordosis achieved after LLIF.[11] Despite these advantages, there are nuanced differences in the prone technique that a surgeon must master to perform LLIF successfully with the patient in the prone position. The aims of this article are to discuss the performance of LLIF with the patient in the lateral decubitus position and highlight key differences encountered when LLIF is performed through the transpsoas approach with the patient in the prone position.

PREOPERATIVE PLANNING
Indications for and Benefits of Lateral Lumbar Interbody Fusion

The indications for LLIF are similar to those for traditional posterior fusion and include degenerative pathologic conditions, such as spinal stenosis, spondylolisthesis, degenerative disc disease, and degenerative scoliosis.[4,12] The lateral transpsoas approach allows for a larger corridor through the disc space and the placement of a much larger interbody cage than would be possible with a posterior lateral interbody fusion or transforaminal lateral interbody fusion. A lateral approach also avoids disrupting the posterior musculature and ligaments. A large interbody cage placed via a lateral transpsoas approach reconstitutes disc height and foraminal height, providing indirect decompression of the neural elements.

Preoperative Imaging

Standing scoliosis radiographs should be obtained before surgery to identify sagittal or coronal imbalance and spinopelvic mismatch. The degree of sagittal imbalance influences the degree of segmental lordosis needed and the type of lordotic cage to place. The degree of coronal deformity is a crucial factor in determining the side of the approach. The coronal angle at the level of interest

will often make one side more favorable than the other for approach. This difference is especially notable at L4/5, which is more easily accessed on the concave side of the lumbar curve, with the iliac crest making the opposite side extremely difficult to access in some patients.

Computed tomography (CT) is beneficial for preoperative planning because it gives insight into bone quality, shows lateral osteophytes that can limit access to a particular side, and clearly shows the pedicles at each level for cases that require supplemental posterior fixation. The degree of disc degeneration and collapse or the presence of vacuum disc phenomenon help guide decision-making because patients with these findings on CT are more likely to benefit from indirect decompression and restoration of disc and foraminal heights.

MRI identifies the levels with central or foraminal stenosis that may be targeted for surgery. MRI can also reveal pathologic conditions such as large disc extrusions or synovial cysts that can cause symptoms but would not be effectively treated with LLIF. The position of the great vessels and the anatomy of the psoas muscle guide decision-making about whether a lateral transpsoas approach is feasible (ie, whether the great vessels are in a lateral position) and which side presents the easiest approach.

PITFALLS TO PERFORMING LATERAL LUMBAR INTERBODY FUSION

- Patients with earlier retroperitoneal surgery
- Lateral position of the great vessels
- High-riding iliac crest
- Presence of transitional psoas or "Mickey Mouse" sign appearance of psoas muscles on MRI (**Fig. 1**). This sign indicates a ventrally displaced lumbar plexus at L4/5.
- Pathology above T12/L1 or below L4/5.

Approach Side

Approaching from the side of the concavity is preferred for a multitude of reasons. First, placing the patient in the lateral position with the convex side of the curve against the operating table promotes some correction of the coronal deformity, which will be further corrected with the LLIF. Additionally, the trajectories of each disc space on the concave side converge toward a single point, often facilitating a single incision in patients who would require multiple incisions if the disc space were approached on the convex side. There is typically a greater degree of foraminal stenosis, collapse, and degeneration on the concave side,

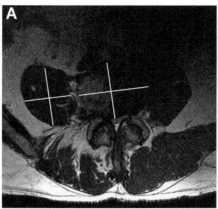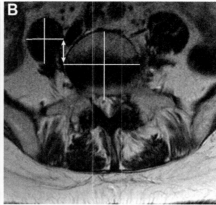

Fig. 1. Axial MRI showing center-to-center distance measured between the psoas muscle and the endplate at L4/5. (*A*) The normal psoas position. (*B*) Transitional psoas, which is also referred to as the "Mickey Mouse" sign. (Used with permission from Barrow Neurological Institute, Phoenix, Arizona.)

and approaching from this side offers access to the location where decompression is most needed.

PROCEDURE
Lateral Decubitus Position

Positioning
Traditional LLIF is performed with the patient in the lateral decubitus position. The patient's arm closest to the bed should be laid onto an arm board, with an axial roll underneath the torso. The other arm should be placed on an elevated armrest and bent at a 90° angle. It is important to have the patient's knees flexed to prevent the lumbar plexus from migrating forward into the dissection plane. The iliac crest should be centered over the break in the bed. The patient is taped tightly to the bed by taping around the pelvis, then along the patient's thigh and lower leg in a "figure-of-eight" pattern. The patient's upper body is securely taped across the torso and under the bed. Once the patient is taped and secured, the bed is retroflexed to open the space between the iliac crest and the 12th rib. This retroflexion of the table also tightens the skin and opens the lateral disc space.

Operation
Step 1: Once the patient is positioned in the lateral decubitus position, fluoroscopy is used to plan the incision. The C-arm should be placed on the side of the patient that is opposite the side on which the surgeon is working. True anterior-posterior (AP) and lateral images should be obtained, with the endplates perfectly aligned to ensure accuracy. The specific rotation of the C-arm in each direction can be marked at this time to ensure ease in returning to these true AP and lateral images later in the case. Lateral fluoroscopy should be used to locate and mark the center of the disc space at each level, along with the trajectory of the disc space. For single-level cases, a 3-cm incision is made along the trajectory of the marked disc space. For multilevel cases, a longer incision in the rostral-caudal direction is made to incorporate the center of the disc space previously marked for each desired level.

Step 2: After making the incision, dissection should be performed down to the fascia using a hemostat in each hand to spread the abdominal muscle apart. One hemostat should spread in the AP direction, and the other should spread in the rostral-caudal direction until the fascia is reached. An incision should be made along the fascia in the same direction as the skin incision with monopolar electrocautery. A finger should be used to probe down to the psoas muscle, which should feel like violin strings as the finger moves across it. The peritoneum should be felt anteriorly, and the transverse process of the vertebra should be identified posteriorly.

Step 3: A finger should be used to protect the abdominal contents anteriorly while the first dilator is inserted through the psoas muscle and onto the disc space below. Lateral radiographs should be obtained to ensure that the dilator is docked in the desired position, most commonly the third quartile of the disc space. Once the correct positioning is confirmed, a Kirschner wire (K-wire) is inserted through the dilator into the disc space. The subsequent dilators are inserted, and directional electromyography (EMG) is used to stimulate in the anterior, caudal, posterior, and rostral directions after the addition of each dilator to ensure there is no nerve involvement and to protect the lumbar plexus. The retractor is then inserted, docked, and attached to the retractor arm; fluoroscopy is used to ensure the retractor position has not moved. The retractor arm should be attached to the opposite side of the bed from the side on which the surgeon is working. When looking down through the retractor, no muscle should protrude from underneath the retractor blades. Once in the correct position, a posterior shim is malleted into the disc space, and the retractor blades are opened away from the posterior shim to protect the femoral nerve.

Step 4: A discectomy is performed by first using an 11-blade for the annulotomy, cutting a rectangle along the visualized disc space. A pituitary rongeur is then used to remove the annulus and underlying disc. Next, a Cobb elevator is used to unroof the annulus from the superior and inferior endplates. The Cobb elevator should be placed parallel to the endplate and can be malleted until it breaks through the contralateral annulus. This step should be performed under fluoroscopy to ensure the instrument does not breach too far through the contralateral side. This step is repeated for the inferior endplate as well. Next, the rest of the disc should be removed using a combination of a box chisel, rasp, rongeur, angled ring curettes, pituitary rongeur, and various scrapers to remove any remaining disc material.

Step 5: Once the disc space has been prepared, implant trials can be inserted. Preoperative imaging can be used to estimate the needed dimensions. It is better to start with a thinner trial because this can help complete the annular release on the contralateral side. AP fluoroscopy should again be used to verify proper positioning while inserting the trials or cage. The degree of resistance while placing each trial will determine the optimal size. The trial with the proper height will fit snugly while not offering too much resistance, which can lead to violation of the endplate with insertion or rupture of the anterior longitudinal ligament.

Step 6: The final dimensions of the cage are relayed to the scrub technician, who prepares the interbody cage on the back table by packing the cage with allograft and connecting it to the applicator. Graft containment guides should prevent any allograft from falling out during insertion. Once the interbody cage is partially inserted, the graft containment guides are removed, and the implant is malleted into place. Intermittent AP fluoroscopy is used to ensure that the implant is being inserted parallel to the endplates and to determine when it has been fully inserted.

Step 7: Once the implant is in the desired position, the surgical field is copiously irrigated. The posterior shim is removed, and the retractor

blades are released. The retractor should be slowly withdrawn, allowing the tissue to fall back into place. While withdrawing the retractor, any areas of bleeding should be cauterized with bipolar electrocautery before further removing the retractor. The fascial layer should be closed tightly with 0-0 sutures. The subcutaneous layer can be closed with 3-0 sutures, and a subcuticular running monofilament suture with surgical glue can be used for the skin.

Prone Position

Positioning
To perform a single-position LLIF, the surgical team places the patient in the prone position on a radiolucent Jackson table to ensure that the abdomen hangs freely in the opening. Hip pads are placed underneath the posterior-superior iliac spine for support. These pads can also be placed slightly below the posterior-superior iliac spine to maximize lordosis. Similar to the lateral decubitus position, the prone position requires that the pelvis and the upper torso be securely taped to the bed. When LLIF is performed with the patient in the prone position, taping the lateral chest by pulling upward toward the head and taping the pelvis by pulling downward toward the feet create further separation between the pelvis and the lower ribs, as well as tightening the skin. In addition to this taping, a bolster is placed contralateral to the approach side, which provides resistance, while inserting the lateral interbody graft and acts similarly to breaking the bed in the lateral position.

Operation
The basic steps for performing LLIF are the same with the patient in the prone or lateral decubitus position. However, critical nuances must be understood to perform LLIF successfully with the patient in the prone position.[13] In this section, we review the steps for the transpsoas approach (**Fig. 2**) and highlight the differences encountered when performing this approach with the patient in the prone position.

Step 1: Intraoperative fluoroscopy should be used to plan the lateral incision, similar to the procedure used for the lateral decubitus position. During this step, the posterior incision should also be planned by delineating the midline and localizing the incision to the appropriate levels. If navigation is used for percutaneous pedicle screw placement, the navigation reference is fixated on the posterior-superior iliac spine. Pedicle screws should be placed before the interbody graft when using navigation to ensure the integrity of image guidance.

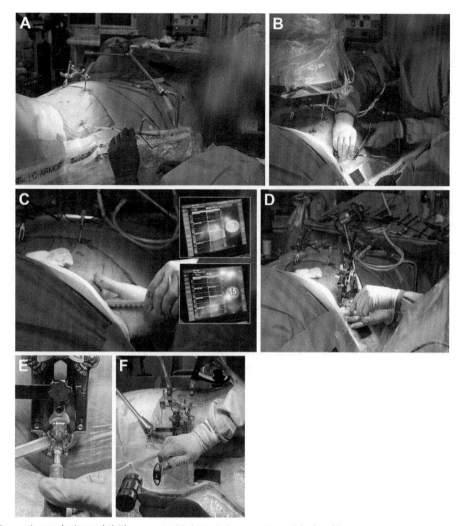

Fig. 2. Operative technique. (*A*) The surgeon is in a sitting position. (*B*) The dilator is placed. (*C*) Sequential dilators are placed, with the performance of running and triggered electromyography (*insets*). (*D*) A retractor is attached to the arm ipsilateral to the incision. (*E*) The disc is visualized, and a discectomy is performed. (*F*) An interbody graft is placed with the surgeon standing to provide a more ergonomic angle. (Used with permission from Godzik J, Ohiorhenuan IE, Xu DS, et al. Single-position prone lateral approach: cadaveric feasibility study and early clinical experience. Neurosurg Focus 2020 Sep;49(3):E15.)

Step 2: Dissecting down and traversing the psoas is more difficult with the patient in the prone position because the depth of the field is greater than with the traditional lateral decubitus position, in which gravity helps pull the tissue down. This nuance is most exaggerated in patients with significant obesity. The surgical assistant can provide counterpressure on the contralateral side to help push the spine closer to the surgeon at this stage. The surgeon should be able to palpate the psoas muscle, the transverse process of the vertebra, and the peritoneum anteriorly during this step.

Step 3: In a similar manner to the procedure for the lateral position, a dilator is placed through the psoas and onto the disc space using intraoperative fluoroscopy to confirm correct placement. A K-wire is inserted into the disc space, and larger dilators are sequentially placed. Electromyographic stimulation is done after the addition of each dilator to ensure there is no nerve involvement and to protect the lumbar plexus. Once the retractor is ready to be placed, the surgeon should be mindful of the tendency to dock the retractor more anteriorly than desired with the patient in the prone position because gravity tends to pull the soft tissue and retractor downward. From the placement of the first dilator until the final retractor is docked, the surgeon should be conscious of the need to aim posteriorly to compensate for the tendency of instruments to be pulled in an anterior direction.

Step 4: The surgeon will notice a significant difference in the ergonomics of performing the discectomy and placing the interbody graft compared with the ergonomics of performing the procedure with the patient in the lateral decubitus position. The surgeon must often hunch over the retractor to visualize the operative field. The surgeon's position is further complicated by the need to extend their neck if they wear surgical loupes designed to look downward. They can sit on a stool and raise the bed closer to eye level to maintain a more neutral posture. However, this position also requires the surgeon to operate with their arms raised for extended periods, which is often unsustainable. Alternatively, the bed can be rotated 15° to 20° to improve the ergonomics of the operation. When the bed is rotated, the C-arm also needs to be rotated such that fluoroscopy shows the endplates are again parallel. Failure to confirm that the endplates are perfectly parallel after the bed is rotated increases the risk of intraoperative subsidence when performing the discectomy and placing the interbody cage.

Steps 5 and 6: Placing the trial and the final interbody cages requires the use of a mallet to insert the trial or cage into the disc space. When the patient is in the lateral decubitus position, the bed provides counterpressure during these steps; however, this counterpressure is lost when the patient is in the prone position. The force of the mallet has the propensity to migrate the retractor anteriorly with each strike and can risk injury to the major vessels or the anterior longitudinal ligament. To prevent this migration, the assistant surgeon can hold the retractor in place when the mallet is used. If the retractor is displaced during these steps, the surgeon must take the retractor out and reinsert the K-wire to find the disc space again.

Step 7: The retractor is slowly pulled out at the end of the procedure to ensure that there are no areas of bleeding as the tissue falls back into place. The various layers are closed as described for the lateral decubitus position.

Intraoperative Monitoring

The implementation of real-time directional EMG monitoring has led to a decrease in postoperative neurologic complications from 30% to less than 1%.[14,15] We advocate for the use of directional EMG for all transpsoas cases, regardless of whether the lateral or prone position is used. Current dilators used in the transpsoas approach incorporate triggered EMG (tEMG) and provide discrete threshold results for nerves of the lumbar plexus. After each sequential dilation, unidirectional tEMG should be used to stimulate in

the anterior, posterior, cranial, and caudal directions. Thresholds less than 5 mA indicate stimulation directly on a nerve; thresholds between 5 and 10 mA indicate close proximity, with a small amount of soft tissue between instrumentation and the nerve; and thresholds greater than 11 mA demonstrate greater distance between instrumentation and the nerve. The directional capabilities and spatial information allow for surgeons to easily understand where to best adjust the instrumentation to avoid injury to the nerve.[16] As a general rule, with thresholds of 10 mA or less, the surgeon should adjust the instruments further from the nerve to prevent neurologic injury.

Intraoperative Navigation of the Interbody

The use of CT-based image-guided navigation systems for placing interbody cages during the transpsoas approach has been advocated, with the goal of increasing placement accuracy, improving workflow, and reducing the radiation exposure associated with traditional fluoroscopy. Although earlier reports have demonstrated the relative safety and accuracy of this technique,[17] the role of navigated placement of interbody cages with the transpsoas approach is still debated. We urge caution when considering navigated interbody cage placement because navigation should be considered a supplemental technology and not a replacement for fluoroscopy. Live imaging with intraoperative fluoroscopy remains the gold standard for understanding and navigating each patient's anatomy to perform this procedure safely. The most significant limitation associated with navigated interbody cages is the lack of a reliable reference to ensure the accuracy of navigation. For open posterior approaches, bony anatomy can be used to verify the calibration of image guidance; however, the lateral transpsoas approach does not provide the same bony landmarks. Without a reliable method of verifying the accuracy of navigation, the surgeon may be unknowingly operating blind. Additionally, the accuracy of navigation is diminished during multilevel cases because the placement of each additional interbody changes the anatomy.

There is an argument for using navigation during interbody placement in prone transpsoas cases where navigation is already being used for the pedicle screw placement. The limitations described above also apply to the prone position. However, for cases in which navigation is planned, a technique in which a 16-guage spinal needle is placed in the spinous process before cross-sectional imaging has been previously described.[18] This technique provides the surgeon with an internal reference point to verify the accuracy of navigation that can help mitigate the risk of errant instrumentation placement.

COMPLICATIONS
Neurological

A common finding in the immediate postoperative period is mild transient hip flexor weakness, which is likely secondary to trauma to the psoas muscle during the approach. In almost all cases, weakness has resolved by the 3-month postoperative follow-up.[19] However, rates of persistent motor weakness and sensory deficits at 18 months of follow-up are approximately 3% and 9%, respectively.[20,21] Femoral nerve injury is an especially serious complication that can result from either direct laceration or focal compression and retraction of the nerve. The risk of this complication is greatest at the L4/5 level. Femoral nerve injury resulting in persistent motor weakness of 3/5 or worse on the Medical Research Council Scale for Muscle Strength at 6 weeks of follow-up has been reported in approximately 2.6% of patients.[19] Stimulation with directional EMG and a reduction in total retraction time can help to prevent femoral nerve injury, especially when working at the L4/5 level.

Vascular

One of the advantages of the lateral approach over an anterior approach is that the great vessels can be avoided. Although the positioning of the great vessels is of greater significance for the anterior lumbar interbody fusion and antepsoas approaches given the nature of those surgical corridors, the positioning of these vessels should still be assessed before performing the transpsoas approach. The preoperative MRI should be carefully reviewed to ensure that the aorta, vena cava, and iliac arteries and veins are not laterally displaced. The laterality of the great vessels is one factor that can help determine the most suitable side of approach. However, a left-sided approach is often preferred because the common iliac vein is more prominent on the right side, and this approach also avoids retraction on the liver and injury to the vena cava. Although the incidence of vascular injury is very low, with reports ranging from 0.03% to 0.4%, there have been reports of severe complications from vascular injury related to unfixed retractor blades and postoperative

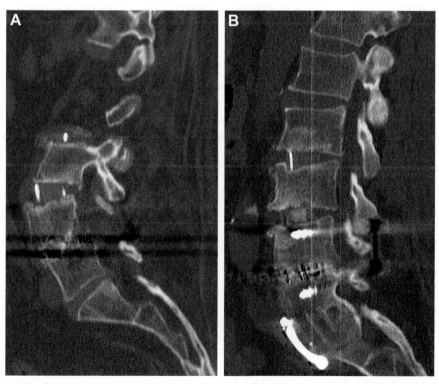

Fig. 3. Sagittal CT of interbody subsidence at L3–4 (*A*) and L2–3 (*B*). In both cases, the interbody graft has subsided into the inferior endplate of the grafted level. (Used with permission from Ohiorhenuan IE, Walker CT, Zhou JJ, Godzik J, Sagar S, Farber SH, Uribe JS. Predictors of subsidence after lateral lumbar interbody fusion. J Neurosurg Spine. 2022;37:183–187.)

anterior cage migration.[22,23] Finally, careful inspection of the tissue as the retractor is being withdrawn to ensure that there is no bleeding is critical to prevent postoperative psoas hematomas that present as worsening weakness or hemorrhagic shock in severe cases.

Visceral

As is the case for vascular injury, the risk of bowel injury or perforation is low but care should be taken during the operation to ensure protection of the viscera, which includes the complete development of the retroperitoneal space during the approach. Additionally, the surgeon should protect the peritoneum anteriorly with their finger when inserting dilators and the retractor to prevent injury.

Subsidence

Subsidence is a well-known phenomenon that can occur in patients undergoing LLIF and is characterized by the settling of the interbody cage into the endplates (**Fig. 3**). The loss of disc and foraminal height from subsidence effectively offsets the indirect decompression achieved with surgery and can cause a return of the patient's symptoms. Subsidence occurs in approximately 11% of patients who undergo LLIF.[24,25] Multiple studies have reported that higher rates of subsidence are associated with interbody cages with an 18-mm width, as opposed to those with 22-mm or 26-mm widths.[25,26] Using wider cages is thought to increase the total surface area the cage spans across the endplates, with a larger portion of the cage residing along the strong epiphyseal ring. Additionally, great care should be taken during the operation to always insert instruments into the disc space parallel to the endplate. This technique prevents violation of the endplate and intraoperative subsidence.

CLINICS CARE POINTS

- Aligning the intraoperative image to be perpendicular to the endplates is paramount. Otherwise, the surgeon could violate the endplate during the procedure and cause graft subsidence.

- Retraction time is exceedingly critical to prevent postoperative neuropraxia or permanent deficits due to ischemia of the lumbar plexus. This principle is especially important at the L4/5 level to prevent femoral nerve injury. We aim for approximately 15 minutes of retraction time per level.

- Do not use grafts that are too large. Although restoration of disc height is the primary goal of surgery, being too aggressive with the interbody cage height can increase the risk of endplate injury and subsidence.

- Interbody cages with a width of at least 22 mm should be used when possible to reduce the risk of cage subsidence.

DISCLOSURE

Dr J.S. Uribe serves as a consultant for Viseon, Inc (Irvine, CA); Misonix, Inc (Farmingdale, NY); SI-BONE (Santa Clara, CA); and AlphaTec Holdings, Inc (San Diego, CA). He receives royalties from SI-BONE, and he has stock and receives stock options and research support from AlphaTec Holdings.

FINANCIAL SUPPORT

None.

ACKNOWLEDGMENTS

The authors thank the staff of Neuroscience Publications at Barrow Neurological Institute for assistance with article preparation.

REFERENCES

1. McAfee PC, Regan JJ, Geis WP, et al. Minimally invasive anterior retroperitoneal approach to the lumbar spine. Emphasis on the lateral BAK. Spine 1998;23(13):1476–84.
2. Ozgur BM, Aryan HE, Pimenta L, et al. Extreme Lateral Interbody Fusion (XLIF): a novel surgical technique for anterior lumbar interbody fusion. Spine J 2006;6(4):435–43.
3. Grant JP, Oxland TR, Dvorak MF. Mapping the structural properties of the lumbosacral vertebral endplates. Spine 2001;26(8):889–96.
4. Kwon B, Kim DH. Lateral lumbar interbody fusion: indications, outcomes, and complications. J Am Acad Orthop Surg 2016;24(2):96–105.
5. Lehmen JA, Gerber EJ. MIS lateral spine surgery: a systematic literature review of complications, outcomes, and economics. Eur Spine J 2015; 24(Suppl 3):287–313.
6. Pereira EA, Farwana M, Lam KS. Extreme lateral interbody fusion relieves symptoms of spinal stenosis and low-grade spondylolisthesis by indirect decompression in complex patients. J Clin Neurosci 2017; 35:56–61.
7. Turner JD, Akbarnia BA, Eastlack RK, et al. Radiographic outcomes of anterior column realignment

for adult sagittal plane deformity: a multicenter analysis. Eur Spine J 2015;24(Suppl 3):427–32.

8. Leveque JC, Yanamadala V, Buchlak QD, et al. Correction of severe spinopelvic mismatch: decreased blood loss with lateral hyperlordotic interbody grafts as compared with pedicle subtraction osteotomy. Neurosurg Focus 2017;43(2):E15.

9. Bhatti AUR, Cesare J, Wahood W, et al. Assessing the differences in operative and patient-reported outcomes between lateral approaches for lumbar fusion: a systematic review and indirect meta-analysis. J Neurosurg Spine 2022;1–17. https://doi.org/10.3171/2022.2.SPINE211164.

10. Walker CT, Farber SH, Cole TS, et al. Complications for minimally invasive lateral interbody arthrodesis: a systematic review and meta-analysis comparing prepsoas and transpsoas approaches. J Neurosurg Spine 2019;1–15. https://doi.org/10.3171/2018.9.SPINE18800.

11. Walker CT, Farber SH, Gandhi S, et al. Single-Position Prone Lateral Interbody Fusion Improves Segmental Lordosis in Lumbar Spondylolisthesis. World Neurosurg 2021;151:e786–92.

12. Mobbs RJ, Phan K, Malham G, et al. Lumbar interbody fusion: techniques, indications and comparison of interbody fusion options including PLIF, TLIF, MI-TLIF, OLIF/ATP, LLIF and ALIF. J Spine Surg 2015;1(1):2–18.

13. Alan N, Kanter JJ, Puccio L, et al. Transitioning from lateral to the prone transpsoas approach: flatten the learning curve by knowing the nuances. Neurosurg Focus Video 2022;7(1):V8.

14. Wang MY, Mummaneni PV. Minimally invasive surgery for thoracolumbar spinal deformity: initial clinical experience with clinical and radiographic outcomes. Neurosurg Focus 2010;28(3):E9.

15. Rodgers WB, Gerber EJ, Patterson J. Intraoperative and early postoperative complications in extreme lateral interbody fusion: an analysis of 600 cases. Spine 2011;36(1):26–32.

16. Uribe JS, Vale FL, Dakwar E. Electromyographic monitoring and its anatomical implications in minimally invasive spine surgery. Spine 2010;35(26 Suppl):S368–74.

17. Joseph JR, Smith BW, Patel RD, et al. Use of 3D CT-based navigation in minimally invasive lateral lumbar interbody fusion. J Neurosurg Spine 2016;25(3):339–44.

18. Rudy RF, Farber SH, Godzik J, et al. Technique for validation of intraoperative navigation in minimally invasive spine surgery. Oper Neurosurg (Hagerstown) 2023;24(4):451–4.

19. Abel NA, Januszewski J, Vivas AC, et al. Femoral nerve and lumbar plexus injury after minimally invasive lateral retroperitoneal transpsoas approach: electrodiagnostic prognostic indicators and a roadmap to recovery. Neurosurg Rev 2018;41(2):457–64.

20. Tohmeh AG, Rodgers WB, Peterson MD. Dynamically evoked, discrete-threshold electromyography in the extreme lateral interbody fusion approach. J Neurosurg Spine 2011;14(1):31–7.

21. Salzmann SN, Shue J, Hughes AP. Lateral lumbar interbody fusion-outcomes and complications. Curr Rev Musculoskelet Med 2017;10(4):539–46.

22. Aichmair A, Fantini GA, Garvin S, et al. Aortic perforation during lateral lumbar interbody fusion. J Spinal Disord Tech 2015;28(2):71–5.

23. Assina R, Majmundar NJ, Herschman Y, et al. First report of major vascular injury due to lateral transpsoas approach leading to fatality. J Neurosurg Spine 2014;21(5):794–8.

24. Ohiorhenuan IE, Walker CT, Zhou JJ, et al. Predictors of subsidence after lateral lumbar interbody fusion. J Neurosurg Spine 2022;1–5. https://doi.org/10.3171/2022.1.SPINE201893.

25. Agarwal N, White MD, Zhang X, et al. Impact of endplate-implant area mismatch on rates and grades of subsidence following stand-alone lateral lumbar interbody fusion: an analysis of 623 levels. J Neurosurg Spine 2020;1–5. https://doi.org/10.3171/2020.1.SPINE19776.

26. Lang G, Navarro-Ramirez R, Gandevia L, et al. Elimination of subsidence with 26-mm-wide cages in extreme lateral interbody fusion. World Neurosurg 2017;104:644–52.

Antepsoas Approaches to the Lumbar Spine

Travis S. CreveCoeur, MD[a], Colin P. Sperring, BS[a], Anthony M. DiGiorgio, DO, MHA[b],
Dean Chou, MD[c], Andrew K. Chan, MD[d],*

KEYWORDS

- Lumbar interbody fusion (LIF) • Anterior to the psoas (ATP) approach
- Oblique lateral interbody fusion (OLIF) • Minimally invasive • Pre-psoas

KEY POINTS

- The ATP approach provides favorable clinical and radiographical outcomes in well-selected cases, while sparing the psoas muscle and, for many surgeons, obviating the need for neuromonitoring.
- The ATP approach is associated with a relatively low complication rate. Transient leg weakness and sensory changes are the most common complications after surgery. Unique complications—although rare—include vascular injury, ureteral injury, and sympathetic chain injury.
- Recent advancements such as navigation and robotic assistance improve the safety and efficiency of the ATP approach.

INTRODUCTION/HISTORY/DEFINITIONS/BACKGROUND

Lumbar interbody fusion (LIF) has been a cornerstone of treatment for patients with degenerative disease pathology for decades. For the majority of its existence, LIF has been accomplished via posterior-approach surgery. However, as LIF became an increasingly common method of lumbar arthrodesis, there has been growing interest in less invasive approaches, leading to innovations in the techniques used for LIF. These advancements, such as the transforaminal, lateral (ie, transpsoas), and oblique [i.e., anterior to psoas (ATP)] approaches, have added to the more traditional anterior and posterior approaches.

Originally described by Capener in 1932, anterior lumbar interbody fusion (ALIF) is an alternative to the posterior approach as it avoids extensive parasinal muscle dissection and permits the implanation of taller cages with larger footprints.[1,2] The anterior approach offers (1) a direct, wide visualization of the disc space, facilitating more complete discectomy and end-plate preparation and (2) the ability to place taller, lordotic cages to aid in better restoration of disc height and segmental lordosis.[3] By avoiding a posterior dissection, it may lead to less postoperative axial back pain and a reduced risk of adjacent segmental disease.[4] However, the anterior approach necessitates the dissection and mobilization of the peritoneum and prevertebral vessels, which may require an access surgeon to perform the approach and a risk of injury to the vessels and nearby structures (eg, ureter, sympathetic plexus).[5–8]

In 1997, Mayer modified the ALIF approach to include an anterolateral approach.[1] ATP interbody fusion has become an increasingly popular alternative to ALIF, offering a minimally invasive approach for interbody fusion from L1-S1.[1,9] The lumbar spine is accessed via the anterior oblique

[a] Department of Neurological Surgery, Neurological Institute of New York, Columbia University College of Physicians and Surgeons, 710 West 168th Street, New York, NY 10033, USA; [b] Department of Neurological Surgery, University of California San Francisco, San Francisco, CA 94143, USA; [c] Department of Neurological Surgery, Neurological Institute of New York, Columbia University College of Physicians and Surgeons, 5141 Broadway, New York, NY 10034, USA; [d] Department of Neurological Surgery, Neurological Institute of New York, Columbia University College of Physicians and Surgeons, 5141 Broadway, 3FW, Room 20, New York, NY 10034, USA

* Corresponding author. NewYork-Presbyterian Och Spine Hospital, 5141 Broadway, New York, NY 10034.
E-mail address: akc2136@cumc.columbia.edu

Neurosurg Clin N Am 34 (2023) 619–632
https://doi.org/10.1016/j.nec.2023.06.009
1042-3680/23/© 2023 Elsevier Inc. All rights reserved.

approach, which avoids the psoas muscle and the abdominal vessels. Its advantages include the sparing of the psoas muscle and lumbar plexus, access to L4-L5 and L5-S1 regardless of the anatomy of the iliac crest, and direct visualization of critical structures.[10–12] Further, with avoidance of a transpsoas approach—and thereby, risk of injury to the lumbar plexus—there is a decreased need for neuromonitoring.[13] A summary of all the approaches are pictured in **Fig. 1**.[14]

Both ATP interbody fusion and ALIF are techniques that may provide indirect decompression. Indirect decompression allows for decompression of the spinal canal and foramina by restoring disk height, reducing spondylolisthesis, and stabilizing the vertebral segment, without directly removing the compressive bony or discoligamentous tissue (ie, direct decompression).[15]

In this article, we will cover the indications of ATP approaches for spinal fusion, its relevant anatomy, preprocedural and intraoperative preparation, outcomes, recovery, complications, and future directions.

INDICATIONS AND CONTRAINDICATIONS

The ATP approach for fusion is suitable for a number of diverse pathologies including degenerative spondylosis, lateral olisthesis, spondylolisthesis (Meyerding Type 1, 2, or 3 in certain cases), mild to moderate spinal central, lateral recess, or foraminal stenosis, and scoliosis.[16–19] It may be used to treat more extensive central, lateral recess, or foraminal stenosis if combined with a

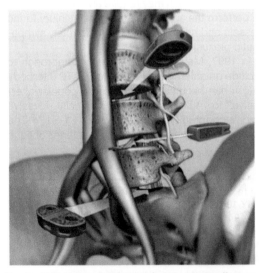

Fig. 1. ALIF, LLIF and ATP, TLIF fusion; Minimally invasive interbody approaches: anterior (ALIF), lateral (LLIF, and ATP), and osterior (TLIF). Copyright to Praveen V. Mummaneni.

direct decompression. The ATP approach for spinal fusion offers the ability to achieve both sagittal and coronal corrections, especially for those patients with degenerative lumbar scoliosis with lateral-olisthesis or lateral ostephytes.[14,16,20]

Patients with spontaneous autofusion of the interverbal space or posterior facet joint ankylosis are not generally not candidates for ATP interbody fusion, as they require a three column osteotomy to achieve correction. Following the minimally invasive spinal deformity (MISDEF) classification system, these patients are classifed as Type III, and may require a more extensive spinal fusion for stablization after the osteotomy.[21] Furthermore, spondylolisthesis greater than Meyerding grade II is also technically difficult due to the overlap of the segmental endplates that may not be sufficient enough to support an interbody disc, as well as the spondylolistehsis obscuring the surgical corridor secondary to the anteriorly displaced femoral plexus.[16,22]

Subsidence can occur due to poor bone mineral density (T values < -1) or violation during endplate preparation. The fragility of the endplate is tied to patient bone quality. Thus, standalone constructs should be avoided in patients with osteoporosis. Rather, these patients should receive bilateral transpedicular screw fixation or avoid fusion surgery altogether until bone density can reach satisfactory levels.[23]

ANATOMY

At incision, the first muscle layers encountered are the external oblique, internal oblique, and transversus abdominis muscles, covered by the transversalis fascia.

The ATP approach uses a retroperitoneal oblique corridor between the psoas major muscle and the great vessels (when accessing L2-L5) and between the bifurcated iliac vessels (when accessing L5-S1).[24] The psoas muscle is positioned laterally, while the vessels are positioned medially.[9] The ATP approach should only be performed from the left side; as it cannot easily be performed from the right side due to the position of iliac vessels and the presence of the inferior vena cava on the right side which can easily tear with manipulation. Thus the left sided approach offers an easier and safer corridor between the aorta and the psoas muscle. A left-sided approach is also used given its larger area (see **Fig. 1**) and fewer anatomic variations.[9] The corridor itself can be as wide as 16 mm at L2-L3, but narrows to 10 mm at more caudal levels.[25] However, this corridor can be expanded with careful dissection and mobilization of the vessels and psoas muscle.

In cadaveric studies conducted by Davis and colleagues,[9] the average width of operation windows from L2-L5 range from 24.45 to 27.00 mm with mild retraction on the psoas muscle. In a recent study by Deng and colleagues, they found the average width of the operative window to be narrower, ranging from 16.6 to 20.27 mm. Specifically, at L4-L5, the average width was 16.6 mm and increased to 26 mm with the retraction of the psoas major.[20,26]

The lumbar plexus lies within the psoas major, and caution must be given when retracting the muscle. The plexus starts more posterior at proximal levels and then moves more anterior distally.[27,28] This plexus is a collection of nerves arising from a contribution of the subcostal nerve, the anterior divisions of the first three lumbar nerves, and the greater part of the fourth lumbar nerve. It is a retroperitoneal structure which is situated posteriorly, anterior to the transverse processes of then lumbar vertebrae, and within the psoas major muscle.[29]

From a lateral decubitus position, the lumbar plexus is located in the posterior fourth of the vertebral body and dorsally. The nerves pass obliquely outward from the vertebral body, then behind and through the psoas muscle. While passing through the psoas, nerves distribute filaments within the muscle. Distal members of the plexus have been shown to marginate anteriorly as they descend within the muscle at descending disc spaces.[29] For example, the femoral nerve, the largest branch of the lumbar plexus and formed by roots of L2, L3 and L4, is found deep within the psoas muscle moving in a posterior-to-anterior trajectory as it reaches the L4–5 disc space. As it continues to descend, it travels between the psoas and iliacus muscles, under the inguinal ligament and into the upper leg, where it splits into the anterior cutaneous and muscular branches.[29]

The sensory nerves arising from L1, the ilioinguinal and iliohypogastric, as well as the lateral femoral cutaneous nerve arising from L2 and L3 emerge from the posterolateral border of the psoas major. They then travel obliquely into the retroperitoneal space, crossing in front of the quadratus lumborum and the iliacus muscles eventually reaching the iliac crest The ilioinguinal and iliohypogastric nerves, coming off of the L1 nerve root, may cross deep to the internal oblique at the L4-L5 level and should be avoided during dissection. The genitofemoral nerve, arising from L1 and L2, is the exception. Starting at its origin, it travels obliquely through the psoas, traveling across the L2-3 disc space and then emerging at the medial border anterior and superficial at the L3-L4 level. Next, it descends along the surface of the psoas and on the anterior quarter of the L4 and L5 vertebral bodies. It splits into the spermatic and lumboinguinal nerves, which innervate the skin around the inguinal and genital region as well as the anterior and medial portion of the upper thigh respectively.[29]

Further, Uribe and colleagues[29] created an anatomical zoning system, which provides safe zones relative to disc spaces to prevent nerve injuries during the transpsoas approach which is tantamount in understanding relative anatomy in the ATP approach. They found that all of the nerve roots could be found within Zone IV, the posterior fourth of the vertebral body. Specifically, at levels L1-L2, all of the respective nerve roots (the L1 root, iliohyopgastric and ilioinguinal) were found posteriorly in Zone IV. At levels L2-L3, all of the nerve roots (L2 root) were found within Zone IV, except for the genitofemoral nerve, which was found in Zone II, the middle anterior quarter. At levels L3-L4, all of the never roots (L2 division, L3 root, and the lateral cutaneous nerve) were found within Zone IV. However, the genitofemoral nerve was found within Zone I, the anterior quarter. At levels L4-L5, the L2 and L3 divisions as well as the L4 root, which together make up the femoral nerve, the obturator nerve and the branches to the psoas were found within both Zone IV and Zone III, the posterior middle quarter.[29]

While there typically are not any major vessels encountered, they should be repected to avoid injury. The positions of the abdominal aorta and the IVC may vary in different individuals and segments. There have been some reports that these large vessels are not entirely in front of the anterior tangent of the vertebral body. The position of the abdominal aorta at L1–5 may occasionally cover part of Zone I, while on the right side of the vertebral body, the inferior vena cava trunk may also partly cover Zone I.

The shape and relationship of the psoas muscle to nearby structures affects the approach used. The psoas major muscle is divided into 2 parts: the superficial and deep parts. The superficial psoas major originates from T12-L4 and the neighboring intervertebral discs. The deep psoas major originates from the transverse processes of L1-4. Fibers of psoas major are oriented inferolateral and come together as a common tendon that descends over the pubis and shares a common insertion with the iliacus muscle on the lesser trochanter of the femur.

In patients with aberrant anatomy such as in patients with scoliosis, the space between the vessels and the psoas muscle may vary. When the psoas major muscle rises laterally or anteriorly at the L4-5 disc level and detaches from the most posterior aspect of the L4-5 disc space despite the absence of transitional vertebrae, this instance is called the "rising psoas sign."[30] The rising psoas sign is related to a higher pelvic incidence and lumbar scoliosis.[31] The space between the psoas muscle and the quadratus lumbourm muscle may increase in some patients, which could lead to mistaking this gap for cooridor between the artery and the psoas muscle. Different positions have an influence on the shape of the psoas muscle. In the right decubitus position, the left psoas major muscle is affected by gravity and is closer to the vertebral body. Hip flexion and knee flexion will also relax the psoas major muscle, thus increasing the cross-sectional area of the psoas major muscle.[21] In contrast, a neutral hip position will decrease the cross-sectional area of the psoas major muscle and widen the corridor between the psoas muscle and the artery.

Mai and colleagues,[32] reviewing magnetic resonance (MR) imaging from 180 patients, set out to define some of the anatomic variations among patients undergoing a lateral LIF. They found that vascular anatomy on the right side was significantly more variant than anatomy on the left. Thus, giving more reasons why the ATP approach is preferably performed from the left. Additionally, age was associated with increased variability of vascular anatomy bilaterally, and the presence of bowel within the operative corridor correlated with BMI. Lastly, amongst age-disturbed patients who underwent lumbar MR imaging, the rising psoas sign was seen in 26.1% of patients.[32]

PRE-operative/Pre-PROCEDURE PLANNING

In pre-procedural planning, lumbar arterial and venous vessels should first be identified on MR imaging to confirm a safe corridor. Their posterior and lateral migration on the side contralateral to the approach should also be appreciated.[33] Each patient may present with unique local anatomy, thus careful assessment of the imaging is crucial. Wang and colleagues reviewed MR imaging of the lumbar region of 300 patients. They found that the location of the left major psoas and major vasculature varied widely across a number of vertically and horizontally defined zones at L2-L3, L3-L4, and L4-L5.[34] The size of corridor can be measured from the psoas anteriorly and the left lateral border of the anterior vessels. However, one must remember that the retraction of the psoas muscle allows for a more flexible corridor size.[3] Corridor distance has been shown to vary by side, age, and disc level.[35] Mean widths of the corridor narrows at lower lumbar disc levels. Left-sided corridors are wider at all lumbar levels, and widths increase with age.[35]

One the advantages of the ATP approach is its reduced rate of lumbar plexus injury,[10–12] However, it is still paramount to appreciate lumbar plexus anatomy when reviewing MR imaging especially in cases of abbrent anatomy. The lumbar plexus often migrates anteriorly in patients with transitional vertebrae, especially at L5-L6 in the instances of patients with 6 lumbar vertebrae. Therefore, for risk management, it is important to evaluate the psoas major, especially for a rising psoas, and its surrounding structures before.[31]

Typically, the visualization of an unobstructed corridor in the pre-operative MR imaging is required to proceed with the ATP approach.[36] However, this assessment is often subjective and can change based on the surgeon experience.[37] Molinares and colleagues,[25] reviewing previous MR imaging, set out to define the safe corridors across patient populations. They found that 90% of cases involving L2-L5 and 69% of cases involving L5-S1 have a safe operative corridor.[25] The major vessels that overlie the intervertebral disc at L5-S1 may contribute towards the discrepancy in safety.[38] Additionally, the right lateral decubital position, and its associated downward migration of the left common iliac vein, may further decrease this corridor.[39] Pictured in **Fig. 2** are the pre-operative films showing an appropriate window for L4-5 ATP approach for fusion.

In 2003, Moro and colleagues[40] set out to define anatomical parameters to clarify safety zones in retroperitoneal endoscopic surgery. The classification name has been aptly named Moro's classification and divides the lumbar intervertebral space into six zones starting with A (anteriorly), I, II, II, IV and P (posteriorly).[40] In 2020, Ng and colleagues[41] modified Moro's to objectively measure the feasibility of the ATP approach at the L4-L5 level. In their system, the corridor was graded from 0 to 3, where 0 is considered no corridor. Psoas classification was included to clarify difficult to pass anatomy (ie high-rising psoas). They proposed that an inoperable corridor was defined as either having a corridor score of 0 or a high riding psoas. Applying this methodology to their patient cohort, they found that 10.5% of patients did not have a measurable corridor, confirming similar results from Molinares and colleagues.[25] Further, 20% of patients had a high-rising psoas. Together, they found that 25% of patients did not have corridor appropriate for the ATP approach. Follow-up studies have examined the reliability of the modified Moro's classification system, and gradings were found to be consistent and highly reliable.[37]

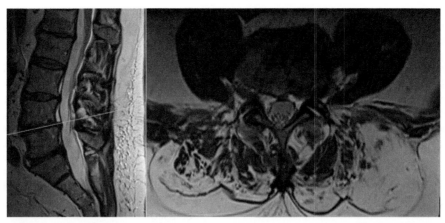

Fig. 2. *MR imaging of corridor window;* MR sagittal and axial cuts of a patient who underwent ATP fusion to L4-5. There is lateral listhesis at L4-5. There is vacuum change in L4-5 disc space, as well as up-down foraminal stenosis at L4-5 (not pictured on parasagittal views) as well as auto-fusion at L5-S1. There are no no vessels obstructing the corridor to access the L4-5 disc space. This patient underwent successful fusion with percutaneous posterior fusion.

Liu and colleagues[42] proposed an alternative methodology where, at each vertebral level, intervertebral space anatomy is categorized into the following sections: the vascular window, bare window, psoas major window, ideal operative window, and actual operative window. Ultimately, they found that, at the L4-L5 level, 6.7% of their population did not have an appropriate corridor, a smaller proportion when compared to Ng and colleagues and Molinares and colleagues.[25,41,42] Together, these studies indicate that despite attempts at objective classification systems, intra-reliability among systems remains inconsistent.

Vascular structures should be assessed using axial and sagittal MR imaging, and the following features should be considered: location of the left common iliac vein, size of the vascular corridor, and the presence of a fat plane (best viewed on T1 imaging) between the left common iliac vein and the intervertebral disc.[24,38] Segmental artery anatomy must also be appreciated. Segmental arteries specifically at the L5 level have a high rate of adjacency to the intervertebral disc, interfering with the surgical site and increasing the risk of hemorrhage.[43]

Alternatives to an ATP approach should be considered if the left common iliac vein crosses the midline, if the vascular corridor is narrow or if a fat plane is absent.[24,38,44] Lastly, accessing the L5-S1 level is not possible when the angle of L5-S1 intervertebral disc in the sagittal plane goes underneath the symphysis bone.[24,38] Similarly, when planning the approach for L4-L5, extra consideration must be paid as the corridor may be obstructed by vascular vessels or a high-riding psoas muscle.[41] In this circumstance, the corridor may be improved by an optimized incision site and placement of the patient in the lateral decubitus position.

Cage subsidence can lead to poor clinical and radiological outcomes, and may be a sequelae of poor bone quality or endplate injury.[24,45] Pre-operative bone density scan may be helpful in preventing this complication. Additionally, hounsfield units (HUs) from preoperative CT imaging can be used to estimate the strength of the endplates. Studies have found that low HUs at the ipsilateral epiphyseal ring were an independent risk factor for endplate violation, and low HUs at the central endplate were associated with delayed cage subsidence.[46,47] Thus, bone density and HUs of the endplate are strong predictors of intraoperative endplate violation and delayed cage subsidence, and should be considered in preprocedural planning, preoperative optimization with anabolic agents for osteoporosis, and during endplate preparation. Observation of modic changes on endplates, or preoperative endplate sclerosis, can also help prevent cage subsidience.[48]

ATP approaches with stand-alone cages, and without posterior fixation, have been shown to be a reasonably safe and effecacious option for a group of well-selected patients.[49] However, a number of studies have reported instances where ATP fusion with stand-alone cages was insufficient.[50,51] Guo and colleagues[51] compared range-of-motion (ROM), stress of the cage and stress of fixation among the stand-alone model, the lateral rod-screw model, the lateral rod-screw plus contralateral translaminar facet screw model, the unilateral pedicle screw model, and the bilateral pedicle screw (BPS) model. They found that bilateral pedicle screw (BPS) fixation had the lowest ROM, stress of the cage, and stress of fixation, and thus provided the greatest stability. Meanwhile, the stand-alone model had the greatest ROM and cage stress, which they ultimately decided was insufficient and placed the cage at risk for subsidence.[51] Song and colleagues[52] similarly showed the superiority of BPS in both normal and osteoporotic vertebrae. Thus, stand-alone constructs may be less appropriate for patients with heightened risk of subsidence, such as those with poor bone quality.

PREP AND PATIENT POSITIONING

ATP approach to spinal fusion should be performed with the patient placed in the right lateral decubitus position. Once again, the ATP approach should only be performed from the left side, as a right sided ATP approach would be too high risk to manipulation to the right-sided position of the inferior vena cava.[1,53,54] The ipsilateral leg can be extended at the hip-knee to stretch the psoas and reduce its girth, thereby potentially reducing the need for retraction.[55] Kotheeranurak and colleagues found that the surgical corridor in the neutral hip position was significantly larger than the flexed position at all levels. Further, anterior thickness and cross-sectional area of the psoas muscle were minimized in the neutral position.[56]

The table should be radiolucent for radiographic visualization and arranged in a slight Trendelenburg. The patient's bony prominences should be padded and body fastened with adhesive drapes to avoid manipulation. A 270-degree prep and drape should be used to allow for both abdominal and posterior access if needed.[57] Anterior-posterior (AP) and lateral fluoroscopic projections should be confirmed to be working effectively before starting the surgery in the given set up. The bed should be positioned so that true AP and lateral images are obtained. Such imaging can also be used to mark the anterior, midpoint, and posterior of the intervertebral space of interest on the skin. The levels of the disc spaces should also be marked following fluoroscopic confirmation.[58] The iliac crest, anterior superior iliac spine, and twelfth rib should also be marked. A typical patient set up is pictured in **Fig. 3**, performed at our institution.

PROCEDURAL APPROACH

- 4 to 6 cm incision should be made following splitting dissection of externaloblique, internal oblique and transversalis.[55,57]

- Transversalis should be split carefully posteriorly to anteriorly to avoid injury to the peritoneum.
- Iliohypogastric and ilioingual nerves may also be present below the internal oblique, and should be avoided.
- Retroperitoneal fat is identified, peritoneum is pushed anteriorly with tonsil sponges, and the psoas major belly is exposed. The psoas major will be the lateral border of the surgical corridor.
- Perivascular fat of the major vessels anterior to the psoas is identified. The surgical corridor is created with blunt and gentle dissection. Tonsil sponges and bipolar cautery may also be used.
- Typically, for cases involving levels L1-L4, ligation of segmental vessels is not necessary.
- The appropriate target level is confirmed by imaging.
- The discectomy is performed, while making sure to preserve the vertebral endplates.
- The endplates are prepared, with extreme care to avoid endplate violation.
- The anterior longitudinal ligament should not be released to avoid anterior "spitting out" of the cage. Intentional ALL release has different indications described elsewhere.
- Appropriate cage dimensions should be determined based on intraoperative trial sizing and preoperative measurement or planning.
- Graft material is added to the cage and the cage is inserted with the aid of imaging.
- Once the cage is confirmed to be in the correct place by imaging, the retroperitoneal space should be evaluated for any active bleeding and major structures should be examined to ensure integrity. The abdominal muscles and soft tissue can then be closed in layers.
- For posterior fixation, the patient can then placed prone on a Jackson frame table or simultaneous or sequential single position surgery, also in the lateral position, may be chosen.
- The pedicle screw-rods system is placed, a direct decompression may be completed as well from the posterior approach along with a posterolateral arthrodesis if desired

Pictured later in discussion in **Fig. 4** are pre-operative and post-operative standing films of the patient undergoing an ATP approach for fusion at L4-5.

RECOVERY, POST-PROCEDURE CARE, AND REHABILITATION/MANAGEMENT

Several studies have shown that the ATP approach may have lower complications rates when

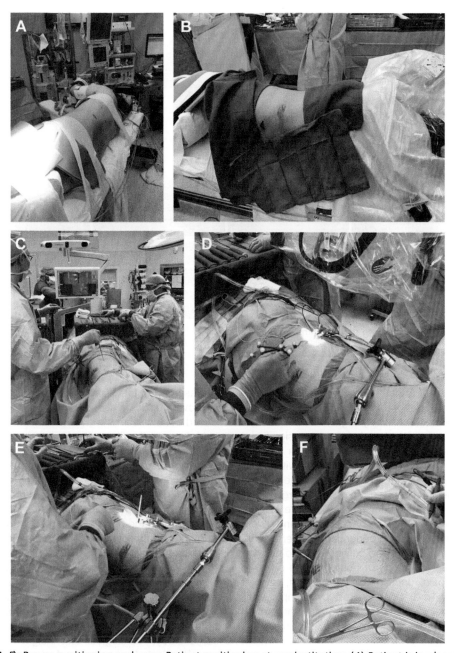

Fig. 3. (A–F): Pre-op positioning and prep; Patient positioning at our institution: (A) Patient is in placed in right lateral decubitus position, all pressure points appropriately padded and patient is strapped in. The incision is marked. (B) The patient is sterily drapped, with the appropriate marking of the intervertebral space of interst isted. (C) Navigation is used to confirm the levels of interest (D) After incision and retroperitoneal dissection, a retractor access system is used, navigation is once again used to confirm location. (E) Subsequent disckectomy is performed (F) Patient is closed in usual multilayer cosure, the patient is then turned prone for posterior instrumented fusion.

compared to transpsoas LLIF and ALIF.[55,59] Specifically, ATP fusion may have lower rates of peritoneal laceration and sensory nerve injury.[59] However, deep vein thrombosis (DVT) and lower extremity atrophy have been reported to occur following ATP fusion.[60]

Wang and colleagues[60] compared patients with ATP fusion who underwent lower extremity rehab for three months to patients with ATP fusion who did not receive any postoperative rehab. They found that within the first two weeks, patients undergoing rehab had lower total pain and lower

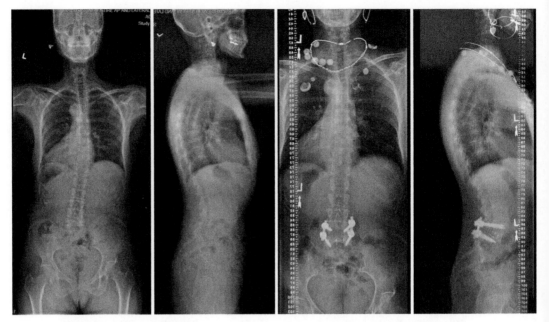

Fig. 4. Pre and poststanding scoliosis films.

back pain compared to the control patients. However, after one month of rehab, they no longer experienced a statistically significant advantage. Those same patients also had a significant improvement in disability scores, but for only the first week. DVTs were lower in those with rehab at both one week after surgery and three months after surgery. At three months after surgery, the decrease in the incidence of DVTs were statistically significant. Lastly, those who underwent postoperative rehab experienced greater patient satisfaction.[60] Wang and colleagues also demonstrated the importance of postoperative rehab in improving pain, function, and satisfaction, but their study may have been limited by sample size. Further studies are required to better understand the necessary duration of lower extremity rehabilitation.

OUTCOMES

A number of clinical studies have reported ATP fusion to be a safe and effective option for LLIF. Ohtori and colleagues[61] examined patients receiving ATP fusion for degenerated lumbar spinal kyphoscoliosis. They found pain and balance scores were significantly improved after surgery, and fusion rates were 90%. Among the 12 patients, there were no major complications. Similarly, in a separate study, Ohtori and colleagues, reviewing 35 patients with spinal degeneration

disease, found that pain scores were significantly improved following surgery and no patient experienced a major complication.

More recently different groups have compared ATP fusion to other approaches of lumbar interbody approaches. Compared to transpsoas LLIF, ATP fusion's hypothetical advantages are avoidance of direct injury to the psoas muscle and, thus, decreased risk of lumbar plexus injury. However, injury to the plexus still can occur due to the retraction of the psoas.[27,29,62,63] A meta-analysis by Li and colleagues,[64] comprised of 56 studies, found that visual analog scale (VAS) and Oswestry Disability Index (ODI) were more improved in ATP fusion compared to transpsoas LLIF. Psoas injury, and the associated anterior thigh syndrome, were thought to contribute to these differences. In this same study, radiological disc height restoration was identical. However, the fusion rate among ATP fusion was 96.9%, while the fusion rate was 91.6% among transpsoas LLIF. Similar trends in fusion rates were reported in another meta-analysis by Souslian and Patel.[65] Further, Walker and colleagues[66] found that operation times were significantly shorter with ATP fusion when compared to transpsoas LLIF.

ATP fusion and ALIF are comparable options for L5-S1 fusion.[67,68] ALIF fusion involves a retro- or transperitoneal approach in the supine position to access L5-S1, while ATP involves a retroperitoneal approach from the lateral decubitus position.

Studies have reported conflicting benefits when comparing these two approaches, and no definitive conclusion can be made.[67,68]

COMPLICATIONS

The most common complications following ATP fusion are transient leg weakness and numbness most likely secondary to the retraction of the psoas muscle and sensory nerves. Fujibayashi and colleagues[59] set out to elucidate the complications associated with LLIF across institutions in Japan. Among 992 patients who underwent ATP fusion, 3.5% of patients experienced sensory nerve injury. The majority of these injuries were transient. Additionally, 3% experienced postoperative psoas weakness.[59] Digorgio and colleagues[69] found a similar rate of transient leg numbness, 6.1%, among their patient 49-pateint cohort. There have been reports of symptoms associated with anterior thigh syndrome–sensory deficit, hip flexion weakness, and pain, however studies have shown this can resolves after three to six months.[70]

Another complication, although less common, is vascular injury. In their study, Fujibayashi and colleagues[59] found that only 1 of the 992 patients experienced a major vascular injury. Tannoury and colleagues,[55] who retrospectively reviewed the complications of 940 patients with ATP fusion, found no major vascular injury. Mehren and colleagues,[71] having reviewed 812 patients, found only 3 instances of major vascular injury. Kim and colleagues,[24] reviewing 752 ATP fusion cases, similarly showed that only 3 cases involved major vascular injury. Preoperative planning involving the identification of major vessels and their proximity to the surgical corridor is paramount to avoid injury to the major vessels. Additionally, segmental arteries can also be injured and cause bleeding intraoperatively. Fujibayashi and colleagues reported an incidence of 0.7% among their 992 patients.[59]

Although intraoperative vascular injuries are rare in ATP fusion, patients remain at risk for deep vein thrombosis (DVT) of the lower extremities after surgery. Wang and colleagues[60], studying the effects of lower limb training during the postoperative period, reported a DVT rate of 16% within 1 week of surgery. Xi and colleagues[72], focusing only on patients who underwent ATP fusion with navigation, reported a much lower rate of DVT, 0.93%. Similarly, Oh and colleagues reported 0 incidences of DVT across 143 ATP fusion surgeries.[73] This reason for the discrepancy is unclear, but the reduced rate of DVT recorded in studies by Xi and

colleagues and Oh and colleagues may be due to poor patient follow-up after surgery.

The ureter may be encountered during the retroperitoneal approach as it is attached to the posterior wall of the peritoneum. Injury to the ureter has been reported in several case reports.[75,76] Fujibayashi and colleagues[59] reported a 0.3% incidence of ureteral injury. While, similar large cohort studies reported 0% incidence.[55] To avoid injury, the ureter should be swept anteriorly with the peritoneum, which should be directly visualized.

Direct bowel injury is extremely rare following ATP fusion.[55,59,77] Although not a direct injury, Tannoury and colleagues[55] reported one incidence of a major bowel complication due to superior mesenteric ischemia leading to eventual partial colectomy. Fujibayashi and colleagues[59] noted no instances of bowel injury in their 992-patient ATP fusion cohort. Similarly, postoperative abdominal wall hernias are rarely reported with a rate of 0% to 0.3%.[55,59,77]

Postoperative ileus (POI) remains a common complication in ATP.[55,71,77,78] In their 460-pateint study, Park and colleagues[78] reported a 3.9% rate of POI. Among these patients, intraoperative administration of remifentanil and inadvertent endplate fracture were identified as independent risk factors for POI. Additionally, POI increased length of stay.[78] Postoperative pain following fracture may stimulate inhibitory neurons and contribute to POI. Further, the release of cytokine and other inflammatory mediators following fracture may have effects on the nearby lumbar plexus.[24,78] Other studies have reported rates of POI ranging from 0.9% to 2.9%.[55,71,77,79]

Reported incidences of lesions to the sympathetic chain are varied across the literature. The "safety corridor" enclosed by the anterior longitudinal ligament medially and the psoas muscle laterally is lined with fibers of the sympathetic chain.[71] Varying rates of reported incidence could be due to slight inter-institutional differences. However, the clinical effects of the injuries are unclear as it has been reported that the sacrifice of the sympathetic chain only produced a "warming" of the affected leg that was unnoticed by the patient.

Cage subsidence is another debilitating complication of ATP fusion that may be associated with poor clinical and radiological outcomes, including the reduction of segmental lordosis, reversal of indirect decompression, and clinical recurrence of radiculopathy.[24,45] Among a 79-patient cohort, Cheng and colleagues[18] reported 10% experienced cage subsidence. For those patients with intraoperative violation of the endplates, the risk of subsidence increases to 18.7%.[74] Despite reported poor clinical and radiological measurements, leg pain, risk of revision surgery, and risk of pseudoarthrosis were found to not significantly increase when comparing ATP fusion with cage subsidence versus ATP without cage subsidence.[79–84] Large cohort studies are required to better understand that impact of cage subsidence in ATP fusion. To avoid endplate violation, and subsequent cage subsidence, bone quality should be assessed preoperatively and the disc space must be prepared with caution, employing serial implant trials and avoiding any excessive force along the endplate.[46,74]

FUTURE DEVELOPMENTS

Spinal navigation assistance systems have become an increasingly popular alternative to fluoroscopy in ATP fusion.[69,79,85] Xi and colleagues,[79] having reviewed over 200 cases with navigated ATP fusion, reported a high accuracy rate of 94.86%. Only one patient returned for revision surgery, and the rate of transient neurologic symptoms was 10.28%, within the normal expectations of ATP fusion surgery.[79] Navigated assistance was shown to be safe and effective. Further, its use reduces exposure to harmful radiation to the surgeon and operative staff. Additionally, the ATP approach allows for two sets of surgeons to perform ATP fusion and posterior fixation simultaneously during single-position surgery. Ouchida and colleagues[86] found that single-position ATP fusion led to less blood loss, time spent in the operating room and surgery time, while exhibiting comparable clinical outcomes.

Diaz-Aguilar and colleagues,[87] recently published the first instance of robot-assisted single-position ATP fusion with posterior fixation. They reported their procedures to have accurate screw placement of 95%, a shortened OR time of 112 minutes, and no major complications. However, a larger study comparing robot-assisted to more traditional ATP fusion is warranted to fully understand its benefits. This is especially important as surgeons embark on the learning curve.

Lastly, in select cases, spinal endoscopy has been added to the ATP approach to assist surgeons treating disk herniation and seeking direct decompression.[88] Without endoscopy, direct removal of these damaged particles may be inhibited by interference of tubular retractor or difficult-to-access deeply located disk. Further, blind removal of these particles cannot be safely performed. By adding a spinal endoscope, fragments can be removed directly under endoscopic visualization.

SUMMARY

ATP fusion is a safe and effective method of LLIF that has applications across a diverse array of pathologies including degenerative spondylosis, spondylolisthesis, spinal stenosis, and scoliosis.[16–19] Its advantages over alternative lumbar interbody fusion methods include avoiding transgression of the psoas muscle and avoiding the lumbar plexus, and possible increased accessibility to L4-5 compared to the transpsoas approach.[10–13] Before the procedure, it is critical that vasculature is identified and bone density is evaluated. Although it can only be performed from the left, it is an alternative to the transpsoas approach.

CLINICS CARE POINTS

- ATP interbody fusion is a minimally invasive lateral, retroperitoneal approach for performing lumbar interbody arthrodesis.
- The advantages of the ATP interbody approach is that it avoid transgression of the psoas muscle when performing an LLIF.
- Patients with severe central canal stenosis may require an additional direct (posterior) decompression.
- The size of the corridor, as well as the location of key vascular structures, should be identified on preoperative imaging, while bone density should be evaluated prior to surgery.
- Transient leg weakness and sensory loss are the most common complications following ATP interbody fusion.
- Intraoperative navigation, robotic-assistance, and single-position surgery are emerging additions to the ATP interbody approach that may potentially improve workflow and efficiency.

DISCLOSURES

The authors have nothing to disclose.

REFERENCES

1. Mayer HM. A new microsurgical technique for minimally invasive anterior lumbar interbody fusion. Spine 1997;22(6):691–9 [discussion: 700].
2. Capener N. Spondylolisthesis. BJS Br J Surg 1932; 19(75):374–86.
3. Quillo-Olvera J, Lin GX, Jo HJ, et al. Complications on minimally invasive oblique lumbar interbody fusion at L2–L5 levels: a review of the literature

and surgical strategies. Ann Transl Med 2018;6(6): 101.

4. Choi KC, Kim JS, Shim HK, et al. Changes in the adjacent segment 10 years after anterior lumbar interbody fusion for low-grade isthmic spondylolisthesis. Clin Orthop 2014;472(6):1845–54.

5. Rajaraman V, Vingan R, Roth P, et al. Visceral and vascular complications resulting from anterior lumbar interbody fusion. J Neurosurg 1999;91(1 Suppl):60–4.

6. Hijji FY, Narain AS, Bohl DD, et al. Lateral lumbar interbody fusion: a systematic review of complication rates. Spine J 2017;17(10):1412–9.

7. Tannoury C, Das A, Saade A, et al. The antepsoas (ATP) surgical corridor for lumbar and lumbosacral arthrodesis: a radiographic, anatomic, and surgical investigation. Spine 2022;47(15):1084–92.

8. Phillips FM, Isaacs RE, Rodgers WB, et al. Adult degenerative scoliosis treated with XLIF: clinical and radiographical results of a prospective multicenter study with 24-month follow-up. Spine 2013; 38(21):1853–61.

9. Davis TT, Hynes RA, Fung DA, et al. Retroperitoneal oblique corridor to the L2-S1 intervertebral discs in the lateral position: an anatomic study. J Neurosurg Spine 2014;21(5):785–93.

10. Hussain NS, Hanscom D, Oskouian RJ. Chyloretroperitoneum following anterior spinal surgery. J Neurosurg Spine 2012;17(5):415–21.

11. Morr S, Kanter AS. Complex regional pain syndrome following lateral lumbar interbody fusion: case report. J Neurosurg Spine 2013;19(4):502–6.

12. Anand N, Baron EM. Urological injury as a complication of the transpsoas approach for discectomy and interbody fusion. J Neurosurg Spine 2013;18(1):18–23.

13. Fujibayashi S, Hynes RA, Otsuki B, et al. Effect of indirect neural decompression through oblique lateral interbody fusion for degenerative lumbar disease. Spine 2015;40(3):E175–82.

14. Mobbs RJ, Phan K, Malham G, et al. Lumbar interbody fusion: techniques, indications and comparison of interbody fusion options including PLIF, TLIF, MI-TLIF, OLIF/ATP, LLIF and ALIF. J Spine Surg 2015;1(1):2–18.

15. Park D, Mummaneni PV, Mehra R, et al. Predictors of the need for laminectomy after indirect decompression via initial anterior or lateral lumbar interbody fusion. J Neurosurg Spine 2020. https://doi.org/10.3171/2019.11.SPINE19314.

16. Xu DS, Walker CT, Godzik J, et al. Minimally invasive anterior, lateral, and oblique lumbar interbody fusion: a literature review. Ann Transl Med 2018; 6(6):104.

17. Chang SY, Nam Y, Lee J, et al. Impact of preoperative diagnosis on clinical outcomes of oblique lateral interbody fusion for lumbar degenerative disease in a single-institution prospective cohort. Orthop Surg 2019;11(1):66–74.

18. Cheng C, Wang K, Zhang C, et al. Clinical results and complications associated with oblique lumbar interbody fusion technique. Ann Transl Med 2021; 9(1):16.

19. Tong YJ, Liu JH, Fan SW, et al. One-stage debridement via oblique lateral interbody fusion corridor combined with posterior pedicle screw fixation in treating spontaneous lumbar infectious spondylodiscitis: a case series. Orthop Surg 2019;11(6):1109–19.

20. Wang K, Zhang C, Wu H, et al. The anatomic characteristics of the retroperitoneal oblique corridor to the I1-s1 intervertebral disc spaces. Spine 2019; 44(12):E697–706.

21. Mummaneni PV, Shaffrey CI, Lenke LG, et al. The minimally invasive spinal deformity surgery algorithm: a reproducible rational framework for decision making in minimally invasive spinal deformity surgery. Neurosurg Focus 2014;36(5):E6. https://doi.org/10.3171/2014.3.FOCUS1413.

22. Rodgers WB, Lehmen JA, Gerber EJ, et al. Grade 2 spondylolisthesis at L4-5 treated by XLIF: safety and midterm results in the "worst case scenario.". Sci World J 2012;2012:1–7.

23. Li R, Li X, Zhou H, et al. Development and application of oblique lumbar interbody fusion. Orthop Surg 2020;12(2):355–65.

24. Kim H, Chang BS, Chang SY. Pearls and pitfalls of oblique lateral interbody fusion: a comprehensive narrative review. Neurospine 2022;19(1):163–76.

25. Molinares DM, Davis TT, Fung DA. Retroperitoneal oblique corridor to the L2-S1 intervertebral discs: an MRI study. J Neurosurg Spine 2016;24(2): 248–55.

26. Deng D, Liao X, Wu R, et al. Surgical safe zones for oblique lumbar interbody fusion of L1-5: a cadaveric study. Clin Anat 2022;35(2):178–85.

27. Benglis DM, Vanni S, Levi AD. An anatomical study of the lumbosacral plexus as related to the minimally invasive transpsoas approach to the lumbar spine: Laboratory investigation. J Neurosurg Spine 2009; 10(2):139–44.

28. Davis TT, Bae HW, Mok JM, et al. Lumbar plexus anatomy within the psoas muscle: implications for the transpsoas lateral approach to the L4-L5 disc. J Bone Jt Surg Am 2011;93(16):1482–7.

29. Uribe JS, Arredondo N, Dakwar E, et al. Defining the safe working zones using the minimally invasive lateral retroperitoneal transpsoas approach: an anatomical study: laboratory investigation. J Neurosurg Spine 2010;13(2):260–6.

30. Voyadzis JM, Felbaum D, Rhee J. The rising psoas sign: an analysis of preoperative imaging characteristics of aborted minimally invasive lateral interbody fusions at L4-5. J Neurosurg Spine 2014;20(5): 531–7.

31. Tanida S, Fujibayashi S, Otsuki B, et al. Influence of spinopelvic alignment and morphology on deviation in the course of the psoas major muscle. J Orthop Sci 2017;22(6):1001–8.

32. Mai HT, Schneider AD, Alvarez AP, et al. Anatomic considerations in the lateral transpsoas interbody fusion: the impact of age, Sex, BMI, and scoliosis. Clin Spine Surg 2019;32(5):215–21.

33. Regev GJ, Kim CW. Safety and the anatomy of the retroperitoneal lateral corridor with respect to the minimally invasive lateral lumbar intervertebral fusion approach. Neurosurg Clin N Am 2014;25(2): 211–8.

34. Wang Z, Liu L, he Xu X, et al. The OLIF working corridor based on magnetic resonance imaging: a retrospective research. J Orthop Surg 2020;15(1): 141.

35. Julian Li JX, Mobbs RJ, Phan K. Morphometric MRI imaging study of the corridor for the oblique lumbar interbody fusion technique at L1-L5. World Neurosurg 2018;111:e678–85.

36. Hu WK, He SS, Zhang SC, et al. An MRI study of psoas major and abdominal large vessels with respect to the X/DLIF approach. Eur Spine J 2011; 20(4):557–62.

37. Kaliya-Perumal AK, Ng JPH, Soh TLT, et al. Reliability of the new modified Moro's classification and oblique corridor grading to assess the feasibility of oblique lumbar interbody fusion. J Orthop 2020; 21:321–5.

38. Orita S, Shiga Y, Inage K, et al. Technical and conceptual review on the L5-S1 oblique lateral interbody fusion surgery (OLIF51). Spine Surg Relat Res 2020; 5(1):1–9.

39. Choi J, Rhee I, Ruparel S. Assessment of great vessels for anterior access of L5/S1 using patient positioning. Asian Spine J 2020;14(4):438–44.

40. Moro T, Kikuchi S ichi, Konno S ichi, et al. An anatomic study of the lumbar plexus with respect to retroperitoneal endoscopic surgery. Spine 2003; 28(5):423–8 [discussion: 427-428].

41. Ng JPH, Kaliya-Perumal AK, Tandon AA, et al. The oblique corridor at L4-L5: a radiographic-anatomical study into the feasibility for lateral interbody fusion. Spine 2020;45(10):E552.

42. Liu L, Liang Y, Zhang H, et al. Imaging anatomical research on the operative windows of oblique lumbar interbody fusion. PLoS One 2016;11(9): e0163452.

43. Orita S, Inage K, Sainoh T, et al. Lower lumbar segmental arteries can intersect over the intervertebral disc in the oblique lateral interbody fusion approach with a risk for arterial injury: radiological analysis of lumbar segmental arteries by using magnetic resonance imaging. Spine 2017;42(3):135–42.

44. Ng JPH, Scott-Young M, Chan DNC, et al. The feasibility of anterior spinal access: the vascular corridor at the L5-S1 level for anterior lumbar interbody fusion. Spine 2021;46(15):983–9.

45. Chang SY, Nam Y, Lee J, et al. Clinical significance of radiologic improvement following single-level oblique lateral interbody fusion with percutaneous pedicle screw fixation. Orthopedics 2020;43(4): e283–90.

46. Xi Z, Mummaneni PV, Wang M, et al. The association between lower Hounsfield units on computed tomography and cage subsidence after lateral lumbar interbody fusion. Neurosurg Focus 2020;49(2):E8.

47. Wu H, Cheung JPY, Zhang T, et al. The role of hounsfield unit in intraoperative endplate violation and delayed cage subsidence with oblique lateral interbody fusion. Glob Spine J 2021. https://doi.org/10. 1177/21925682211052515. 21925682211052516.

48. Liu J, Ding W, Yang D, et al. Modic Changes (MCs) associated with endplate sclerosis can prevent cage subsidence in oblique lumbar interbody fusion (OLIF) stand-alone. World Neurosurg 2020;138:e160–8.

49. Huo Y, Yang D, Ma L, et al. Oblique lumbar interbody fusion with stand-alone cages for the treatment of degenerative lumbar spondylolisthesis: a retrospective study with 1-year follow-up. Pain Res Manag 2020;2020:9016219.

50. Fang G, Lin Y, Wu J, et al. Biomechanical comparison of stand-alone and bilateral pedicle screw fixation for oblique lumbar interbody fusion surgery-a finite element analysis. World Neurosurg 2020;141: e204–12.

51. Guo HZ, Tang YC, Guo DQ, et al. Stability evaluation of oblique lumbar interbody fusion constructs with various fixation options: a finite element analysis based on three-dimensional scanning models. World Neurosurg 2020;138:e530–8.

52. Song C, Chang H, Zhang D, et al. Biomechanical evaluation of oblique lumbar interbody fusion with various fixation options: a finite element analysis. Orthop Surg 2021;13(2):517–29.

53. Silvestre C, Mac-Thiong JM, Hilmi R, et al. Complications and morbidities of mini-open anterior retroperitoneal lumbar interbody fusion: oblique lumbar interbody fusion in 179 patients. Asian Spine J 2012;6(2):89–97.

54. Ohtori S, Orita S, Yamauchi K, et al. Mini-open anterior retroperitoneal lumbar interbody fusion: oblique lateral interbody fusion for lumbar spinal degeneration disease. Yonsei Med J 2015;56(4):1051–9.

55. Tannoury T, Kempegowda H, Haddadi K, et al. Complications associated with minimally invasive anterior to the psoas (ATP) fusion of the lumbosacral spine. Spine 2019;44(19):E1122–9.

56. Kotheeranurak V, Singhatanadgige W, Ratanakornphan C, et al. Neutral hip position for the oblique lumbar interbody fusion (OLIF) approach increases the retroperitoneal oblique corridor. BMC Musculoskelet Disord 2020;21:583.

57. Makhni MC, Lin JD, Lehman RA. The ante-psoas approach for lumbar interbody fusion. In: O'Brien JR, Kalantar SB, Drazin D, et al, editors. The resident's guide to spine surgery. Cham, Switzerland: Springer International Publishing; 2020. p. 177–85. https://doi.org/10.1007/978-3-030-20847-9_21.

58. Mehren C, Korge A. Minimally invasive anterior oblique lumbar interbody fusion (OLIF). Eur Spine J 2016;25(Suppl 4):471–2.

59. Fujibayashi S, Kawakami N, Asazuma T, et al. Complications associated with lateral interbody fusion: nationwide survey of 2998 cases during the first 2 years of its use in Japan. Spine 2017;42(19): 1478–84.

60. Wang H, Huo Y, Zhao Y, et al. Clinical rehabilitation effect of postoperative lower-limb training on the patients undergoing olif surgery: a retrospective study. Pain Res Manag 2020;2020:1065202.

61. Ohtori S, Mannoji C, Orita S, et al. Mini-open anterior retroperitoneal lumbar interbody fusion: oblique lateral interbody fusion for degenerated lumbar spinal kyphoscoliosis. Asian Spine J 2015;9(4): 565–72.

62. Grunert P, Drazin D, Iwanaga J, et al. Injury to the lumbar plexus and its branches after lateral fusion procedures: a cadaver study. World Neurosurg 2017;105:519–25.

63. Gragnaniello C, Seex K. Anterior to psoas (ATP) fusion of the lumbar spine: evolution of a technique facilitated by changes in equipment. J Spine Surg 2016;2(4):256–65.

64. Li HM, Zhang RJ, Shen CL. Differences in radiographic and clinical outcomes of oblique lateral interbody fusion and lateral lumbar interbody fusion for degenerative lumbar disease: a meta-analysis. BMC Musculoskelet Disord 2019;20:582.

65. Souslian FG, Patel PD. Review and analysis of modern lumbar spinal fusion techniques. Br J Neurosurg 2021;1–7. https://doi.org/10.1080/02688697.2021.1881041.

66. Walker CT, Farber SH, Cole TS, et al. Complications for minimally invasive lateral interbody arthrodesis: a systematic review and meta-analysis comparing prepsoas and transpsoas approaches. J Neurosurg Spine 2019;1–15. https://doi.org/10.3171/2018.9.SPINE18800.

67. Chung HW, Lee HD, Jeon CH, Chung NS. Comparison of surgical outcomes between oblique lateral interbody fusion (OLIF) and anterior lumbar interbody fusion (ALIF). Clin Neurol Neurosurg 2021;209: 106901.

68. Xi Z, Burch S, Mummaneni PV, et al. Supine anterior lumbar interbody fusion versus lateral position oblique lumbar interbody fusion at L5-S1: A comparison of two approaches to the lumbosacral junction. J Clin Neurosci 2020;82(Pt A):134–40.

69. DiGiorgio AM, Edwards CS, Virk MS, et al. Stereotactic navigation for the prepsoas oblique lateral lumbar interbody fusion: technical note and case series. Neurosurg Focus 2017;43(2):E14.

70. Pumberger M, Hughes AP, Huang RR, et al. Neurologic deficit following lateral lumbar interbody fusion. Eur Spine J 2012;21(6):1192–9.

71. Mehren C, Mayer HM, Zandanell C, et al. The oblique anterolateral approach to the lumbar spine provides access to the lumbar spine with few early complications. Clin Orthop 2016;474(9):2020–7.

72. Xi Z, Chou D, Mummaneni PV, et al. The Navigated Oblique Lumbar Interbody Fusion: Accuracy Rate, Effect on Surgical Time, and Complications. Neurospine 2020;17(1):260–7.

73. Oh BK, Son DW, Lee SH, et al. Learning curve and complications experience of oblique lateral interbody fusion : a single-center 143 consecutive cases. J Korean Neurosurg Soc 2021;64(3):447–59.

74. Abe K, Orita S, Mannoji C, et al. Perioperative complications in 155 patients who underwent oblique lateral interbody fusion surgery: perspectives and indications from a retrospective, Multicenter Survey. Spine 2017;42(1):55–62.

75. Yoon SG, Kim MS, Kwon SC, et al. Delayed ureter stricture and kidney atrophy after oblique lumbar interbody fusion. World Neurosurg 2020;134:137–40.

76. Lee HJ, Kim JS, Ryu KS, et al. Ureter injury as a complication of oblique lumbar interbody fusion. World Neurosurg 2017;102. 693.e7-693.e14.

77. Woods KRM, Billys JB, Hynes RA. Technical description of oblique lateral interbody fusion at L1–L5 (OLIF25) and at L5–S1 (OLIF51) and evaluation of complication and fusion rates. Spine J 2017;17(4): 545–53.

78. Park SC, Chang SY, Mok S, et al. Risk factors for postoperative ileus after oblique lateral interbody fusion: a multivariate analysis. Spine J 2021;21(3): 438–45.

79. Hu Z, He D, Gao J, et al. The influence of endplate morphology on cage subsidence in patients with stand-alone oblique lateral lumbar interbody fusion (OLIF). Glob Spine J 2021. https://doi.org/10.1177/2192568221992098. 2192568221992098.

80. Marchi L, Abdala N, Oliveira L, et al. Radiographic and clinical evaluation of cage subsidence after stand-alone lateral interbody fusion. J Neurosurg Spine 2013;19(1):110–8.

81. Malham GM, Parker RM, Blecher CM, et al. Assessment and classification of subsidence after lateral interbody fusion using serial computed tomography. J Neurosurg Spine 2015;23(5):589–97.

82. Okano I, Jones C, Rentenberger C, et al. The association between endplate changes and risk for early severe cage subsidence among standalone lateral lumbar interbody fusion patients. Spine 2020; 45(23):E1580–7.

83. Tempel ZJ, McDowell MM, Panczykowski DM, et al. Graft subsidence as a predictor of revision surgery following stand-alone lateral lumbar interbody fusion. J Neurosurg Spine 2018;28(1):50–6.

84. Rentenberger C, Okano I, Salzmann SN, et al. Perioperative risk factors for early revisions in stand-alone lateral lumbar interbody fusion. World Neurosurg 2020;134:e657–63.

85. Choy W, Mayer RR, Mummaneni PV, et al. Oblique lumbar interbody fusion with stereotactic navigation: technical note. Glob Spine J 2020;10(2 Suppl):94S–100S.

86. Ouchida J, Kanemura T, Satake K, et al. Simultaneous single-position lateral interbody fusion and percutaneous pedicle screw fixation using O-arm-based navigation reduces the occupancy time of the operating room. Eur Spine J 2020;29(6): 1277–86.

87. Diaz-Aguilar LD, Shah V, Himstead A, et al. Simultaneous robotic single-position surgery (SR-SPS) with oblique lumbar interbody fusion: a case series. World Neurosurg 2021;151:e1036–43.

88. Heo DH, Choi WS, Park CK, et al. Minimally invasive oblique lumbar interbody fusion with spinal endoscope assistance: technical note. World Neurosurg 2016;96:530–6.

Anterior Column Realignment
Adult Sagittal Deformity Treatment Through Minimally Invasive Surgery

Gregory M. Mundis Jr, MD[a,b], Robert Kenneth Eastlack, MD[a,b], Amber LaMae Price, MD[a,b],*

KEYWORDS

- Anterior column release • Lateral lumbar interbody fusion • Spinal deformity
- Anterior longitudinal ligament • Lordosis • Sagittal imbalance • Minimally invasive spine surgery

KEY POINTS

- Lordotic gains from the anterior column realignment procedure can depend on the use of posterior release/osteotomy.
- It is critical to measure preoperative sagittal parameters, intended lordotic goals, and anticipated correction combined with intraoperative assessment of intradiscal angle to allow for appropriate correction of sagittal deformity.
- Vascular and neurologic injuries are the most concerning risks of the procedure. They are best avoided by critical evaluation of the preoperative vascular anatomy, patient selection and exclusion, meticulous dissection, and presence of appropriate safety measures in the event of unintentional violation.
- Proximal junctional kyphosis is proportional to the amount of correction needed and achieved; patients are at higher risk when overcorrection of sagittal parameters occurs.

INTRODUCTION

Treatment of adult spinal deformity requires a complex decision-making process aimed at achieving the reestablishment of spinopelvic equilibrium and restoration of sagittal and coronal spinal balance. Multiple studies have evaluated the direct link between health-related quality of life data and its relation to adult spinal deformity surgery.[1,2] As demonstrated by Glassman and colleagues, the severity of symptoms is clearly related to progressive sagittal imbalance. The authors demonstrated that patients with a positive sagittal balance had worse scores in pain and they concluded that positive sagittal balance is the most important and reliable radiographic predictor of worsened clinical health parameters.[1]

Traditionally, posterior-based osteotomies (posterior column and pedicle subtraction) have been used in realignment of the spinal column to achieve appropriate sagittal spinal alignment. Technological advancements have ultimately shifted the surgical approach to less-invasive techniques in an effort to decrease the historic perioperative complication rates and morbidity of traditional osteotomies while still allowing for decompression of the neural anatomy, realignment of the spine column, and solid arthrodesis.[3,4] Anterior column realignment (ACR) is a novel, minimally invasive technique that uses a retroperitoneal approach to the lumbar spine in combination with lateral lumbar interbody fusion (LLIF) to allow for transection of the anterior longitudinal ligament (ALL) and achieve larger focal and regional

a Scripps Clinic, Department of Spine Surgery, 10666 North Torrey Pines Road, La Jolla, CA 92037, USA; b San Diego Spine Foundation, Suite 212, 6190 Cornerstone Ct. East, San Diego, CA 92121, USA
* Corresponding author.
E-mail address: ambpriceSDSF@gmail.com

Neurosurg Clin N Am 34 (2023) 633–642
https://doi.org/10.1016/j.nec.2023.06.010
1042-3680/23/

corrections of lumbar lordosis to restore sagittal alignment.

PATIENT SELECTION
Indications

Multiple factors must be evaluated to appropriately select patients that may benefit from a less-invasive procedure to correct sagittal malalignment. These include the number of levels involved (focal vs regional vs global sagittal deformity), severity of deformity, prior surgical interventions, region of spinal deformity, and the flexibility of the spinal segment. In general, T12 and L5 disc segments can be accessed from the lateral approach but level selection should be dictated by where the major lordosis correction is desired. Mummaneni and colleagues[5] outlined an algorithm for determining the deformity patient population that is most amenable for an minimally invasive surgery (MIS) treatment. These criteria include an sagittal vertical axis (SVA) less than 6 cm unless their deformity is flexible, pelvic tilt less than 25°, pelvic incidence to lumbar lordosis (PI-LL) mismatch between 10° and 30°, maximum coronal cobb angle less than 20°, and thoracic kyphosis less than 60°. The presence of a vacuum disc phenomenon is a positive indicator of an open disc space amenable to interbody correction and fusion.[6]

Contraindications

When evaluating patients for potential ACR, anatomic considerations are critical. MRI and or computed tomography (CT) should be scrutinized to determine the feasibility of retroperitoneal approach and access to the prevertebral space behind the great vessels. Assessment of this space is focused on the presence of fat between the vessels and the most ventral aspect of the disc, which signifies a safe plane for dissection. Additionally, large anterior osteophytes that disallow a linear dissection between vessels and annulus represent a heightened danger in navigating the plane, and perhaps an outright contraindication. Evaluation for vascular anomalies such as retrocaval renal veins and duplication should be undertaken. Psoas position should also be considered. Ventral displacement of the psoas relative to the disc space has been correlated with migration of the lumbosacral plexus anteriorly and a higher incidence of the iliac vasculature being located adjacent to the anterior third of the disc space, particularly at L4-5 disc space.[7]

History of earlier solid fusion is a contraindication, and preoperative CT should be used to evaluate potential fusion of the segment. It should be noted that ACR can be performed in patients with an earlier posterior fusion alone with an open disc space. This requires a posterior column osteotomy before the ACR being performed.[8] Further relative contraindications to the ACR procedure include infection, radiation treatment, and/or peritonitis that may have resulted in adhesions, and low excursion of the great vessels resulting in a high vascular risk. Increased subsidence rates have been seen in patients in the setting of osteoporotic or osteopenia, as well. Subsidence can result in local kyphosis and inability to achieve or retain correction in the sagittal plane.

PREOPERATIVE PLANNING
Determining the Grade of Osteotomy/Release

Preoperative planning in determining appropriateness of ACR is critical in the success of the procedure. Technically, this procedure is intended to manipulate an open disc space to achieve the desired improvement in segmental lordosis. Thus, a thorough knowledge of patient global spinal alignment, distribution of segmental lordosis, and age-directed spinal parameter goals are crucial.[9] The minimally invasive surgical decision-making algorithm (MISDEF2) was iterated by a panel of deformity surgeons to dictate and classify deformities that could reasonably respond to MIS approaches.[10] Patients were classified into 4 separate categories. The first class of patients met no major sagittal malalignment criteria and were amenable to MIS decompression or fusion modalities. The second class of patients demonstrated moderate sagittal deformity as defined by a sagittal vertical axis greater than 6 mm, a pelvic tilt greater than 25°, lateral listhesis greater than 6 mm, coronal cobb angle greater than 20°, or PI-LL mismatch between 10° and 30°. This group was thought to benefit from lordosis correction via interbody technique. Patients in the third class were found to present with the most severe deformities. These patients were found to have similar malalignment criteria as the second class; however, there was also evidence of a fixed deformity, thoracic kyphosis greater than 60°, or PI-LL mismatch greater than 30°. Surgical recommendations for this group included open posterior surgery with osteotomies and extension of the fusion into the thoracic spine. To provide further clinical context, Uribe and colleagues developed an osteotomy classification for ACR. Based on the classification, the amount of segmental correction will vary significantly with the ACR depending on how much posterior bone is resected. Five levels of osteotomies were described as demonstrated in **Fig. 1**: Grade 1 ACR: ALL Release with

ACR Classification	Construct	Schwab Modifier	Approach Modifier
Grade A	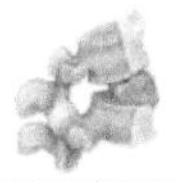 (illustration)	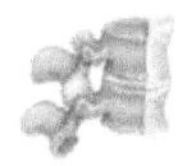 (illustration) 0	Lateral or Anterior
Grade 1	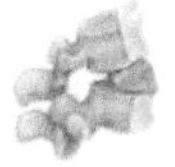 (illustration)	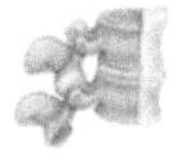 (illustration) 1	
Grade 2	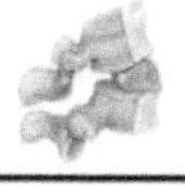 (illustration)	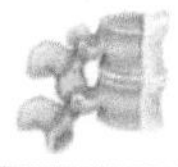 (illustration) 2	Lateral or Anterior or Posterior
Grade 3	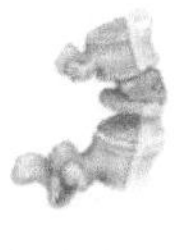 (illustration)	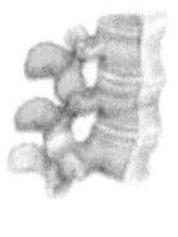 (illustration) 3	
Grade 4	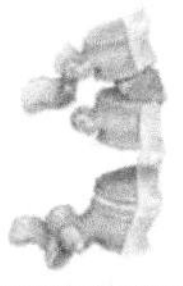 (illustration)	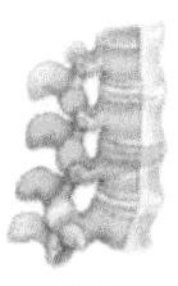 (illustration) 4	
Grade 5	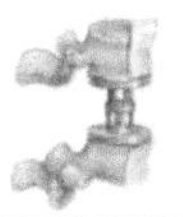 (illustration)	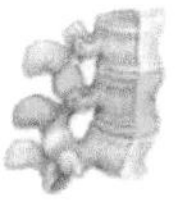 (illustration) 5	

Fig. 1. ACR classification from Uribe and colleagues demonstrating the Schwab osteotomy classification correlate for each ACR construct. (Used with permission from Barrow Neurological Institute, Phoenix, Arizona.).

Hyperlordotic Cage and Inferior Facetectomy (Schwab Grade 1), Grade 2 ACR: ALL Release with Hyperlordotic Cage and Posterior Osteotomies (PCO, Schwab Grade 2), Grade 3 and ACR: ALL Release with Hyperlordotic Cage and 3 Column Osteotomy (Schwab Grades 3 and 4), and Grade 5 ACR: Vertebrectomy with ALL Release. ACR in combination with Schwab Grade 2 osteotomies generally produce sagittal lordosis correction on average of 23°. If greater than or equal to 30° of correction is desired, using a higher grade osteotomy should be considered.[11]

Side of Approach

The initial factor that should be considered when determining the side of the approach is the anatomic location of the vasculature with respect to the disc space. The inferior vena cava can present a significant risk if present on the contralateral side and not visible during the sectioning of the ligament or the contralateral annulus. Specific considerations can be made in the setting of scoliosis correction. Generally, the authors prefer to approach from the concavity because it allows for more release of the collapsed side and it provides a corridor to access 3 to 4 levels through a smaller and/or singular incision. Additionally, the tilt of the

L4-5 disk space often favors an approach from the concavity. Advantages of approaching from the convexity include a more open disc space allowing for easier entry, as well as a shorter reach to the spine, but more incisions may be necessary to access all levels to be addressed. Axial rotation of the spine can also be factored into the approach. Generally approaching the disc space is more direct when the ventral aspect of the disc is rotated toward the side of the approach. Consideration of the iliac crest height and tilt of the disc space relative to the pelvis is critical if an L4-5 ACR is to be performed.

SURGICAL TECHNIQUE

In 2005, the first ACR procedure was performed and was subsequently reported first by Dr Behrooz Akbarnia.[12] Since that time, significant advances in the technique have evolved and are often used in conjunction with those seen in the LLIF procedure.[13] The procedure involves sectioning of the ALL to facilitate the placement of a hyperlordotic implant.

Anterior Column Realignment Anatomy

The ALL is a robust ligament that spans from the clivus to the sacrum. It is composed of 3 layers.

The superficial layer spans 4 to 5 vertebral bodies while the intermittent layer spans 2 to 3 vertebral bodies. The deepest layer of the ALL connects adjacent vertebral bodies and is considered intersegmental. These fibers lie just ventral to the periosteum along the ventral body wall and to the annulus the level of the disc space. Running adjacent to the ALL is the sympathetic plexus. It is located primarily between the ligament and the medial border of the psoas. The great vessels lie just to the left and right of the vertebral bodies themselves: the aorta centrally and the inferior vena cava to the right. The aortic and iliac bifurcations typically occur at the level of L4. Variations in the anatomy include the presence of the bifurcation of both great vessels into iliac vessels at the L5 level.[14,15] The lumbar segmental arteries originate from the abdominal aorta and course dorsolaterally along the midpoint of the vertebral body toward the intervertebral foramen, deep to the sympathetic plexus and to the tendinous arches of the psoas. Careful consideration must be used when scrutinizing preoperative MRI to localize these branching vessels because injury can result in substantial bleeding intraoperatively. Lumbar plexus anatomy is also critical to consider when approaching the disc spaces at the different lumbar levels. In traditional LLIF, Regev and colleagues published a retrospective study of 100 human MRIs where they measured the average percent distance from posterior border of the disc space to the motor nerves. They then proceeded to define a "safe zone" for each respective disc level. These safe zones were found to be largest at the L1-2 level and proceeded to become narrower because the nerves traveled distally to the more caudal disc spaces. This study demonstrated the progressive ventral trajectory of the lumbosacral plexus because it travels from cranial to caudal.[16]

Patient Positioning

Before positioning, the operating room table must be evaluated to ensure that unobstructed imaging may be obtained with the C-arm. Patient is positioned in the lateral decubitus position with the approach side up. The iliac crests are positioned at the level of the table break. The hips are flexed 30° to relax the psoas muscle and lumbar plexus, and flexion of the knees to 90° further contributes to limiting tension on the lumbar plexus.[17] An axillary roll is placed in the axilla to decompress the brachial plexus. The patient is stabilized by taping of the patient's chest and iliac crests to the table. The C-arm should be brought in to obtain true anteroposterior (AP) and lateral imaging. Adjustments should be made to obtain a perfect AP image indicated by a midline spinous process and symmetric pedicles. Adjustment should not be made to the C-arm but rather to the table via rotation until the appropriate view is obtained. The arm should then be transitioned to a 90° angle to the floor to obtain a true lateral image. True lateral indicators include linear endplates, linear posterior cortex, and superimposed pedicles. Again, the table should be adjusted in a Trendelenburg fashion to obtain the perfect lateral view. In multilevel cases, the surgeon will likely need to readjust the table for an optimal image at each level.

Approach

Standard LLIF approach is used. The retroperitoneal space may be obtained either via a single-flank incision or a 2-incision technique.[18,19] The incision is opened with a scalpel and electrocautery is used to expose the fascia of the external oblique. Using a combination of Metzenbaum scissor and gentle finger dissection, access to the retroperitoneum is gained by traversing the 3 lateral muscle layers including the external oblique, internal oblique, and transversus abdominis. The transversalis fascia must then be traversed to enter the retroperitoneal space. As described by Dakwar and colleagues,[20] there are 4 main nerves that travel outside the psoas: subcostal, iliohypogastric, ilioinguinal, and lateral femoral cutaneous nerve. In addition, the subcostal nerves travel along the inferior borders of the 12th rib and the ventral aspect of the quadratus lumborum. The iliohypogastric and ilioinguinal nerves originate at the most cephalad position of the psoas muscle and course obliquely through the retroperitoneum. The lateral femoral cutaneous nerve exits the lateral portion of the psoas at L4 and travels along the iliacus muscle. Care should be taken to prevent damage to these nerves during the dissection. Access is then gained into the retroperitoneal space and finger dissection is used to sweep the peritoneal structures anteriorly and guide the surgeon's digit to the superficial surface of the psoas muscle. Directly medial to the transverse process is the psoas. The peritoneum is swept away from the psoas to ensure a clear path for the dilators. The initial dilator is then guided down to the psoas muscle with the utilization of surgeon's digit and lateral fluoroscopy. Directional dynamically triggered electromyography (t-EMG) is used to guide the initial dilator through the psoas. This device provides information regarding both the direction and the proximity of the lumbosacral plexus.[21,22] If a threshold of less than 5 mA is obtained, the dilator may be in contact with the nerve.[23,24] The dilator is then rotated 360° to provide information regarding the location of the nerves. After confirming appropriate position of the initial dilator using t-EMG and lateral fluoroscopy, the K-wire can be placed through the dilator into the disc space. Sequential dilators are then used over the initial dilator. The retractor is then guided in place over the dilators and secured to an articulating arm. The operative field is finally interrogated with direct visual inspection and a triggered EMG probe to verify the absence of neural elements within the field. An intradiscal shim is then placed to secure the posterior blade into the disc space. Once the retractor is in its desired position, it is expanded to allow for preparation of the disc space. At this time, the ACR can be performed.

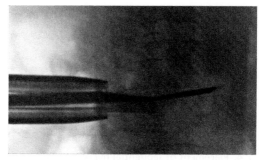

Fig. 2. Cobb is used to release contralateral annulus.

Procedural Steps for Performing Anterior Longitudinal Ligament Release

1. Define the plane that exists anteriorly to the ALL and posterior to the major vessels and sympathetic autonomic plexus. This step is performed with the use of Penfield dissectors. Tactile feedback is necessary to ensure that the appropriate plane is identified. Minimal resistance should be met when performing the dissection. Once a plane is defined, a ventral anterior retractor blade is placed across to the contralateral side of the disc space to protect both vessels.

2. Perform the channel discectomy initially, with release of the contralateral annulus, and while preserving the ALL. The maintenance of the ALL during this time allows for a safe and effective discectomy.

3. Cobb elevators are used to directly release the disc material from the superior and inferior endplates in a subchondral fashion. Care should be taken to avoid endplate violation. Intraoperative fluoroscopy can be used as necessary to help ensure correct trajectories are taken. Once the contralateral annulus is contacted with the Cobb elevator, a mallet is used to release both the superior and inferior endplates (**Fig. 2**). Pituitaries can be used to remove residual disc.

4. The author's preferred technique is to use a box cutter to debulk the disc space. This is an optional step. Fluoroscopy should be used throughout the duration of this step to ensure that the box chisel is orthogonal to the disc space. Particular attention should be paid to appropriate seating of the box cutter within the disc space to prevent unintentional release of the ALL.

5. Direct visualization of the ALL is obtained. Resection is carried out in an anterior to posterior fashion to minimize the potential risk of injury to the ventral vasculature. The ALL is incised until two-thirds has been released (**Fig. 3**). Various instruments can be used to divide the ALL including a long-handled scalpel or box cutter chisel. We avoid sharp dissection of the contralateral one-third of the ALL and contralateral anterior corner of the annulus due to inadequate visualization and potential risk to the major vessels. Gradual distraction of the disc space is then performed to slowly release the remaining portion of ALL and annulus using trials or an expandable mechanism.

6. Sequential hyperlordotic interbody trials are then placed into the disc space under fluoroscopy to evaluate for optimal intradiscal angle and segmental lordosis correction based on preoperative planning (**Fig. 4**). Care should be taken to select an implant with appropriate posterior height to maintain foraminal height.

7. Once the appropriate interbody device has been determined, endplate preparation is carried out. This is performed using rasps and stirrup curets with the goal of removing any residual cartilage and disc material.

8. The interbody graft is then delivered into the appropriate anterior/posterior location. An

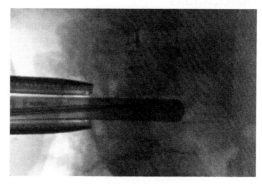

Fig. 3. Completion of the ALL release.

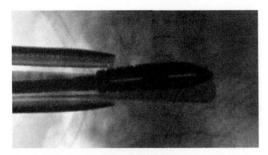

Fig. 4. Placement of sequential hyperlordotic trials.

integrated device or fixation is desirable, so that the cage is well secured and unable to migrate during prone repositioning and posterior column osteotomies/releases (**Fig. 5**).

Posterior Construct

The release of the ALL results in significant destabilization of the motion segment, particularly when combined with posterior releases, because the combination represents a 3-column destabilization. Appropriate stabilization is required to prevent instrumentation failure and subsequent pseudarthrosis. A study performed by Januszewski and colleagues[25] evaluated the amount of rod stress experienced after a pedicle subtraction osteotomy (PSO) versus an ACR. A 3-dimensional finite element model was used to compare a 25° PSO at L3 to an L3-4 ACR with placement of a 30° hyperlordotic interbody implant and posterior column osteotomy. The study demonstrated that rod stress was similar between PSO with adjacent interbody support and ACR. Both ACR and PSO had approximately 50% rod stress reduction in flexion with the placement of additional satellite rods. Given the above data and need to reduce potential pseudarthrosis and motion segment instability, the authors recommend placing a 4-rod spanning construct similar to those used for 3-column posterior osteotomies.

COMPLICATIONS

The International Spine Study Group performed a critical analysis of sagittal plane deformity correction in 2017.[26] In the study, 17 ACR patients were matched with 17 PSO patients by their respective PI, LL, and thoracic kyphosis. Rates of major intraoperative and perioperative complications were found to be similar between patients with ACR and patients with PSO (25.3% vs 41.2%, respectively). One vascular injury was reported in a patient with ACR but did not occur during the resection of the ALL. Three of the patients within the ACR group developed motor weakness with 2 experiencing full recovery.

Vascular Injury

Injury to the major vessels is one of the most potentially devastating complications that can occur during the ACR procedure. Various steps should be taken to avoid vascular injury including appropriate preoperative planning and patient selection as stated above. Before the surgical procedure, the patients should be typed and crossed for 2 units of packed red blood cells and hemostatic agents should be available and open in the operating room. Intraoperatively, if the surgeon is unable to safely develop the plane between the ALL and retroperitoneal vasculature, the procedure should be aborted. Direct visualization of the ipsilateral ALL is critical to allow for safe incision with the scalpel in anteroposterior fashion. Finally, the use of distraction maneuvers to release the final third of the ALL provides a much safer method than incision as visualization is poor in this area. If vascular injury is encountered, hemostatic and packing agents should be placed and manual compression should be carried out while awaiting evaluation by the vascular surgeon. In 2015, Uribe and colleagues provided a large survey study and literature review for complications associated with LLIF.[27] In this study, vascular injuries were reported to occur 0.1% of the time. Walker and colleagues further reviewed non-ACR lateral interbody fusion procedures from both transpsoas and prepsoas approaches.[28] Their reported risk of vascular injury was 0.4% and 1.8%, respectively. Due to the nature of defining the plane adjacent to the great vessels and resecting the ALL in close proximity to the vessels

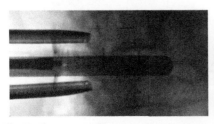
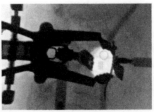
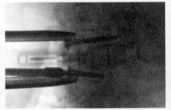

Fig. 5. Placement of hyperlordotic implant and fixation with screws.

(although protected by the retractor), there is a theoretic increased vascular injury risk during ACR; however, a recent review of published ACR studies suggests that major vascular injuries were quite rare and occurred most often in the setting of revision surgery.[29]

Motor/Neurologic Deficit

As demonstrated in the traditional LLIF, the most common complication following ACR technique is ipsilateral iliopsoas weakness (0.7%–33.6%).[30] Murray and colleagues performed a review of neurologic deficits following MIS ACR for adult spinal deformity.[31] The study included 31 patients that underwent 47 ACR procedures. The major reported complications were 8 patients with iliopsoas weakness and one patient with retrograde ejaculation. Of the 8 patients that experienced iliopsoas weakness, 75% had fully recovered at 3 months postop. Saigal and colleagues[13] evaluated 26 patients who underwent ACR with a mean follow-up of 2.8 years. They found that neurologic complications occurred in 32% patients. One patient experienced both motor and sensory loss. New thigh numbness or paresthesia developed in 3 patients but only one persisted at the latest follow-up. A total of 6 patients developed a new motor deficit with 4 having persistent weakness at follow-up. The previously mentioned ISSG study[26] found that the majority of motor deficits occur at the level of L4-5.[26] Two main factors may contribute to this finding. With regards to anatomy, the lumbar plexus courses its way

ventrally because it moves cranially to caudally. It is found in its most ventral position at the level of L4/5, making it more susceptible to injury. In particular, the femoral nerve (formed by the L2, L3, and L4 nerve roots) is susceptible to injury at the posterior third of the L4-5 disc space. In addition, the ACR technique requires additional time for psoas and plexus retraction, leading to an increased risk to the neural elements at this level.

Foraminal height should also be considered. There is a known inverse relationship between the amount of lordosis correction and the foraminal height. As lordosis increases, foraminal height diminishes. Due to the hyperlordotic implants, the foraminal height in ACR may be decreased compared with traditional LLIF.[32] As such, implants with adequate posterior heights must be selected to prevent foraminal stenosis and impingement of the exiting nerve root.

Proximal Junctional Kyphosis

Proximal junctional kyphosis (PJK) is known common complication that occurs postoperatively in patients undergoing correction for adult sagittal plane deformities. No current studies have compared ACR and PCO directly although its incidence with the ACR technique is comparable to that of the open correction. Gandhi and colleagues evaluated the incidence of PJK and proximal junctional failure in patients undergoing sagittal plane correction with LLIF and ACR.[33] They found that patients treated with LLIF without sagittal plane correction did not incur any PJK and PJF.

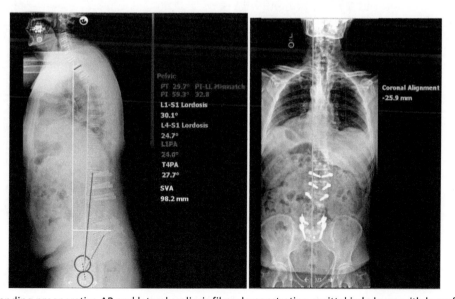

Fig. 6. Standing preoperative AP and lateral scoliosis films demonstrating sagittal imbalance with loss of lumbar lordosis.

Table 1
Baseline sagittal parameters with surgical goals and postoperative assessment

Parameter	Baseline	Goal	Postop
PI	59	59	59
LL (L1-S1)	30	65	54
LL (L4-S1)	24	40	24
LPA	9.5	24	16
TPA	28	9.5 ± 5	17
PI-LL mismatch	33	<9	7
SVA	9.8	<4	5.2

However, an increase incidence of PJK/PJF was seen with increased sagittal plane correction. Following ACR, PJK and PJF occurred in 30% and 11% of patients, respectively. When ACR was combined with a PCO, the incidence of PJK and PJF increased to 42.9% and 40%, respectively. Several risk factors were identified in this study, including patient age, severity of the patient's deformity, and overcorrection of deformity based on age-adjusted goals. Given these findings, the risk of proximal junctional pathology is considerably high and routine postoperative surveillance is recommended.

OUTCOMES OF ANTERIOR COLUMN REALIGNMENT

The radiographic results of the first case series study of 17 patients demonstrated a mean motion segment angle of 9° preoperatively, improving to 19° after ACR, 26° after posterior instrumentation and maintained at 23° at the latest follow-up. The mean lumbar lordosis was 16° preoperatively, improving to 38° after ACR and 45° after posterior instrumentation and maintained at 51° at the latest follow-up. Pelvic tilt averaged 34° before ACR and improved to 24° after ACR and posterior instrumentation and maintained at 25° at the latest follow-up. Patients with preoperative negative T1 spinopelvic inclination (T1SPI) corrected from 6° to 2° and those with 0 or positive T1PSI corrected from 5° to 3° after ACR at the latest follow-up.[12] Turner and colleagues also performed a multicenter analysis of radiographic outcomes of patients who underwent ACR.[34] A total of 34 patients were included that had an ACR performed at 58 levels. Spinopelvic and sagittal parameters were evaluated at preop, 3 months postop, and 1-year postop. These included PI, LL, T1 spinopelvic inclination (T1SPi), PT, and intradiscal angle (IDA). PI-LL mismatch improved from a mean of 29.4 to 6.6. PT improved from 28.3 to 22.1. In a

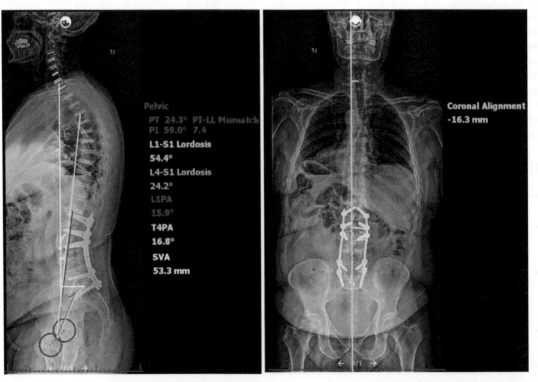

Fig. 7. Standing postoperative AP and lateral scoliosis films demonstrating restoration of sagittal balance parameters after ACR.

propensity matched study, Mundis and colleagues found that at 1-year follow-up, patients with ACR had a significant improvement in all radiographic measures including PI, LL, and TK. ACR and PSO groups did not differ with regards to improvement in LL (34.6 vs 26.1), PI-LL (33.5 vs 24.9), T1 spino-pelvic inclination (3.9 vs 8.1), and T1 pelvic angle (13.3 vs 11.4) at 1-year postop.[26] ACR was found to be superior to PSO in correcting pelvic tilt (8.8 vs 2.6). A retrospective review performed by Leveque compared the outcomes of 12 ACRs and 14 PSO ASD patients.[35] The 2 groups were matched with regards to baseline demographics and severity of PI-LL mismatch. Correction of LL was 35° in the PSO group and 31° in the ACR group. Total operative time and length of stay were similar. Patients with ACR were found to have significantly less operative blood loss than patients with PSO (1466 vs 2910 mL).

CASE EXAMPLE

A 70-year-old man who initially presented with L5 radiculopathy and underwent a selective fusion via ALIF to partially correct sagittal alignment below an earlier 4 level reconstruction that included posterolateral fusion L4-5, pseudarthrosis of a posterolateral attempted fusion at L3-4, and dynamic stabilization L1-3. Ultimately, the patient developed foraminal compromise and radiculopathy at the levels of dynamic stabilization, and in the setting of persistent sagittal malalignment (Fig. 6). Appropriate surgical parameters were calculated to establish normal sagittal parameters (Table 1). He was therefore taken for a definitive revision MIS reconstruction that included LLIF at L1-2 and L3-4 (to treat the pseudarthrosis), along with an ACR at L2-3 for sagittal realignment. Postoperative parameters are demonstrated in Fig. 7.

CLINICS CARE POINTS

- ACR is a powerful MIS technique that allows for correction of segmental and regional lumbar lordosis to restore sagittal balance.
- Patient selection: Evidence of anterior column fusion is a contraindication to the procedure. Patients remain candidates when posterior fusion is present but disc spaces remain open.
- Surgical Technique: Direct visualization of the ALL is critical during the resection portion of the procedure. Resection should be carried out in an anterior to posterior fashion to minimize risk to the ventral vasculature. Sharp dissection of the the contralateral one

third of the ALL is avoided. Gradual distraction of the disc space with slow release of the ALL is preferred.
- Complications: Some studies have demonstrated the majority of motor deficits after surgery occur at the L4/5 level. This is due to the anatomical position of the lumbar plexus. ACR requires additional time for retraction which can lead to an exacerbation of this risk.

DISCLOSURE

The San Diego Spine Foundation supplied resources for completion of this review.

REFERENCES

1. Glassman SDB K, Dimar JR, Horton W, et al. The impact of positive sagittal balance in adult spinal deformity. Spine 2005;30:2024–9.
2. Pellise FV-C,A, Ferrer M, Domingo-Sabat M, et al. .: Impact on health related quality of life of adult spinal deformity (ASD) compared with other chronic conditions. Eur Spine J 2015;24:3–11.
3. Bao H, Yan P, Qiu Y, et al. Coronal imbalance in degenerative lumbar scoliosis: Prevalence and influence on surgical decision-making for spinal osteotomy. Bone Joint Lett J 2016;98-b:1227–33.
4. Yilgor C, Sogunmez N, Yavuz Y, et al. Relative lumbar lordosis and lordosis distribution index: individualized pelvic incidence-based proportional parameters that quantify lumbar lordosis more precisely than the concept of pelvic incidence minus lumbar lordosis. Neurosurg Focus 2017;43:E5.
5. Mummaneni PV, Hussain I, Shaffrey CI, et al. The minimally invasive interbody selection algorithm for spinal deformity. J Neurosurg Spine 2021;34:741–8.
6. Yen CP, Beckman JM, Vivas AC, et al. Effects of intradiscal vacuum phenomenon on surgical outcome of lateral interbody fusion for degenerative lumbar disease. J Neurosurg Spine 2017;26:419–25.
7. Louie PK, Narain AS, Hijji FY, et al. Radiographic Analysis of Psoas Morphology and its Association With Neurovascular Structures at L4-5 With Reference to Lateral Approaches. Spine 2017;42: E1386–92.
8. Hills JM, Yoon ST, Rhee JM, et al. Anterior Column Realignment (ACR) With and Without Pre-ACR Posterior Release for Fixed Sagittal Deformity. Int J Spine Surg 2019;13:192–8.
9. Yilgor C, Sogunmez N, Boissiere L, et al. Global Alignment and Proportion (GAP) Score: Development and Validation of a New Method of Analyzing Spinopelvic Alignment to Predict Mechanical Complications After Adult Spinal Deformity Surgery. J Bone Joint Surg Am 2017;99:1661–72.

10. Mummaneni PV, Park P, Shaffrey CI, et al. The MIS-DEF2 algorithm: an updated algorithm for patient selection in minimally invasive deformity surgery. J Neurosurg Spine 2019;32(2):221–8.

11. Uribe JS, Schwab F, Mundis GM, et al. The comprehensive anatomical spinal osteotomy and anterior column realignment classification. J Neurosurg Spine 2018;29:565–75.

12. Akbarnia BA, Mundis GM Jr, Moazzaz P, et al. Anterior column realignment (ACR) for focal kyphotic spinal deformity using a lateral transpsoas approach and ALL release. J Spinal Disord Tech 2014;27: 29–39.

13. Saigal RM, G M, Eastlack R, et al. Anterior Column Realignment (ACR) in Adult Sagittal Deformity Correction: Technique and Review of the Literature. Spine 2016;41(Suppl 8):S66–73.

14. Agur DA, Grant JCB. Grant's atlas of anatomy. Philadelphia, PA: Wolters Kluwer Health/Lippincott Williams & Wilkins; 2013.

15. FH N. Atlas of human anatomy. Philadelphia, PA: Elsevier Health Sciences; 2010.

16. Regev GJ, Chen L, Dhawan M, et al. Morphometric analysis of the ventral nerve roots and retroperitoneal vessels with respect to the minimally invasive lateral approach in normal and deformed spines. Spine 2009;34:1330–5.

17. O'Brien J, Haines C, Dooley ZA, et al. Femoral nerve strain at L4-L5 is minimized by hip flexion and increased by table break when performing lateral interbody fusion. Spine 2014;39:33–8.

18. Ozgur BM, Aryan HE, Pimenta L, et al. Extreme Lateral Interbody Fusion (XLIF): a novel surgical technique for anterior lumbar interbody fusion. Spine J 2006;6:435–43.

19. Yen CP, Uribe JS. Procedural Checklist for Retroperitoneal Transpsoas Minimally Invasive Lateral Interbody Fusion. Spine 2016;41(Suppl 8):S152–8.

20. Dakwar E, Vale FL, Uribe JS. Trajectory of the main sensory and motor branches of the lumbar plexus outside the psoas muscle related to the lateral retroperitoneal transpsoas approach. J Neurosurg Spine 2011;14:290–5.

21. Berjano P, Lamartina C. Minimally invasive lateral transpsoas approach with advanced neurophysiologic monitoring for lumbar interbody fusion. Eur Spine J 2011;20:1584–6.

22. Tohmeh AG, Rodgers WB, Peterson MD. Dynamically evoked, discrete-threshold electromyography in the extreme lateral interbody fusion approach. J Neurosurg Spine 2011;14:31–7.

23. Calancie B, Madsen P, Lebwohl N. Stimulus-evoked EMG monitoring during transpedicular lumbosacral spine instrumentation. Initial clinical results. Spine 1994;19:2780–6.

24. Maguire J, Wallace S, Madiga R, et al. Evaluation of intrapedicular screw position using intraoperative evoked electromyography. Spine 1995;20:1068–74.

25. Januszewski J, Beckman JM, Harris JE, et al. Biomechanical study of rod stress after pedicle subtraction osteotomy versus anterior column reconstruction: A finite element study. Surg Neurol Int 2017;8:207.

26. Mundis GM Jr, Turner JD, Deverin V, et al. A Critical Analysis of Sagittal Plane Deformity Correction With Minimally Invasive Adult Spinal Deformity Surgery: A 2-Year Follow-Up Study. Spine Deform 2017;5:265–71.

27. Uribe JS, Deukmedjian AR. Visceral, vascular, and wound complications following over 13,000 lateral interbody fusions: a survey study and literature review. Eur Spine J 2015;24(Suppl 3):386–96.

28. Walker CT, Farber SH, Cole TS, et al. Complications for minimally invasive lateral interbody arthrodesis: a systematic review and meta-analysis comparing prepsoas and transpsoas approaches. J Neurosurg Spine 2019;30(4):1–15.

29. Cheung ZB, Chen DH, White SJW, et al. Anterior Column Realignment in Adult Spinal Deformity: A Case Report and Review of the Literature. World Neurosurg 2019;123:e379–86.

30. Ahmadian A, Deukmedjian AR, Abel N, et al. Analysis of lumbar plexopathies and nerve injury after lateral retroperitoneal transpsoas approach: diagnostic standardization. J Neurosurg Spine 2013;18: 289–97.

31. Murray G, Beckman J, Bach K, et al. Complications and neurological deficits following minimally invasive anterior column release for adult spinal deformity: a retrospective study. Eur Spine J 2015; 24(Suppl 3):397–404.

32. Uribe JSS DA, Dakwar E, Baaj AA, et al. Lordosis restoration after anterior longitudinal ligament release and placement of lateral hyperlordotic interbody cages during the minimally invasive lateral transpsoas approach: a radiographic study in cadavers. J Neurosurg Spine 2012;17:476–85.

33. Gandhi SV, Januszewski J, Bach K, et al. Development of Proximal Junctional Kyphosis After Minimally Invasive Lateral Anterior Column Realignment for Adult Spinal Deformity. Neurosurgery 2019;84: 442–50.

34. Turner JD, Akbarnia BA, Eastlack RK, et al. Radiographic outcomes of anterior column realignment for adult sagittal plane deformity: a multicenter analysis. Eur Spine J 2015;24(Suppl 3):427–32.

35. Leveque J-C, Yanamadala V, Buchlak QD, et al. Correction of severe spinopelvic mismatch decreased blood loss with lateral hyperlordotic interbody grafts as compared with pedicle subtraction osteotomy. Neurosurgical Focus FOC 2017;43:E15.

Minimally Invasive Transforaminal Lumbar Interbody Fusion
Strategies for Creating Lordosis with a Posterior Approach

Teerachat Tanasansomboon, MD[a,b,c], Jerry E. Robinson III, MD[d,1], Neel Anand, MD[a],*

KEYWORDS

- MIS-TLIF • Minimally invasive transforaminal lumbar interbody fusion • Lumbar lordosis • Sagittal
- Spinopelvic parameter • Spinal alignment

KEY POINTS

- MIS-TLIF has comparable results in restoring the lumbar lordosis to open TLIF and other lumbar interbody fusion procedures.
- The effectiveness of MIS-TLIF for restoring lumbar lordosis may be varied depending on the surgical techniques reported in the literature.
- The appropriate patient positioning, optimizing disc space preparation, maximizing disc space height, placement of the cage anteriorly, and reducing spondylolisthesis are the crucial steps for creating lumbar lordosis during the MIS-TLIF procedure.

INTRODUCTION

The minimally invasive transforaminal lumbar interbody fusion (MIS-TLIF), an evolution of the open TLIF, has recently gained popularity among spine surgeons worldwide.[1] MIS-TLIF minimizes the muscle retraction and soft tissue damage while providing the benefit of direct decompression of the neural elements. The interbody implant allow spinal fusion from within the disc space. Furthermore, It facilitates disc height (DH) restoration, and correction of the lumbar lordosis (LL).[2]

Currently, there is no established definition of MIS-TLIF, and the heterogeneity of how to perform this procedure remains substantial.[3] Commonly, open paramedian incisions are planned to avoid detaching the paraspinal musculature from their midline origins. Likewise, various muscle-splitting tubular retractors have been used to create a surgical window for reaching the targeted facet joint and disc space. Furthermore, multiple methods of intraoperative imaging have been advocated for this procedure, including fluoroscopy-assisted or navigation-assisted systems.[4,5] In addition, a visualization device, such as a microscope, is usually used during the procedure for magnification and lighting.[6] Even with variation in surgical techniques, MIS-TLIF has demonstrated superior clinical outcomes to open TLIF with lower

a Department of Orthopedic Surgery, Cedars-Sinai Medical Center, 444 South San Vicente Boulevard, Suite 901, Los Angeles, CA 90048, USA; b Board of Governors Regenerative Medicine Institute, Cedars-Sinai Medical Center, Los Angeles, CA, USA; c Department of Orthopedics, Center of Excellence in Biomechanics and Innovative Spine Surgery, Faculty of Medicine, Chulalongkorn University, Bangkok, Thailand; d University of Pittsburg Medical Center (UPMC), Harrisburg, PA, USA
1 Present address: 820 Sir Thomas Ct, Harrisburg, PA 17109.
* Corresponding author.
E-mail address: neelanand@mac.com

Neurosurg Clin N Am 34 (2023) 643–651
https://doi.org/10.1016/j.nec.2023.06.014
1042-3680/23/© 2023 Elsevier Inc. All rights reserved.

postoperative pain scores, lower blood loss, and a shorter length of hospital stay.[7,8] In addition, the fusion rates were more than 90% and comparable with open TLIF.[9–11]

Despite these proven benefits, the reported outcomes concerning the restoration of global and segmental LL from the MIS-TLIF technique is limited and varied.[12] The purpose of this article is to review the outcomes concerning the restoration of LL after the MIS-TLIF and to present the strategies to create LL by using this MIS posterior approach.

MINIMALLY INVASIVE TRANSFORAMINAL LUMBAR INTERBODY FUSION OUTCOMES REGARDING LUMBAR LORDOSIS RESTORATION

The restoration and maintenance of sagittal spinal alignment, especially LL, is important as it leads to sustained favorable postoperative clinical results and decreases the risk of adjacent segment degeneration (ASD).[13–15] Several studies demonstrated that LIF procedures, including open TLIF, MIS-TLIF, lateral lumbar interbody fusion (LLIF), and anterior lumbar interbody fusion (ALIF), preserve and restore global and segmental LL for degenerative lumbar spinal pathology.[16,17] However, there is a lack of consensus as to which LIF technique is best for creating and sustaining both global and segmental LL.[18]

Several studies reported that MIS-TLIF has similar radiographic outcomes in terms of LL restoration compared to the open TLIF.[19,20] However, Li and colleagues showed that open TLIF had better segmental LL improvement compared to the MIS-TLIF.[21] The open TLIF approach may offer a better restoration of LL due to its ability to perform bilateral facetectomies at the operated spinal level.

The anterior lumbar interbody fusion (ALIF) is shown to improve the global and segmental LL by $10.6 \pm 12.5°$ and $6.7 \pm 3.5°$, respectively.[22] In contrast, MIS-TLIF procedure could provide $5.2 \pm 5.9°$ (range -7 to 15) and $2.1 \pm 1.7°$ (0–8) global and segmental LL correction respectively.[12] Although ALIF demonstrates a superior ability for LL correction, vascular complications and availability of an access surgeon may limit its widespread adoption. In addition, MIS-TLIF can be performed at any lumbar spinal level, while ALIF is usually limited to the lower lumbar segments.

Isaacs and colleagues compared MIS-TLIF and extreme lateral interbody fusion (XLIF) in a randomized control trial (RCT) and found a nonsignificant difference in the global LL improvement between these 2 techniques, in which MIS-TLIF

and XLIF gained 3.9°, and 1.8°, respectively, from the preoperative to the 2-year postoperative period.[23] In contrast, a recent meta-analysis by Wang and colleagues demonstrated that the oblique lateral interbody fusion (OLIF) achieved better LL correction than MIS-TLIF.[24] The OLIF gained 17.73°, while MIS-TLIF could restore the LL about 2.61° when comparing the preoperative to postoperative time point.

Given these discrepancies, several factors could affect LL correction during an MIS-TLIF. Kim and colleagues reported an increase in segmental LL likely results from an anteriorly positioned interbody cage and lower preoperative segmental lordosis at the operative level.[25] Cage characteristics could also influence sagittal alignment after MIS-TLIF. Lawless and colleagues found significantly better improvement in global LL with a static lordotic cage ($2.95° \pm 7.2°$) compared to a non-lordotic titanium cage ($-0.3° \pm 7.1°$) in one- and two-level MIS-TLIF. However, improvements in segmental LL were similar between both groups.[26] A meta-analysis by Alvi and colleagues demonstrated that using an expandable interbody cage in MIS-TLIF could provide better segmental LL at the operated level, but did not demonstrate a difference in terms of the global LL restoration when compared to static cages.[27] Choi and colleagues conducted an RCT to compare the use of banana-shaped cages to straight cages in MIS-TLIF and found no significant difference between postoperative global and segmental LL at the final follow-up.[28]

STRATEGIES FOR CREATING LUMBAR LORDOSIS BY USING MINIMALLY INVASIVE TRANSFORAMINAL LUMBAR INTERBODY FUSION

During the MIS-TLIF surgery, several surgical steps and techniques could help surgeons restore a greater degree of lumbar lordosis starting with appropriately positioning the patient to maximize their physiologic lordosis.[29] Prone positioning can prove to be a powerful tool for restoring LL prior to any incision, especially in patients with preoperative hypolordosis.[30] We recommend positioning the patient in the standard prone position on a Jackson frame while maintaining the hips in an extension (neutral) position.[31] It is unnecessary to apply the reverse jackknife (lumbar hyperextension) position on the frame as this has been associated with vertebral fracture adjacent to the TLIF construct.[32]

Concerning intraoperative neurophysiological monitoring (IONM), its routine use as an adjunct for non-complex lumbar spinal surgeries is still

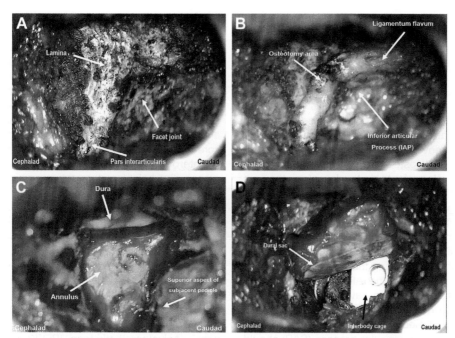

Fig. 1. Intraoperative images illustrate (A) the bony landmarks of interest before performing the ipsilateral bony decompression, (B) the initial osteotomy cut from the caudal edge of the lamina through the pars interarticularis, (C) the posterior annulus identification, and (D) an interbody cage placement in the disc space.

controversial.[33] Several authors reported that IONM provided no additional benefit for 1- or 2-level MIS-TLIF or posterior lumbar fusion procedures.[34,35] However, the senior author (NA) usually uses the IONM for the MIS-TLIF procedure. It could help with the early detection and mitigation of neurologic injury with minimal additional risk, particularly in patients who need deformity correction.[36,37]

Localization and Incision Planning

The laterality for the interbody placement usually corresponds to the most symptomatic side. This maximizes the direct decompression for the symptomatic nerve roots.

After appropriate positioning, the operative site is prepped and draped in a standard sterile fashion. We fluoroscopically localized the pedicles entry points on the side of the planned interbody placement. These entry points are marked on the skin and 1-inch paraspinal incision, which connects the points, is performed for single-level MIS-TLIF. Electrocautery is used to dissect through subcutaneous fat until the lumbar fascia is encountered. On the contralateral side, two small 1 cm (cm) stab incisions are utilized for a single-level posterior percutaneous instrumentation. We prefer vertically oriented stab incisions as these are potentially extensile if needed.

Pedicle Cannulation and Guide Wire Placement

The percutaneous pedicle screw heads and extension sleeves are often bulky and can lead to decreased visualization during an MIS-TLIF. Therefore, we prefer to cannulate and insert a guide wire into each pedicle and secure the free ends of the wires away from the surgical field until cage insertion is completed. Once the cage placement is complete, we can place cannulated percutaneous pedicle screws over the appropriately placed guide wires. It should be noted that guide wires and/or percutaneous pedicle screws placement can be performed after cage insertion if desired (Case example later in discussion). However, surgeons should exercise caution when doing so, as the exposed dura is now at risk of injury during the posterior instrumentation.

Exposure and Bony Decompression

The ipsilateral lumbar fascia bridging the two wires is sharply cut with cautery, and the paraspinal muscular interval between the multifidus muscle medially and the longissimus muscle laterally is identified. The muscular interval is dissected deeply to identify the underlying bony landmarks of interest; the facet joint and pars interarticularis (**Fig. 1**A). We do not perform dissection lateral to the facet joint as we do not routinely perform a posterolateral fusion as part of our MIS-TLIF technique. This is in alignment with other technical reports of the procedure.[11]

The bony decompression in MIS-TLIF is usually limited to an ipsilateral hemilaminectomy and unilateral facetectomy on the symptomatic side; however, if a central decompression is needed, an "over the top" decompression can be performed via the unilateral hemi-laminectomy.[38] The authors prefer to remove the inferior articular process (IAP) via a right-angle osteotomy through the pars interarticularis. We prefer to do this low along the pars (close to the IAP) to avoid an inadvertent injury to the exiting nerve root (**Fig. 1**B). While others may advocate for identifying the exiting nerve root, we do not routinely perform this step. Described later, our technique allows us to safely enter the disc space without identifying the exiting nerve root.

After the removal of the IAP, the underlying ligamentum flavum will be revealed. This is then removed to reveal the lateral edge of the dural sac, the most medial boundary for the MIS-TLIF. Next, the superior articular process (SAP) should be partially resected. Care should be taken not to remove too much of the SAP. Doing so may weaken the superior cortex of the subjacent pedicle, leading to pedicle screw loosening or iatrogenic fracture during any potential interpedicular compression or distraction maneuvers.[31]

With successful partial removal of the SAP, the superior aspect of the subjacent pedicle can be palpated. This structure can be followed downward, leading directly to the disc space. Sweeping soft tissue structures (epidural veins or fat) superiorly from the inferior pedicle will reveal the annulus of the targeted disc space (**Fig. 1**C). In this way, we can safely identify the disc space without dissecting and identifying the exiting nerve root.

Discectomy and Endplate Preparation

The discectomy and endplate preparation are also important steps aiding the restoration of LL from an MIS-TLIF. Wong and colleagues recommended using angled instruments to obtain even greater segmental release and to ensure 60% to 80% disc space preparation for arthrodesis.[39] Care is taken to remove the cartilaginous endplates meticulously during this step to avoid bony endplate injuries. We prefer rounded disc space shavers to sharp ones as these have less chance for inadvertent endplate violation. Intermittent medial retraction of the thecal sac can be utilized for further disc space preparation or for dealing with central disc herniation. Constant retraction should be avoided as it increases the risk of postoperative radiculopathy or neurologic deficit.[31]

Surgeons may also use sequentially larger blunt interbody dilators to increasingly distract the collapsed disc space or to release and mobilize the vertebral segment.[39] When a low-grade spondylolisthesis is present, Wong and colleagues recommend inserting the contralateral cannulated percutaneous pedicle screws with extension sleeves and rod at the step of pedicle cannulation and guide wire placement. These contralateral screws can be used simultaneously with sequential interbody dilators to distract the disc space, increase disc height, reduce the spondylolisthesis, and restore segmental LL.[39]

Interbody Cage Placement

Once discectomy, endplate preparation, and disc space dilation are complete, an appropriately sized interbody cage, which correspond to the interference fit trial spacer, is selected, and filled with osteobiologic materials. For a single-level MIS-TLIF, the authors prefer a static, curved (banana), polyetheretherketone (PEEK) cage filled with 4 mg (mg) of recombinant human bone morphogenic protein-2 (rhBMP-2) surrounded by 5 mL (mL) of moldable allograft demineralized bone matrix (DBM).[31] The interbody spacer is malleted anteriorly into the disc space under fluoroscopic guidance until it reaches the anterior ring apophysis (**Fig. 1**D). Then, the curved cage is rotated until it is settled within the anterior third of the disc space. This anterior cage position can help restore LL when performing the MIS-TLIF.[25] After successful cage implantation, hemostasis is obtained at the disc and epidural space and the ipsilateral tubular retractor is removed.

Posterior Instrumentation

Regarding posterior instrumentation, several techniques aid in creating LL during the MIS-TLIF. The authors utilize a cantilever reduction maneuver which can reduce spondylolisthesis and help restore LL.[11,31] We perform percutaneous cannulated pedicle screws placement over guide wires after cage insertion. The cannulated screws with rod reduction sleeves are placed over each wire on both sides of the operated spinal segment in a standard fashion. We routinely utilize precontoured lordotic rods of appropriate length, and these are guided down to the rod reduction sleeves on each side. Be sure to assess that both rods are passed below the lumbar fascia and that no intervening muscle or fascia is entrapped under the rod during the insertion. The rod is reduced to the caudal pedicle screw first, followed by the rostral screw.

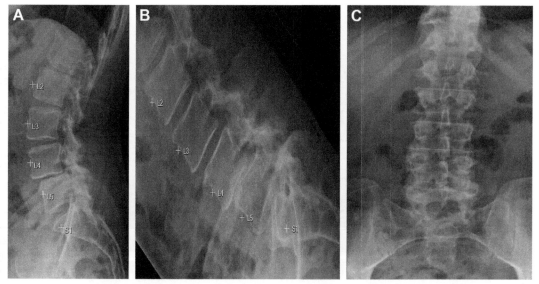

Fig. 2. Preoperative lateral (*A*) extension, (*B*) flexion, and (*C*) anteroposterior plain radiographs.

Wong and colleagues proposed an alternative technique to maximize the restoration of segmental LL during posterior instrumentation.[39] After the rods were inserted and moderately secured with set screws on both sides, they applied a bilateral compression maneuver to the construct before the final locking of set screws. We recognize that this is a commonly employed maneuver to recreate lordosis, but we do not employ it as this maneuver may inadvertently loosen the pedicle screws.

Rajakumar and colleagues reported the rocking technique to reduce various grades of spondylolisthesis and help restore LL and overall sagittal profile.[40] The authors retain the interference fit trial spacer within the disc space after the discectomy and endplate preparation step to keep the disc space distracted as this assist with spondylolisthesis reduction. Then, they applied the percutaneous screws on the contralateral side, and the screw towers were mated. Afterward, the screw system was gently moved back and forth in the craniocaudal direction (rocking) a few times to release the remaining soft tissue attached to the vertebral segment. After finishing the rocking maneuver, the listhesis reduction was evaluated under lateral fluoroscopy and the rod was guided into the screw towers. The screw caps are inserted and tightened using the cantilever reduction technique. The ipsilateral percutaneous pedicle screws are inserted after interbody cage insertion. Again, the screw caps are applied using the cantilever maneuver to reduce any residual spondylolisthesis.

Recently, Park and colleagues proposed the swing technique, a modified version of the rocking

technique.[41] The authors utilized the long tab type percutaneous pedicle screw and rod system for easier manipulation. They inserted percutaneous pedicle screw-rod constructs bilaterally after completing the interbody cage placement. All screw caps were inserted and tightened but not completely locked to maintain slight movement at the screw heads. Then, each unilateral screw/rod construct was gently swung together back and forth several times in the craniocaudal direction until the proper reduction angle was found under lateral fluoroscopy. Final tightening was done for all set screws while the screw tower-rod constructs on both sides were held in the reduced position.

Final Evaluation and Closure

After completing the posterior instrumentation, the final construct is evaluated under anteroposterior (AP) and lateral fluoroscopy. Hemostasis is obtained, and the wounds are closed in standard fashion.

CASE EXAMPLE

A 66-year-old male presented with severe low back pain, neurogenic claudication, and right leg radiculopathy. He had L3-5 micro-decompression 5 years prior and presents to our clinic after exhausting non-operative interventions. He had right-sided numbness and tingling along L4 dermatome with prolonged walking, and his legs feel heavy after walking a mile. He did not have any motor weakness nor any bowel or bladder complaints.

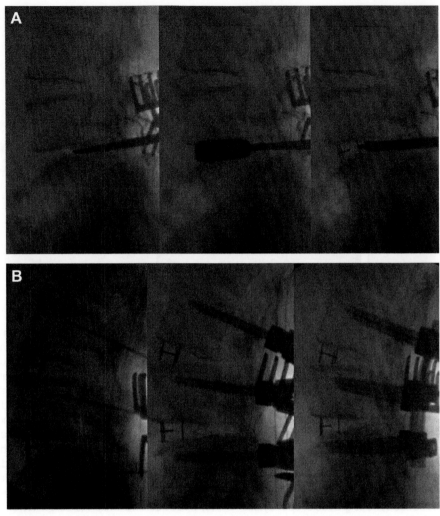

Fig. 3. Intraoperative lateral fluoroscopic images demonstrate (*A*) the disc space preparation, dilation, and interbody cage insertion at the L4/5 level, and (*B*) percutaneous screws and rods placement with cantilever maneuver to reduce the L4/5 spondylolisthesis.

Lumbar flexion/extension plain x-rays demonstrated a mobile spondylolisthesis at L4/L5 level that progresses from grade 1 to grade 2 on the flexion image. A very subtle grade 1 spondylolisthesis at L3/L4 level was likely present as well. There was a vacuum disc phenomenon at the L4/L5 level. Pelvic incidence (PI) is 45° and global L1-S1 lordosis is 50°. Despite the preserved PI-LL relationship, there was a non-physiologic L2/L3 and L3/L4 hyper-lordosis, a compensatory mechanism from L4/L5 hypo-lordosis. There was no coronal deformity (**Fig. 2**).

Lumbar magnetic resonance imaging (MRI) additionally demonstrated a mild to moderate central stenosis at L3/L4, but worst at L4/L5 level. There were severe bilateral foraminal stenosis at L3/L4 and L4/L5 levels. Furthermore, there were disc space degeneration at L3/L4 and L4/L5 levels.

The surgical plan was for MIS-TLIF L3-5 with interbody placement on the patient's right side (side of the radiculopathy). Intra-operative fluoroscopy was utilized and demonstrated on **Fig. 3**.

The patient had great relief from the surgery. The postoperative images are demonstrated in **Fig. 4**. Overall, the global LL has increased from 50° preoperatively to 55° postoperatively, but notice the relaxed, physiologic disc space at L2/L3 level. The L3-5 segmental lordosis was 32° preoperatively and increased to 40° postoperatively. There has been a greater increase in segmental LL, with only a minor increase in global LL. The full relationship between segmental lordosis and global lordosis has yet to be fully understood and the need further investigations.[12]

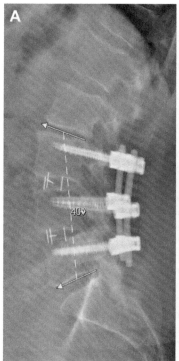
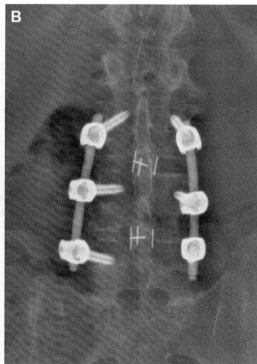

Fig. 4. Postoperative (*A*) lateral, and (*B*) anteroposterior plain radiographs. The yellow arrows and dot line demonstrate the measurement of segmental LL at L3-5 levels.

SUMMARY

MIS-TLIF is an effective MIS lumbar interbody fusion that can achieve lumbar lordosis restoration. Several crucial steps aid in this sagittal profile correction during the MIS-TLIF, including the appropriated prone positioning, optimizing disc space preparation, maximizing disc space height, anterior interbody cage placement, and reducing the spondylolisthesis.

CLINICS CARE POINTS

- MIS-TLIF is an effective MIS procedure to restore lumbar lordosis and has comparable results to open TLIF and other MIS lumbar interbody fusion techniques.

- Due to the heterogeneity of techniques reported in the literature, MIS-TLIF demonstrates variability in its restoration of lumbar lordosis.

- Several crucial steps aid in lumbar lordosis restoration during an MIS-TLIF, and are as follows: appropriate prone positioning, optimizing disc space preparation, maximizing disc space height, anterior interbody cage placement, and reducing spondylolisthesis.

DISCLOSURE

Each author certifies that he has no commercial associations (eg, consultancies, stock ownership, equity interest, patent/licensing arrangements, and so forth) that might pose a conflict of interest in connection with the submitted article.

REFERENCES

1. Prabhu MC, Jacob KC, Patel MR, et al. History and Evolution of the Minimally Invasive Transforaminal Lumbar Interbody Fusion. Neurospine 2022;19: 479–91.
2. Yingsakmongkol W, Jitpakdee K, Varakornpipat P, et al. Clinical and Radiographic Comparisons among Minimally Invasive Lumbar Interbody Fusion: A Comparison with Three-Way Matching. Asian Spine J 2022;16:712–22.
3. Lener S, Wipplinger C, Hernandez RN, et al. Defining the MIS-TLIF: A Systematic Review of Techniques and Technologies Used by Surgeons Worldwide. Global Spine J 2020;10. 151-67s.
4. Phani Kiran S, Sudhir G. Minimally invasive transforaminal lumbar interbody fusion - A narrative review on the present status. J Clin Orthop Trauma 2021; 22:101592.
5. Singhatanadgige W, Pholprajug P, Songthong K, et al. Comparative Radiographic Analyses and

Clinical Outcomes Between O-Arm Navigated and Fluoroscopic-Guided Minimally Invasive Transforaminal Lumbar Interbody Fusion. Int J Spine Surg 2022;16:151–8.

6. Singhatanadgige W, Chamadol H, Tanasansomboon T, et al. Surgical Outcomes of Minimally Invasive Transforaminal Lumbar Interbody Fusion Using Surgical Microscope vs Surgical Loupes: A Comparative Study. Int J Spine Surg 2022;16:625–30.

7. Miller LE, Bhattacharyya S, Pracyk J. Minimally Invasive Versus Open Transforaminal Lumbar Interbody Fusion for Single-Level Degenerative Disease: A Systematic Review and Meta-Analysis of Randomized Controlled Trials. World Neurosurg 2020;133:358–65.e4.

8. Singh K, Nandyala SV, Marquez-Lara A, et al. A perioperative cost analysis comparing single-level minimally invasive and open transforaminal lumbar interbody fusion. Spine J 2014;14:1694–701.

9. Kim CH, Easley K, Lee JS, et al. Comparison of Minimally Invasive Versus Open Transforaminal Interbody Lumbar Fusion. Global Spine J 2020;10. 143-50s.

10. Singhatanadgige W, Tangchitcharoen N, Kerr SJ, et al. A Comparison of Polyetheretherketone and Titanium-Coated Polyetheretherketone in Minimally Invasive Transforaminal Lumbar Interbody Fusion: A Randomized Clinical Trial. World Neurosurg 2022;168:e471–9.

11. Anand N, Hamilton JF, Perri B, et al. Cantilever TLIF with structural allograft and RhBMP2 for correction and maintenance of segmental sagittal lordosis: long-term clinical, radiographic, and functional outcome. Spine (Phila Pa 1976) 2006;31:e748–53.

12. Carlson BB, Saville P, Dowdell J, et al. Restoration of lumbar lordosis after minimally invasive transforaminal lumbar interbody fusion: a systematic review. Spine J 2019;19:951–8.

13. Kepler CK, Rihn JA, Radcliff KE, et al. Restoration of lordosis and disk height after single-level transforaminal lumbar interbody fusion. Orthop Surg 2012;4:15–20.

14. Tian H, Wu A, Guo M, et al. Adequate Restoration of Disc Height and Segmental Lordosis by Lumbar Interbody Fusion Decreases Adjacent Segment Degeneration. World Neurosurg 2018;118:e856–64.

15. Singhatanadgige W, Suranaowarat P, Jaruprat P, et al. Indirect Effects on Adjacent Segments After Minimally Invasive Transforaminal Lumbar Interbody Fusion. World Neurosurg 2022. https://doi.org/10.1016/j.wneu.2022.08.087.

16. Uribe JS, Myhre SL, Youssef JA. Preservation or Restoration of Segmental and Regional Spinal Lordosis Using Minimally Invasive Interbody Fusion Techniques in Degenerative Lumbar Conditions: A Literature Review. Spine (Phila Pa 1976) 2016;41:s50–8.

17. Ahlquist S, Park HY, Gatto J, et al. Does approach matter? A comparative radiographic analysis of spinopelvic parameters in single-level lumbar fusion. Spine J 2018;18:1999–2008.

18. Rothrock RJ, McNeill IT, Yaeger K, et al. Lumbar Lordosis Correction with Interbody Fusion: Systematic Literature Review and Analysis. World Neurosurg 2018;118:21–31.

19. Dibble CF, Zhang JK, Greenberg JK, et al. Comparison of local and regional radiographic outcomes in minimally invasive and open TLIF: a propensity score-matched cohort. J Neurosurg Spine 2022;1–11.

20. Le H, Anderson R, Phan E, et al. Clinical and Radiographic Comparison Between Open Versus Minimally Invasive Transforaminal Lumbar Interbody Fusion With Bilateral Facetectomies. Global Spine J 2021;11:903–10.

21. Li F, Li C, Xi X, et al. Distinct fusion intersegmental parameters regarding local sagittal balance provide similar clinical outcomes: a comparative study of minimally invasive versus open transforaminal lumbar interbody fusion. BMC Surg 2020;20:97.

22. Formica M, Quarto E, Zanirato A, et al. ALIF in the correction of spinal sagittal misalignment. A systematic review of literature. Eur Spine J 2021;30:50–62.

23. Isaacs RE, Sembrano JN, Tohmeh AG. Two-Year Comparative Outcomes of MIS Lateral and MIS Transforaminal Interbody Fusion in the Treatment of Degenerative Spondylolisthesis: Part II: Radiographic Findings. Spine (Phila Pa 1976) 2016;41:s133–44.

24. Wang J, Liu J, Hai Y, et al. OLIF versus MI-TLIF for patients with degenerative lumbar disease: Is one procedure superior to the other? A systematic review and meta-analysis. Front Surg 2022;9:1014314.

25. Kim SH, Hahn BS, Park JY. What Affects Segmental Lordosis of the Surgical Site after Minimally Invasive Transforaminal Lumbar Interbody Fusion? Yonsei Med J 2022;63:665–74.

26. Lawless MH, Claus CF, Tong D, et al. Radiographic and Patient-Reported Outcomes of Lordotic Versus Non-lordotic Static Interbody Devices in Minimally Invasive Transforaminal Lumbar Interbody Fusion: A Longitudinal Comparative Cohort Study. Cureus 2022;14:e21273.

27. Alvi MA, Kurian SJ, Wahood W, et al. Assessing the Difference in Clinical and Radiologic Outcomes Between Expandable Cage and Nonexpandable Cage Among Patients Undergoing Minimally Invasive Transforaminal Interbody Fusion: A Systematic Review and Meta-Analysis. World Neurosurg 2019;127:596–606.e1.

28. Choi WS, Kim JS, Hur JW, et al. Minimally Invasive Transforaminal Lumbar Interbody Fusion Using Banana-Shaped and Straight Cages: Radiological and Clinical Results from a Prospective Randomized Clinical Trial. Neurosurgery 2018;82:289–98.

29. Barrey C, Darnis A. Current strategies for the restoration of adequate lordosis during lumbar fusion. World J Orthop 2015;6:117–26.

30. Harimaya K, Lenke LG, Mishiro T, et al. Increasing lumbar lordosis of adult spinal deformity patients via intraoperative prone positioning. Spine (Phila Pa 1976) 2009;34:2406–12.

31. Anand N, Kong C. Can Minimally Invasive Transforaminal Lumbar Interbody Fusion Create Lordosis from a Posterior Approach? Neurosurg Clin N Am 2018;29:453–9.

32. Saville PA, Anari JB, Smith HE, et al. Vertebral body fracture after TLIF: a new complication. Eur Spine J 2016;25:230–8.

33. Charalampidis A, Jiang F, Wilson JRF, et al. The Use of Intraoperative Neurophysiological Monitoring in Spine Surgery. Global Spine J 2020;10(1 Suppl). 104-14s.

34. Garces J, Berry JF, Valle-Giler EP, et al. Intraoperative neurophysiological monitoring for minimally invasive 1- and 2-level transforaminal lumbar interbody fusion: does it improve patient outcome? Ochsner J 2014;14(1):57–61.

35. Austerman RJ, Sulhan S, Steele WJ, et al. The utility of intraoperative neuromonitoring on simple posterior lumbar fusions-analysis of the National Inpatient Sample. J Spine Surg 2021;7(2):132–40.

36. Lall RR, Lall RR, Hauptman JS, et al. Intraoperative neurophysiological monitoring in spine surgery: indications, efficacy, and role of the preoperative checklist. Neurosurg Focus 2012;33(5):e10.

37. Ament JD, Leon A, Kim KD, et al. Intraoperative neuromonitoring in spine surgery: large database analysis of cost-effectiveness. N Am Spine Soc J 2023; 14:100206.

38. Singhatanadgige W, Promsuwan M, Tanasansomboon T, et al. Is Unilateral Minimally Invasive Transforaminal Lumbar Interbody Fusion Sufficient in Patients with Claudication? A Comparative Matched Cohort Study. World Neurosurg 2021;150:e735–40.

39. Wong AP, Smith ZA, Stadler JA 3rd, et al. Minimally invasive transforaminal lumbar interbody fusion (MI-TLIF): surgical technique, long-term 4-year prospective outcomes, and complications compared with an open TLIF cohort. Neurosurg Clin N Am 2014;25: 279–304.

40. Rajakumar DV, Hari A, Krishna M, et al. Complete anatomic reduction and monosegmental fusion for lumbar spondylolisthesis of Grade II and higher: use of the minimally invasive "rocking" technique. Neurosurg Focus 2017;43:E12.

41. Park B, Noh SH, Park JY. Reduction and monosegmental fusion for lumbar spondylolisthesis with a long tab percutaneous pedicle screw system: "swing" technique. Neurosurg Focus 2019;46:e11.

The MIS PSO

Oliver G.S. Ayling, MD, MSc[a,b], Michael Y. Wang, MD[a,b,*]

KEYWORDS

- Pedicle subtraction osteotomy • Spinal deformity • Minimally invasive spine surgery

KEY POINTS

- The minimally invasive pedicle subtraction osteotomy (MIS PSO) is a hybrid approach combining traditional MIS and open surgical deformity techniques.
- The MIS PSO is associated with decreased morbidity with lower blood loss and less soft tissue disruption.
- The MIS PSO is technically challenging and requires a solid foundation in both MIS and traditional open surgery for adult spinal deformity correction.

INTRODUCTION

Adult spinal deformity is associated with a decreased quality of life secondary to pain and disability. Fortunately, many patients benefit from surgical correction of the spinal deformity leading to clinically significant improvements in functional ability, pain, and quality of life.[1–3] Coinciding with advances in modern medical care there is an increasingly aged population in North America, of which a considerable proportion will develop debilitating symptoms due to degenerative spinal deformity.[4]

Traditional methods of spinal deformity correction have focused on anterior column height restoration or various posterior column osteotomies leading to restoration of spinal balance in the coronal and sagittal planes of the thoracolumbar region.[5–14] Current methods for spinal deformity correction have significant limitations such as, large open subperiosteal exposures, increased blood loss, and potentially multistaged approaches that may preclude patients of more advanced age being considered for surgical intervention.[4] Furthermore, older patients are more likely to have significant medical comorbidities that increase their risk profile of operative and postoperative adverse events, with up 70% of patients of advanced age undergoing spinal deformity surgery experiencing a complication.[15]

Increasingly patients of advanced age are expecting to lead active lives without pain or disability and as such less-invasive approaches, in order to mitigate morbidity, are increasingly being used in spine surgery. Less-invasive approaches most commonly include lateral prepsoas or transpsoas approaches with the possibility of anterior column height restoration to improve coronal and sagittal imbalances.[3,14,16] A major drawback of the lateral approaches for the correction of spinal deformities is that they often require an inherently mobile spinal column and therefore may not be suitable for fixed spinal deformities. Classically the pedicle subtraction osteotomy (PSO) is the method of choice for correction of large fixed deformities in the thoracolumbar spine because it allows for powerful restoration of sagittal balance and subsequent bony fusion.[5] The PSO is discussed in detail other articles within this book. The MIS PSO, a hybrid approach, has been developed to take advantage of the intrinsic value of the open PSO but with the aim of minimizing the morbidly associated with open procedures.[3,4,17] The MIS PSO will be discussed in this article.

SURGICAL TECHNIQUE

The MIS PSO is a hybrid technique where a mini-open subperiosteal exposure is performed at the

a Department of Neurosurgery, University of Miami, Miami, FL, USA; b Department of Neurological Surgery, University of Miami MILLER School of Medicine, 1095 Northwest 14th Terrace (D4-6), Miami, FL 33136, USA
* Corresponding author. Department of Neurological Surgery, University of Miami MILLER School of Medicine, 1095 Northwest 14th Terrace (D4-6), Miami, FL 33136
E-mail address: MWang2@med.miami.edu

Neurosurg Clin N Am 34 (2023) 653–658
https://doi.org/10.1016/j.nec.2023.06.011
1042-3680/23/© 2023 Elsevier Inc. All rights reserved.

level of the planned PSO while all other elements of the surgery are done in true MIS fashion via percutaneous approaches. The key to this method is the combination of open and MIS techniques. This hybrid approach with the mini-open access to the PSO allows for control of blood loss and adequate exposure of the neural elements during the PSO. Subsequently, tissue disruption and blood loss are minimized when performing MIS transforaminal interbody insertions below the PSO or when placing percutaneous pedicle screws and rod insertion. A challenge to any MIS procedure is the placement of a rod across multiple segments of the spine, particularly when passing a highly lordotic rod after sagittal imbalance correction. To circumvent this issue, the MIS PSO uses the 4-rod technique that acts as a cantilever across the PSO site to control the coronal and sagittal correction of the deformity. Moreover, it is easier to pass 2 rods from above and 2 rods from below with the appropriate amount of lordosis and then connect at the central open incision, again taking advantage of the hybrid approach. Furthermore, the ability to manipulate the rod in situ allows for mechanical stabilization of the spine without a temporary rod before PSO closure. An added benefit to the 4-rod construct is the minimization of rod stress during rod bending and contouring because the forces are distributed across the multiple rods but the overall lordosis is equivalent to a single rod.

MIS PSO SURGICAL STEPS

1. Appropriate anesthesia and hemodynamic/ neurological monitoring are established
2. The patient is placed prone on a Jackson spine table, prepped, and draped widely
3. A midline skin incision dorsally to encompass all planned levels (typically thoracic to sacral) and carried down to the subcutaneous fat with the fascia remaining intact. Subsequent percutaneous steps of the operation are performed through the fascia. This technique avoids multiple skin incisions, reduces blood loss, and is preferable cosmetically
4. Traditional MIS transforaminal interbody fusions are performed below the levels of the planned PSO
5. Exposure of the PSO site, most commonly L3. A complete subperiosteal exposure lateral to the transverse processes and cranial-caudal from pedicle to pedicle is performed.
6. At the PSO site a full laminectomy with bilateral facetectomies are performed
7. The exiting and traversing nerve roots at the site of the PSO are completely exposed so

that the pedicle at the PSO site is clearly identified and the neural elements protected
8. The transverse processes are removed bilaterally at the PSO level
9. The pedicles at the PSO site are removed bilaterally with the Leksell rongeurs and made flush with the vertebral body. Hemostasis is continually achieved
10. Cottonoid patties are placed ventrolateral to the vertebral bodies, bilaterally, to dissect soft tissue away from the vertebral bodies and protect adjacent vascular structures
11. Percutaneous pedicle screws are placed at least 3 levels above and 3 levels below the PSO site
12. Fusion above the PSO is achieved by percutaneously drilling the facet joints before pedicle screw insertion and placement of 0.25 mg of recombinant bone morphogenic protein-2 below the pedicle screw head so that it sits between the facet joint and pedicle screw. Alternatively, a subperiosteal exposure unilaterally above the PSO site and an interlaminar fusion can be performed. Fusion below the PSO is achieved via the interbody grafts. Interbody grafts above the PSO may also be considered for additional fusion
13. Via the opening of the pedicle into the vertebral body, from the prior pedicle resection, curettes are used to perform decancellation osteotomies bilaterally. In this manner, progressively enlarging curettes are used to remove cancellous bone from within the vertebral body. Working in a cone-shaped fashion, with the apex of the cone ventral, the cancellous bone is removed at each side and then angled curettes are used to remove cancellous bone from the central vertebral body. Any bone removed is saved for later fusion purposes
14. The posterior longitudinal ligament and posterior wall of the vertebral body are then removed entirely. This step necessitates retraction of the thecal sac sequentially on each side
15. If an extended PSO is planned, then the caudal intervertebral disc can then be removed
16. The 4 rods, with appropriate lordosis, are placed subfascially and passed from cranial and caudal to meet at the open site. Rod-to-rod side connectors are then placed to facilitate eventual rod connection but are left loose at this stage. Setscrews are placed down the reduction tabs so that the rods are in contact with the screw heads but the setscrews are still loose to allow for eventual rod maneuvering during closure of the PSO

17. With the 4 rods in place, the final portion of bone is removed from the lateral cortical walls of the vertebral body on each side using Leksell rongeurs. The bone of the lateral vertebral body wall is removed in a wedge-shaped manner that mirrors the decancellation cones performed earlier

18. Ensure no bone or ligament ventral to the thecal sac remains that may abut the neural elements on osteotomy closure

19. Closure of the PSO occurs by simultaneously applying force to the rod holders so that they are brought together toward the PSO site from cranial and caudal directions. This maneuver creates a greenstick fracture at the osteotomy site and then closure of the PSO with resulting increased lordosis. The side-to-side rod connectors are then attached to each other and tightened, followed by tightening of the pedicle setscrews. Controlling the 4 rods simultaneously allows correction in the coronal and sagittal planes without translation of the spinal column above and below the PSO site (**Figs. 1** and **2**)

20. After closure and securing of the PSO site, the nerves and thecal sac are inspected to ensure no compression has occurred. Hemostasis is achieved

21. Closure in standard fashion

OUTCOMES: CLINICAL AND RADIOGRAPHIC

In a series of 16 patients treated at the University of Miami with a mean follow-up of ~18 months and an average patient age of ~70 years,[3] there were significant improvements in patient-reported outcomes as well as radiographic parameters. There was a mean of 7.6 levels fused, and half of the patients underwent bilateral iliac screw fixation with all constructs spanning the lumbosacral and thoracolumbar junctions. Ten of the 16 patients had a PSO performed at L3, whereas 6 had a PSO at L2. Performing the MIS PSO at L4 is avoided due to an increased risk of nerve injury leading to foot drop. The mean length of operative time was ~350 minutes with an average of ~850 cc of blood loss.

In this series of 16 patients undergoing a MIS PSO for deformity correction, the clinical changes were measured preoperatively and at last follow-up using the VAS back and leg scores, and ODI. VAS leg and back scores improved considerably from 6 to 1 and 8 to 2, respectively. The ODI also improved from a mean of 50 preoperatively to 16 postoperatively. Additionally, postoperative ambulatory distance greatly improved for all patients from a mean of 115 feet to 2100 feet.

Radiographic parameters, based on 36-inch standing scoliosis radiographs, were assessed at

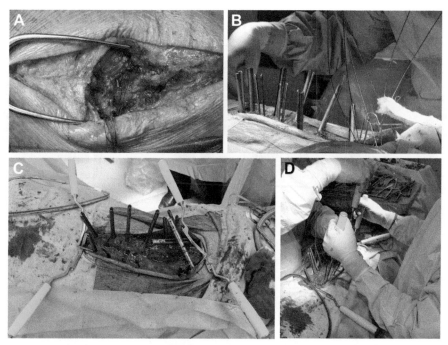

Fig. 1. Intraoperative photographs of the MIS PSO. Midline opening with preservation of the fascia above and below the MIS PSO site (*A*). Placement of percutaneous pedicle screws with reduction towers above and below the PSO (*B*). Placement of the 4 rods before PSO closure (*C*) and performing the initial PSO closure with maneuvering of the rod and setscrew placement via the reduction towers (*D*).

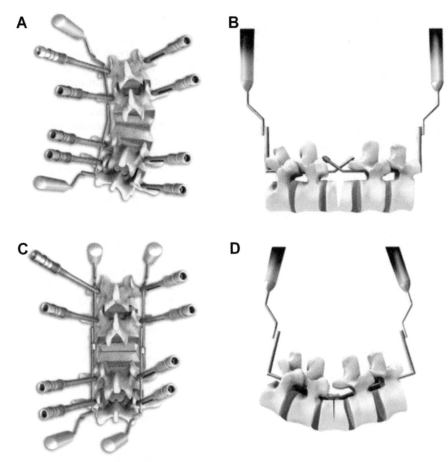

Fig. 2. Artistic rendering of the 4-rod technique for MIS PSO closure. Coronal (*A*) and sagittal (*B*) planes before PSO closure. Coronal (*C*) and sagittal (*D*) planes after PSO closure.

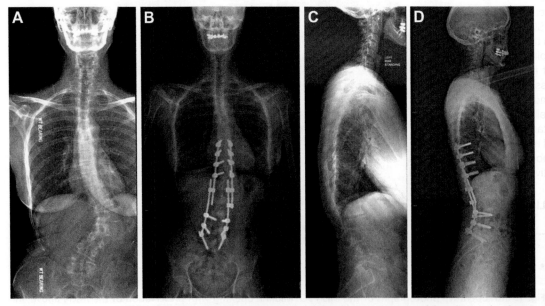

Fig. 3. Standing 36-inch films. Anterior-posterior preoperative (*A*) and postoperative (*B*) radiographs demonstrating improvement in coronal balance after MIS PSO. Lateral preoperative (*C*) and postoperative (*D*) radiographs demonstrating improved sagittal balance in the same patient.

last follow-up, compared with preoperative images. Coronal alignment, lumbar Cobb angle, lumbar lordosis minus pelvic incidence, and the sagittal vertical axis all substantially improved. Overall coronal alignment improved from 28 to 16 mm; the lumbar Cobb angle improved from 40° to 15°; the mean postoperative lumbar lordosis minus pelvic incidence was 8°; sagittal vertical axis improved from 100 to 40 mm (**Fig. 3**). Fusion rates were assessed in 10 patients with CT scanning at 1 year postoperatively, and a solid fusion was present in 8 of these patients at all levels. There were no symptomatic cases of proximal junctional kyphosis.

ADVERSE EVENTS

No cases were converted to completely open operations, and there were no cases of paralysis or death. Overall perioperative adverse events were low in the series from the University of Miami, with 1 durotomy, 1 postoperative wound infection, and 1 case of cerebral infarction. Hardware-related complications included one iliac screw-rod displacement and one interbody dislodgement requiring return to the operating room. There was one case of rod fracture across the PSO site occurring 1 year after surgery.

SUMMARY

The MIS PSO is a hybrid approach using less-invasive surgical approaches combined with traditional open spinal deformity techniques for the treatment of adult spinal deformities. The MIS PSO allows for the correction of spinal deformities in the coronal and sagittal planes, even in the fixed spine, and simultaneously mitigating the morbidity of traditional open surgery by preserving the soft tissues and minimizing blood loss. The treatment and increasingly positive outcomes of adult spinal deformities continues to evolve with our understanding of spinal biomechanics and development of new technologies, with the MIS PSO providing a tool to the spine surgeon to accomplish their operative goals.

CLINICS CARE POINTS

- The MIS PSO is a hybrid approach combining traditional MIS and open surgical deformity techniques.
- The use of the MIS PSO is associated with decreased morbidity with less blood loss and less soft tissue disruption.

- The MIS PSO is technically challenging and requires a solid foundation in both MIS and traditional open surgery for adult spinal deformity correction.

DISCLOSURE

The authors have nothing to disclose.

REFERENCES

1. Smith JS, Klineberg E, Schwab F, et al. Change in classification grade by the SRS-schwab adult spinal deformity classification predicts impact on health-related quality of life measures: prospective analysis of operative and nonoperative treatment. Spine 2013;38(19):1663.
2. Wang MY. Miniopen Pedicle subtraction osteotomy: surgical technique and initial results. Neurosurgery Clinics 2014;25(2):347–51.
3. Wang MY, Bordon G. Mini-open pedicle subtraction osteotomy as a treatment for severe adult spinal deformities: case series with initial clinical and radiographic outcomes. J Neurosurg Spine 2016;24(5):769–76.
4. Wang MY, Madhavan K. Mini-open pedicle subtraction osteotomy: surgical technique. World Neurosurgery 2014;81(5):843.e11–4.
5. Bridwell KH, Lewis SJ, Lenke LG, et al. Pedicle subtraction osteotomy for the treatment of fixed sagittal imbalance. JBJS 2003;85(3):454.
6. Heary RF, Bono CM. Pedicle subtraction osteotomy in the treatment of chronic, posttraumatic kyphotic deformity. J Neurosurg Spine 2006;5(1):1–8.
7. Kim YJ, Bridwell KH, Lenke LG, et al. Results of lumbar pedicle subtraction osteotomies for fixed sagittal imbalance: a minimum 5-year follow-up study. Spine 2007;32(20):2189.
8. Mummaneni PV, Dhall SS, Ondra SL, et al. Pedicle subtraction osteotomy. Neurosurgery 2008;63(3):A171.
9. Ondra SL, Marzouk S, Koski T, et al. Mathematical calculation of pedicle subtraction osteotomy size to allow precision correction of fixed sagittal deformity. Spine 2006;31(25):E973.
10. Chou D, Lau D. The mini-open pedicle subtraction osteotomy for flat-back syndrome and kyphosis correction: operative technique. Operative Neurosurgery 2016;12(4):309.
11. Wang MY, Berven SH. Lumbar pedicle subtraction osteotomy. Operative Neurosurgery 2007;60(2):140.
12. Demirkiran G, Theologis AA, Pekmezci M, et al. Adult spinal deformity correction with multi-level anterior column releases: description of a new surgical technique and literature review. Clinical Spine Surgery 2016;29(4):141.

13. Xu DS, Paluzzi J, Kanter AS, et al. Anterior column release/realignment. Neurosurgery Clinics 2018; 29(3):427–37.

14. Saigal R, Mundis GM, Eastlack R, et al. Anterior column realignment (ACR) in adult sagittal deformity correction. Spine 2016;41(1):S66–73.

15. Smith JS, Shaffrey CI, Glassman SD, et al. Risk-Benefit assessment of surgery for adult scoliosis: an analysis based on patient age. Spine 2011; 36(10):817.

16. Ozgur BM, Aryan HE, Pimenta L, et al. Extreme Lateral Interbody Fusion (XLIF): a novel surgical technique for anterior lumbar interbody fusion. Spine J 2006;6(4):435–43.

17. Voyadzis JM, Gala VC, O'Toole JE, et al. Minimally invasive posterior osteotomies. Neurosurgery 2008; 63(3):A204.

Robotic-Assisted Surgery and Navigation in Deformity Surgery

Christine Park, MS[a],*, Saman Shabani, MD[b], Nitin Agarwal, MD[c],
Lee Tan, MD[a], Praveen V. Mummaneni, MD, MBA[a]

KEYWORDS

- Navigation guidance • Robotics • Advanced technology • Adult spinal deformity • Surgery

KEY POINTS

- As three-dimensional (3D) navigation and robotic-assisted deformity surgery are becoming increasingly popular, there are currently increasing data on the impact of robotics use on patient-related outcomes including instrumentation failure, complication rates, and surgical efficiency.
- Navigation-guided approaches have been developed to maximize screw placement success and minimize injury.
- Despite the potential advantages of 3D navigation and robotics systems, there is limited data available demonstrating superiority of these advanced technology over the traditional freehand fluoroscopy-guided method specifically in the setting of spinal deformity.

INTRODUCTION

Adult spinal deformity (ASD) is characterized by misalignment and imbalance in the sagittal and coronal planes that may result in disability in daily activities of living and significant negative impact in quality of life.[1–3] The current prevalence is estimated to be up to 70% in those of age 60 years or older and is projected to increase with the aging population.[4,5]

The goal of ASD surgery is to correct the deformity based on appropriate spinopelvic parameters. Advances in surgical techniques and perioperative care have increased the pursuit of surgical treatment for ASD with promising potential in improving pain and disability.[6–8] However, surgery is still not without risks. Postoperative complications such as instrumentation failure and infection, blood loss, and long duration of surgery remain challenging issues.

The development of intraoperative navigation and surgical robotics has been rapidly progressing and has made significant advancement in spine surgery in terms of improved preoperative visualization and planning, screw placement accuracy, and reduced postoperative complications.[9–13] As robots are becoming more capable of handling increasingly complex spinal procedures, robotic-assisted surgery is beginning to become more widely adopted in spine procedures including deformity corrections.[14,15]

DISCUSSION
Instrumentation

Pedicle screw placement with intraoperative fluoroscopy is a popular and established technique for reconstructive surgery for deformity. However, the pedicle wall breach rate using the freehand technique can range up to 23%.[16] Factors that can affect accuracy include the surgeon's experience, case complexity, limitations of two-dimensional (2D) imaging, and patient-specific factors. Two-dimensional imaging resulting from

[a] Department of Neurological Surgery, University of California, 505 Parnassus Avenue, San Francisco, CA 94143, USA; [b] Department of Neurological Surgery, Medical College of Wisconsin, 8701 Watertown Plank Road, Milwaukee, WI 53226, USA; [c] Department of Neurological Surgery, 200 Lothrop Street, Pittsburgh, PA 15213, USA
* Corresponding author. 325 Ninth Avenue, Box 359924, Seattle, WA 98104.
E-mail address: christine.park@ucsf.edu

Neurosurg Clin N Am 34 (2023) 659–664
https://doi.org/10.1016/j.nec.2023.05.002
1042-3680/23/Published by Elsevier Inc.

fluoroscopy/plain films has limitations in assessing the true anatomy, which is critical for accurate pedicle screw placement. This is especially pronounced in patients with spinal deformity who have difficult anatomy and yet often require extensive constructs.[17,18] Moreover, about a quarter of all patients who have malpositioned instrumentation may require implant revision or removal, which is associated with high cost and morbidity.[17,19] To this end, three-dimensional (3D) intraoperative imaging techniques such as computed tomography (CT) imaging may improve screw placement accuracy.[17,20–22] Intraoperative 3D imaging allows the surgeon to identify misplaced screws during the procedure and replace these screws before completion of the operation. In addition, CT-guided navigation can provide real-time 3D feedback for the surgeon by using preoperative and/or intraoperative CT scan to digitally reconstruct an anatomic map for the surgeon during the operation. The ability to see the 3D anatomy of the spine may be useful in complex deformity surgery, revision surgery, and pelvic fixation where visualization and understanding of the deformed spine are essential.

In addition to 3D imaging, the integration of robotics into spine surgery has been an integral part of improving the instrumentation accuracy especially in the realm of minimally invasive surgery (MIS) (**Figs. 1** and **2**). For spinal fusion procedures, previous studies have demonstrated numerous advantages of robotic-assisted navigation with accuracy rates up to 98%.[11,23] In addition to increased accuracy, robotic-assisted spine surgery results in minimal intraoperative blood loss and less tissue destruction compared with the conventional freehand technique and MIS.[24–26]

Despite the benefits of navigation- and robotic-guided spine surgery, the currently available evidence demonstrates similar performance for guided navigation and traditional freehand technique.[27–29] Although there are no studies demonstrating a definitive advantage of navigated techniques in the setting of spinal deformity, the use of navigated techniques may be a valuable aid to the surgeons in complex spine cases per their preference.

Sacroiliac Fixation

Successful lumbosacral fusions have been difficult to achieve, with high postoperative complications and pseudoarthrosis rates due to the unfavorable anatomical structure and biomechanical profile of the lumbosacral junction.[30] Bilateral iliac screws were traditionally used to strengthen the caudal end of lumbosacral constructs during posterior

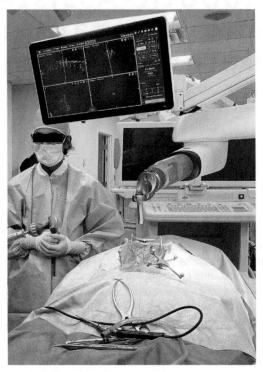

Fig. 1. An example of a surgical robot for spinal fusion surgery.

lumbosacral instrumented fusion.[31,32] Studies have shown that iliac screw fixation increases the biomechanical strength at the lumbosacral junction with good clinical outcomes.[30,32,33] Robotic-assisted iliac screw fixation has been increasingly pursued when considering a minimally invasive

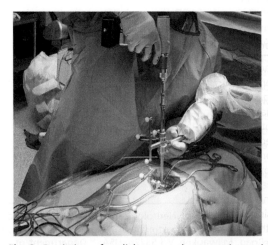

Fig. 2. Depiction of pedicle screw placement in a spinal fusion surgery which involves the robotic arm guidance for pedicle screw placement followed by insertion of pedicle screw in the trajectory defined by the robotic arm.

approach due to the heterogeneity and suboptimal visualization of the pelvic anatomy.[34,35] Iliac screw fixation is critical to a variety of indications including long-segment constructs, high-grade spondylolisthesis, pseudoarthrosis, and deformity correction. Studies have shown that image-guided sacroiliac screw fixation allows for minimally invasive approach without compromising the strength of the sacropelvic fixation that enhances bony fusion.[36–39] Furthermore, navigated sacroiliac surgeries reduce surrounding tissue damage, minimize bleeding, and decrease the risk for wound infection and disunion[40–43] while maintaining accuracy rate as high as 95%.[43–45]

However, due to their lateral positioning relative to the axis of lumbar screws, these iliac screw heads require additional contorting of the rods or needing to be accompanied by an offset connector, both of which contribute to increasing the risk of potential mechanical failure. As an alternative strategy to reduce the need for unnatural rod adjustments and an extra component for instrumentation, bilateral sacroiliac screws were introduced in which the heads of the screws can align with the rest of the lumbosacral screws in a long construct.[36] Particularly, S2 alar-iliac screws demonstrate improved outcomes for pelvic obliquity correction and anchor stability compared with traditional iliac fixation.[46] More recently, studies have shown that image-guided sacroiliac screw fixation allows for minimally invasive approach without compromising the strength of the sacropelvic fixation that enhances bony fusion.[36–39] Furthermore, navigated sacroiliac surgeries may further reduce surrounding tissue damage, minimize bleeding, and decrease the risk for wound infection and disunion.[40,41]

Radiation Exposure

Radiation exposure to the surgeon during spine surgery is another disadvantage of the freehand technique which often requires multiple fluoroscopic images for confirmation. The 3D navigation and robotics systems have been shown to significantly decrease the radiation exposure for the surgeon compared with the freehand technique.[11,12,47–49] However, due to the use of intraoperative CT scan, radiation exposure may not be decreased (and, in some instances, increased) for the patient using the 3D navigation and robotics systems.[50] Although the reduction in radiation exposure for the surgical team is a significant benefit, this may come at the expense of increased radiation to the patient; hence, the surgeon should be aware of this risk when evaluating patients and selecting the most appropriate surgical approach.

Disadvantages

Three-dimensional navigation and robotics have many potential benefits including improved instrumentation accuracy, better appreciation of anatomy, and reduced radiation exposure to the surgical team. Despite these advantages, there still exist significant limitations in fully adopting this technology. First, one of the important limitations is the cost.[14] As novel robotics systems are hitting the market, the cost is also proportionally increasing with the newer models approaching over $1 million US dollars.[51] Currently, there are no studies to date that demonstrate superior cost-effectiveness of these advanced guidance systems in deformity surgery. Second, particularly for senior surgeons with experience and proficiency using freehand fluoroscopy-guided techniques, the addition of 3D navigation or robotic technology may increase operative time without imparting a meaningful clinical benefit in terms of improved patient outcomes due to the learning curve that may be associated with its initial use.[48,52–56] Over time, these advanced instrumentation tools may improve complication and reoperation rates related to malpositioned screws as well as reduce total operative time, particularly in patients with abnormal and complex spine anatomy. Finally, reliance on navigation technology can compromise the anatomy skills of surgeons in training which may lead to suboptimal outcomes in circumstances of technology failure or when technology support is not available (eg, nights and weekends). Hence, surgeons must take caution against relying too heavily on navigational assistance and use it primarily as an assistive tool to augment their understanding of the patient-specific anatomy to allow for safer and more efficient surgeries.

SUMMARY

The use of 3D navigation systems and robotics in deformity surgery is an area of rapid advancement in the treatment of ASD. In spinal fusion surgery, robotics has led to increased intraoperative accuracy for pedicle screw placement while decreasing radiation exposure, complication rates, blood loss, and recovery time for patients. Compared with the historically accepted freehand fluoroscopy-assisted instrumentation, there is currently insufficient evidence suggesting any definitive advantages of robotics over the traditional freehand technique. Most of the studies demonstrating superiority of robotic systems are relatively small and are retrospective given the early stages of these technologies for use in deformity surgery.

Also, the incorporation of these advanced navigation systems can be financially and chronologically costly. Ideally, the surgeon should use this advanced technology as a tool for enhancing their surgical workflow but should not rely on this technology to replace surgical experience, a detailed understanding of spine anatomy, and sound clinical judgment.

CLINICS CARE POINTS

- Robotic-assisted spinal fusion and sacroiliac fixation surgeries have suggested high accuracy rates, minimal intraoperative blood loss, and less injury to surrounding tissue compared with the conventional freehand technique.

- The three-dimensional (3D) navigation and robotics systems have been shown to significantly decrease the radiation exposure for the surgical team compared with the freehand technique; however, due to the use of intraoperative computed tomography scan, radiation exposure may not be significantly decreased for the patient.

- Limitations to 3D navigation and robotics include cost, learning curve, and technology dependence.

- Further evidence is needed to validate the advantages of robotics over the traditional freehand technique in deformity surgery.

DISCLOSURE

C. Park: None; S. Shabani: None; N. Agarwal: Thieme Publishing, Springer Publishing; L. Tan: Medtronic, Stryker Spine, Accelus; P.V. Mummaneni: DePuy Spine, Globus, Nuvasive, Brainlab, BK Medical, Thieme Publishing, Springer Publishing, Spinicity/ISD, AO Spine, ISSG, NREF, PCORI, Alan and Jacqueline Stuart Spine Outcomes Center, Joan O'Reilly Endowed Professorship, NIH/NIAMS.

REFERENCES

1. Schwab F, Lafage V, Farcy JP, et al. Surgical rates and operative outcome analysis in thoracolumbar and lumbar major adult scoliosis: application of the new adult deformity classification. Spine 2007; 32(24):2723–30.

2. Bess S, Line B, Fu KM, et al. The Health Impact of Symptomatic Adult Spinal Deformity: Comparison of Deformity Types to United States Population Norms and Chronic Diseases. Spine 2016;41(3): 224–33.

3. Pellisé F, Vila-Casademunt A, Ferrer M, et al. Impact on health related quality of life of adult spinal deformity (ASD) compared with other chronic conditions. Eur Spine J 2015;24(1):3–11.

4. Schwab F, Dubey A, Gamez L, et al. Adult scoliosis: prevalence, SF-36, and nutritional parameters in an elderly volunteer population. Spine 2005;30(9): 1082–5.

5. Ames CP, Scheer JK, Lafage V, et al. Adult Spinal Deformity: Epidemiology, Health Impact, Evaluation, and Management. Spine Deform 2016;4(4):310–22.

6. Bridwell KH, Baldus C, Berven S, et al. Changes in radiographic and clinical outcomes with primary treatment adult spinal deformity surgeries from two years to three- to five-years follow-up. Spine 2010; 35(20):1849–54.

7. Smith JS, Lafage V, Shaffrey CI, et al. Outcomes of Operative and Nonoperative Treatment for Adult Spinal Deformity: A Prospective, Multicenter, Propensity-Matched Cohort Assessment With Minimum 2-Year Follow-up. Neurosurgery 2016;78(6):851–61.

8. Smith JS, Shaffrey CI, Glassman SD, et al. Risk-benefit assessment of surgery for adult scoliosis: an analysis based on patient age. Spine 2011; 36(10):817–24.

9. Amiot LP, Lang K, Putzier M, et al. Comparative results between conventional and computer-assisted pedicle screw installation in the thoracic, lumbar, and sacral spine. Spine 2000;25(5):606–14.

10. Overley SC, Cho SK, Mehta AI, et al. Navigation and Robotics in Spinal Surgery: Where Are We Now? Neurosurgery 2017;80(3s):S86–99.

11. Kantelhardt SR, Martinez R, Baerwinkel S, et al. Perioperative course and accuracy of screw positioning in conventional, open robotic-guided and percutaneous robotic-guided, pedicle screw placement. Eur Spine J 2011;20(6):860–8.

12. Roser F, Tatagiba M, Maier G. Spinal robotics: current applications and future perspectives. Neurosurgery 2013;72(Suppl 1):12–8.

13. Wang MY, Goto T, Tessitore E, et al. Introduction. Robotics in neurosurgery. Neurosurg Focus 2017; 42(5):E1.

14. Faria C, Erlhagen W, Rito M, et al. Review of Robotic Technology for Stereotactic Neurosurgery. IEEE Rev Biomed Eng 2015;8:125–37.

15. Bertelsen A, Melo J, Sánchez E, et al. A review of surgical robots for spinal interventions. Int J Med Robot 2013;9(4):407–22.

16. Rajasekaran S, Vidyadhara S, Ramesh P, et al. Randomized clinical study to compare the accuracy of navigated and non-navigated thoracic pedicle screws in deformity correction surgeries. Spine 2007;32(2):E56–64.

17. Shillingford JN, Laratta JL, Sarpong NO, et al. Instrumentation complication rates following spine surgery: a report from the Scoliosis Research Society (SRS) morbidity and mortality database. J Spine Surg 2019;5(1):110–5.

18. Li G, Lv G, Passias P, et al. Complications associated with thoracic pedicle screws in spinal deformity. Eur Spine J 2010;19(9):1576–84.

19. Sankey EW, Mehta VA, Wang TY, et al. The medicolegal impact of misplaced pedicle and lateral mass screws on spine surgery in the United States. Neurosurgical Focus FOC 2020;49(5):E20.

20. Gelalis ID, Paschos NK, Pakos EE, et al. Accuracy of pedicle screw placement: a systematic review of prospective in vivo studies comparing free hand, fluoroscopy guidance and navigation techniques. Eur Spine J 2012;21(2):247–55.

21. Van de Kelft E, Costa F, Van der Planken D, et al. A prospective multicenter registry on the accuracy of pedicle screw placement in the thoracic, lumbar, and sacral levels with the use of the O-arm imaging system and StealthStation Navigation. Spine 2012; 37(25):E1580–7.

22. Tian NF, Xu HZ. Image-guided pedicle screw insertion accuracy: a meta-analysis. Int Orthop 2009; 33(4):895–903.

23. Devito DP, Kaplan L, Dietl R, et al. Clinical acceptance and accuracy assessment of spinal implants guided with SpineAssist surgical robot: retrospective study. Spine 2010;35(24):2109–15.

24. Schatlo B, Molliqaj G, Cuvinciuc V, et al. Safety and accuracy of robot-assisted versus fluoroscopy-guided pedicle screw insertion for degenerative diseases of the lumbar spine: a matched cohort comparison. J Neurosurg Spine 2014;20(6):636–43.

25. Jiang B, Pennington Z, Azad T, et al. Robot-Assisted versus Freehand Instrumentation in Short-Segment Lumbar Fusion: Experience with Real-Time Image-Guided Spinal Robot. World Neurosurg 2020;136:e635–45.

26. Staub BN, Sadrameli SS. The use of robotics in minimally invasive spine surgery. J Spine Surg 2019; 5(Suppl 1):S31–40.

27. Verma R, Krishan S, Haendlmayer K, et al. Functional outcome of computer-assisted spinal pedicle screw placement: a systematic review and meta-analysis of 23 studies including 5,992 pedicle screws. Eur Spine J 2010;19(3):370–5.

28. Tjardes T, Shafizadeh S, Rixen D, et al. Image-guided spine surgery: state of the art and future directions. Eur Spine J 2010;19(1):25–45.

29. Liu H, Chen W, Wang Z, et al. Comparison of the accuracy between robot-assisted and conventional freehand pedicle screw placement: a systematic review and meta-analysis. Int J Comput Assist Radiol Surg 2016;11(12):2273–81.

30. Santos ER, Sembrano JN, Mueller B, et al. Optimizing iliac screw fixation: a biomechanical study on screw length, trajectory, and diameter. J Neurosurg Spine 2011;14(2):219–25.

31. Kuklo TR, Bridwell KH, Lewis SJ, et al. Minimum 2-year analysis of sacropelvic fixation and L5-S1 fusion using S1 and iliac screws. Spine 2001;26(18):1976–83.

32. Tsuchiya K, Bridwell KH, Kuklo TR, et al. Minimum 5-year analysis of L5-S1 fusion using sacropelvic fixation (bilateral S1 and iliac screws) for spinal deformity. Spine 2006;31(3):303–8.

33. Cunningham BW, Lewis SJ, Long J, et al. Biomechanical evaluation of lumbosacral reconstruction techniques for spondylolisthesis: an in vitro porcine model. Spine 2002;27(21):2321–7.

34. Shin JH, Hoh DJ, Kalfas IH. Iliac screw fixation using computer-assisted computer tomographic image guidance: technical note. Neurosurgery 2012;70(1 Suppl Operative):16–20. discussion 20.

35. Miller F, Moseley C, Koreska J. Pelvic anatomy relative to lumbosacral instrumentation. J Spinal Disord 1990;3(2):169–73.

36. Kim KD, Duong H, Muzumdar A, et al. A novel technique for sacropelvic fixation using image-guided sacroiliac screws: a case series and biomechanical study. J Biomed Res 2019;33(3):208–16.

37. Turel MK, Kerolus M, Deutsch H. Minimally Invasive Sacroiliac Fixation for Extension of Fusion in Cases of Failed Lumbosacral Fusion. J Neurosci Rural Pract 2018;9(4):574–7.

38. Phan K, Li J, Giang G, et al. A novel technique for placement of sacro-alar-iliac (S2AI) screws by K-wire insertion using intraoperative navigation. J Clin Neurosci 2017;45:324–7.

39. Williams SK, Quinnan SM. Percutaneous Lumbopelvic Fixation for Reduction and Stabilization of Sacral Fractures With Spinopelvic Dissociation Patterns. J Orthop Trauma 2016;30(9):e318–24.

40. Iorio JA, Jakoi AM, Rehman S. Percutaneous Sacroiliac Screw Fixation of the Posterior Pelvic Ring. Orthop Clin North Am 2015;46(4):511–21.

41. Halawi MJ. Pelvic ring injuries: Surgical management and long-term outcomes. Journal of clinical orthopaedics and trauma 2016;7(1):1–6.

42. Hu X, Lieberman IH. Robotic-guided sacro-pelvic fixation using S2 alar-iliac screws: feasibility and accuracy. Eur Spine J 2017;26(3):720–5.

43. Shillingford JN, Laratta JL, Park PJ, et al. Human versus Robot: A Propensity-Matched Analysis of the Accuracy of Free Hand versus Robotic Guidance for Placement of S2 Alar-Iliac (S2AI) Screws. Spine 2018;43(21):E1297–304.

44. Laratta JL, Shillingford JN, Meredith JS, et al. Robotic versus freehand S2 alar iliac fixation: in-depth technical considerations. Journal of spine surgery (Hong Kong) 2018;4(3):638–44.

45. Laratta JL, Shillingford JN, Lombardi JM, et al. Accuracy of S2 Alar-Iliac Screw Placement Under Robotic Guidance. Spine Deform 2018;6(2):130–6.

46. Sponseller PD, Zimmerman RM, Ko PS, et al. Low profile pelvic fixation with the sacral alar iliac technique in the pediatric population improves results at two-year minimum follow-up. Spine 2010;35(20): 1887–92.

47. Lieberman IH, Hardenbrook MA, Wang JC, et al. Assessment of pedicle screw placement accuracy, procedure time, and radiation exposure using a miniature robotic guidance system. J Spinal Disord Tech 2012;25(5):241–8.

48. Gao S, Lv Z, Fang H. Robot-assisted and conventional freehand pedicle screw placement: a systematic review and meta-analysis of randomized controlled trials. Eur Spine J 2018;27(4):921–30.

49. Smith HE, Welsch MD, Sasso RC, et al. Comparison of radiation exposure in lumbar pedicle screw placement with fluoroscopy vs computer-assisted image guidance with intraoperative three-dimensional imaging. J Spinal Cord Med 2008;31(5):532–7.

50. Mendelsohn D, Strelzow J, Dea N, et al. Patient and surgeon radiation exposure during spinal instrumentation using intraoperative computed tomography-based navigation. Spine J 2016;16(3):343–54.

51. Vo CD, Jiang B, Azad TD, et al. Robotic Spine Surgery: Current State in Minimally Invasive Surgery. Global Spine J 2020;10(2 Suppl):34S–40S.

52. Lee KH, Yeo W, Soeharno H, et al. Learning curve of a complex surgical technique: minimally invasive transforaminal lumbar interbody fusion (MIS TLIF). J Spinal Disord Tech 2014;27(7):E234–40.

53. Sharif S, Afsar A. Learning Curve and Minimally Invasive Spine Surgery. World Neurosurg 2018; 119:472–8.

54. Sclafani JA, Kim CW. Complications associated with the initial learning curve of minimally invasive spine surgery: a systematic review. Clin Orthop Relat Res 2014;472(6):1711–7.

55. Hu X, Lieberman IH. What is the learning curve for robotic-assisted pedicle screw placement in spine surgery? Clin Orthop Relat Res 2014;472(6): 1839–44.

56. Li HM, Zhang RJ, Shen CL. Accuracy of Pedicle Screw Placement and Clinical Outcomes of Robot-assisted Technique Versus Conventional Freehand Technique in Spine Surgery From Nine Randomized Controlled Trials: A Meta-analysis. Spine 2020;45(2): E111–9.

Section IV: Postoperative Optimization

Complications and Avoidance in Adult Spinal Deformity Surgery

Joseph R. Linzey, MD, MS[a], Jock Lillard, MD[b], Michael LaBagnara, MD[b], Paul Park, MD[b],*

KEYWORDS

- Complications • Avoidance • Adult spinal deformity surgery • Hardware failure
- Proximal junctional kyphosis

KEY POINTS

- Adult spinal deformity surgery has a high risk for complications.
- The most common intraoperative and postoperative complications include intraoperative cerebrospinal fluid leak, high blood loss, new neurologic defects, hardware failure, proximal junctional kyphosis/failure, surgical site infection, and medical complications.
- There are multiple strategies and surgical techniques for avoiding and/or managing these complications.

INTRODUCTION

Adult spinal deformity (ASD) is a complex disease that can result in significant disability.[1] In patients with refractory symptomatic ASD, studies have reported significant positive benefits from surgical treatment, with improvements in pain, health-related quality of life outcomes, and patient satisfaction.[2,3] This patient population, however, is challenging to manage due to the complexity of the surgeries as well as patient comorbidities.[4,5] Complications from surgical treatment are frequent and have been reported to impact as many as 70% of patients undergoing deformity surgery.[6] Reoperations are also prevalent; in one large multicenter study, 15.4% of patients required early reoperation within 1 year of index surgery for unexpected complications.[5] In addition to the higher risk for complications and its associated additional costs for treatment, ASD surgery itself is costly, with estimates as high as $103,143 per surgical procedure.[7]

Given the high risk and added cost of complications to an already expensive surgery, it is imperative to be aware of the most prominent medical and surgical complications associated with ASD surgery in addition to strategies for avoiding those pitfalls. Our aim is to highlight the more common surgical and medical complications associated with ASD surgery as well as detail clinical pearls to minimize occurrence and/or mitigate the harm of these complications.

SURGICAL COMPLICATIONS
Intraoperative Cerebrospinal Fluid Leak

Intraoperative dural tears resulting in a cerebrospinal fluid (CSF) leak have a varied incidence in the literature, occurring in 0.1% to 12.1% of patients.[8–12] While CSF leaks may cause limited mobility immediately after surgery and thus delayed recovery, they rarely cause long-term sequalae for patients. Specific to the deformity literature, Feng and colleagues[12] reported 8 of 7284 thoracic pedicle screws causing an intraoperative CSF leak, 7 of which were located on the concave side of the scoliosis. In 5 of the 8 cases, there were concomitant intraoperative neuromonitoring changes, with normal neurologic

a Department of Neurosurgery, University of Michigan, 1500 East Medical Center Drive, Ann Arbor, MI 48109, USA; b University of Tennessee & Semmes-Murphey Clinic, Memphis, TN 38120, USA
* Corresponding author. University of Tennessee & Semmes-Murphey Clinic, 6325 Humphreys Blvd., Memphis, TN 38120.
E-mail address: ppark@semmes-murphey.com

Neurosurg Clin N Am 34 (2023) 665–675
https://doi.org/10.1016/j.nec.2023.06.012

function in all 8 patients at 2-year follow-up. For the majority of their CSF leaks, they did not perform direct repair and only sealed the pedicle hole with bone wax. Alternatively, Di Silvestre and colleagues[10,11] recommended direct repair of the CSF leak by performing a hemilaminectomy to visualize the leak and then close the dural tear with suture and fibrin glue.

The etiologies for dural tears are variable, as are the methods for repair. If direct visualization of the dural tear is possible, a combination of (1) primary closure with suture only, (2) sealant only, (3) fat or muscle graft only, (4) suture + sealant, (5) suture + fat or muscle graft, (6) fat or muscle graft + sealant, or (7) suture + fat or muscle graft + sealant can be used depending on the size and extent of the tear.[13–15] A meticulous and layered closure of the surgical incision should follow. The use of subfascial drains after durotomy is controversial. Some literature suggests that subfascial drains can help avoid an increase in epidural fluid pressure and eliminate dead space.[14] There is also debate in the literature regarding the length of time a subfascial drain, if employed, should remain in place, with different studies advocating from 2 to 17 days.[16–18]

Additionally, efforts to optimize CSF mechanics can be used in isolation or in combination with the previously mentioned methods of primary repair.[14] Specifically, the placement of a lumbar drain can decrease the hydrostatic pressure on the repaired dural tear, allowing for more optimal healing.[14] Typically, for the first 2 to 4 days after lumbar drain placement, the patient should remain flat to further decrease hydrostatic pressure.[19]

High Intraoperative Blood Loss

ASD surgery is associated with a risk for extensive blood loss given the size of the surgical incision, extent of muscular dissection, and bony bleeding. White and colleagues[20] found that out of 5805 patients undergoing ASD surgery, 27.1% received a transfusion of blood. This study identified multiple risk factors for high blood loss requiring transfusion, including: patient age, American Society of Anesthesiologists (ASA) score of 3 or greater, cardiac comorbidity, bleeding disorders, posterior approach, pelvic fixation, and whether an osteotomy was performed.[20] Raad and colleagues[21] added arthrodesis of 11 or more levels, malalignment in both coronal and sagittal planes, and osteoporosis as additional risk factors for high blood loss. High blood loss can have a number of negative effects on patients such as hypotension and end-organ ischemia. Additionally, the treatment of high blood loss can have deleterious effects,

including transfusion-related circulatory overload, transfusion-related lung injury, and other transfusion-related reactions.[22–25]

Given the risk of excessive blood loss during ASD surgery, multiple strategies can be employed to minimize blood loss. One recent prospective, randomized controlled trial (RCT) demonstrated that the use of a bipolar sealer device (ie, Aquamantys bipolars) significantly reduced the operative time, blood loss, and need for postoperative transfusions in patients undergoing posterior spinal fusion for scoliosis.[26] Additionally, the use of Cell Saver, a method of intraoperative cell salvage to allow autologous re-infusion of blood, has been demonstrated to be efficient as well as cost-effective for patients with greater than 614 cc of blood loss.[27] A significant amount of research has been pursued regarding the use of tranexamic acid (TXA) on blood loss during ASD surgery.[25,28,29] TXA is an antifibrinolytic agent that prevents conversion of plasminogen to plasmin, the enzyme responsible for the degradation of fibrin within clots.[25] Wong and colleagues[30] performed an RCT and found that TXA significantly reduced perioperative blood loss in thoracic and lumbar fusion surgery, though there was not a significant difference in postoperative transfusion rates. Hariharan and colleagues[31] performed a meta-analysis evaluating the overall effect of TXA and found that TXA was associated with lower blood loss and transfusion volume in patients who underwent ASD surgery.

New Neurologic Deficit

Rates of new neurologic deficits following ASD surgery are relatively low, with most studies estimating less than 10% of patients have new weakness or paralysis.[32–34] However, a prospective study by Kelly and colleagues[35] argued that retrospective studies likely underestimate neurologic deficits in complex ASD surgery. Their prospective study found that neurologic deficits occurred in closer to 18% of patients undergoing complex ASD surgery.

The majority of new neurologic deficits are localized to a single nerve root, though there are also reports of spinal cord injury.[34–36] Causes of nerve injury are diverse and can occur with hardware placement or improper technique. A malpositioned pedicle screw traversing the canal or foramen in addition to interbody cage placement can cause nerve root injury if an insufficient discectomy is performed, there is mechanical damage to the nerve during decompression, via over distraction of the disc space with an interbody cage that is too large.[36,37] Beyond maintaining proper technique, intraoperative diagnostic tools such as intraoperative monitoring have been advocated to prevent neurologic injury.

In patients undergoing three-column osteotomies, the complication rate can be even higher given the degree of focal correction. Bianco and colleagues[38] reported a postoperative rate of new motor deficits or paralysis of 12.1% after three-column osteotomies. This study found that the more extensive the ASD surgery, the higher the complication risk (single vs two osteotomies, thoracic osteotomies, and so forth). Daubs and colleagues[39] found that patients over 60 years old who underwent three-column osteotomies had significantly more neurologic deficits. To minimize this risk, it is important to inspect the foramina and central canal to ensure there is no compression of the neural elements when a three-column osteotomy is closed.

Many of the neurologic deficits encountered in ASD surgery are transient, with a smaller number of permanent deficits. Kim and colleagues[40] found that 11.6% of patients undergoing either posterior vertebral column resection or decancellation osteotomy had transient neurologic deficits, while only 2.6% had a permanent deficit. This study found that patients with preoperative kyphosis, post-tuberculous kyphosis, preoperative neurologic deficits, fusion greater than 5 levels, resection of 2 of more vertebrae, insertion of a vertebrectomy cage, operative time greater than 200 minutes, and blood loss greater than 3 L were significantly more likely to have postoperative neurologic deficits.[40]

Intraoperative neuromonitoring (IONM) is helpful in obtaining early information regarding possible neurologic injury. The main forms of IONM are somatosensory-evoked potentials (SSEPS) which directly monitor the sensory pathways, motor-evoked potentials (MEPs) which monitor motor function via the corticospinal tract and skeletal muscles innervated by alpha-motor neurons, and electromyography (EMG) to monitor at the root level.[36,41] IONM is not perfect; there are reports of false negatives and false positives.[42,43] Ziewacz and colleagues[44] created a checklist for spinal surgeons to use if there are intraoperative changes of IONM to maximize a positive outcome for the patients. For example, if MEPs are altered during a case, the surgeon should stop any current manipulation, assess the field for obvious causes of cord compression, and consider correcting the deformity while the neurophysiologist repeats the MEP and SSEP tests and checks for lead pull out. The anesthesiologist can lighten anesthesia, reduce the inhalation component of the anesthetic in cases of non-pure total intravenous anesthesia (TIVA), check hemoglobin/hematocrit, temperature, ins-and-outs, extremity positioning, and blood pressure, and if MAPs are low, give medications to elevate MAP to 90 to 100. The anesthesiologist should also verify that no neuromuscular blockade had been given. If there is no change with the suggestions listed in the checklist, MAPs should be increased greater than 100, steroids should be administered, and consideration should be given to a wake-up test or aborting the operation.[44]

Hardware Failure

Hardware failure and screw misplacement can be a cause for early return to the operating room (OR) for revision surgery. Núñez-Pereira et al.[6] performed a multi-institution, prospective study that demonstrated that early, unanticipated revision surgery in patients who have undergone ASD surgery has a negative impact on mental health at 6 months and reduces chances of reaching the minimally clinically important difference (MCID) improvement in the Oswestry Disability Index (ODI), Short Form-36 (SF-36), and Scoliosis Research Society-22 (SRS-22) at 2 years.

Dinizo and colleagues[45] found that 9.4% of their study group developed a postoperative complication after ASD surgery, with 67.7% of those patients needing a re-operation. Of that group, 13.4% were due to instrumentation failure, including malpositioned pedicle screws or migration of interbody cages (**Fig. 1**). Spinal navigation or robotic-assisted surgery has been advocated to reduce the misplacement of pedicle screws and interbody cages. In a recent systematic review and meta-analysis of randomized studies comparing robotic or navigated versus freehand pedicle screw placement, accuracy and safety were significantly higher with robotic and navigated guidance.[46] In another study involving primarily pediatric deformity patients, navigated pedicle screw placement resulted in higher accuracy and significantly decreased return to OR for screw malposition compared to fluoroscopic freehand pedicle screw placement.[47]

Rod fracture is another implant-related complication (**Fig. 2**). Smith and colleagues[48] performed a prospective, multicenter assessment of rod fractures and found that, after multivariate regression, the only risk factor associated with rod fracture was pedicle subtraction osteotomy (PSO). In an effort to minimize this complication, there has been a focus on multiple-rod constructs with the addition of either satellite or accessory rods, as well as larger rods made of stronger metals.[49–51] Multiple studies have demonstrated significantly

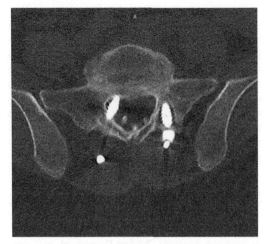

Fig. 1. Axial CT image of a misplaced pedicle screw.

fewer rod fractures, decreased incidence of pseudarthrosis, and fewer re-operations when a multiple-rod construct is used, compared to 2-rod constructs.[49,52,53] Smith and colleagues[54] found that rates of rod fractures were 8.6% for titanium alloy, 7.4% for stainless-steel, and 2.7% for cobalt chromium. On the other hand, in a prospective, multicenter study of patients who underwent a PSO, the rate of rod fracture was significantly higher in patients with cobalt chromium rods than with titanium alloy or stainless-steel rods (33% vs 0%, $P = .010$).[48]

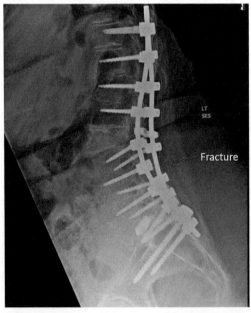

Fig. 2. Sagittal X-ray image of a rod fracture in a thoracolumbar deformity construct.

While there are multiple risk factors for hardware failure, one of the most significant is preoperative osteoporosis. Gupta and colleagues[55] found that patients who were osteoporotic were significantly more likely to need revision surgery secondary to instrumentation failure and postoperative fractures compared to patients without osteoporosis (40.5% vs 28.0%, $P = .01$). Given the significantly increased risk of instrumentation failure in patients with osteoporosis, an appropriate medical work-up should be obtained before offering surgery, including imaging assessments of bone density.[56] There are multiple medical strategies for bone health optimization that can prevent instrumentation failure in this patient group, including bisphosphonates and anabolic medications.[57] Yagi and colleagues[58] found that prophylactic teriparatide therapy improved the volumetric bone mineral density and bone mineral content at upper-instrumented vertebra (UIV+1), with the incidence of proximal junctional kyphosis (PJK) significantly lower in the teriparatide group compared to the control.

Additionally, Chang and colleagues[59] discussed the use of polymethylmethacrylate (PMMA) augmentation of pedicle screws, particularly in patients with osteoporosis, with significant improvements in ODI score, in kyphotic deformity correction, and with minimal screw migration postoperatively. In this study, the average loss of kyphosis correction in these osteoporotic patients was only 3°.[59] A recent study by Kolz and colleagues[60] found that cement augmentation in patients with osteoporosis was associated with a decreased risk of PJK ($P = .009$, OR 0.16).

Multiple RCTs have been performed to evaluate the role of external bone growth stimulators in augmenting fusion rates in ASD surgery. Park and colleagues[61] performed a systematic review and found 6 RCTs that discussed the use of electrical stimulation with a wide range of findings. Given the inconsistent data, it was difficult to conclusively determine the role of electrical stimulation in the postoperative fusion setting. However, Akhter and colleagues[62] conducted a more recent meta-analysis that demonstrated that electrical stimulation increased the odds of a successful fusion by 2.5-fold relative to control (OR = 2.53 95% CI 1.86–3.43, $P < .00001$).

Proximal Junctional Kyphosis

Proximal junctional kyphosis (PJK) is the increase of kyphosis superior to UIV, classically defined as kyphosis of 10 or more degrees greater than preoperative measurements by calculating the angle between the inferior endplate of UIV and the superior endplate of UIV+2 by the sagittal Cobb method.[63,64] Proximal junctional failure (PJF) is the most severe, symptomatic form of this complication and typically requires surgical treatment (**Fig. 3**). Multiple different complications can be encapsulated in PJF, including hardware failure, bony fractures, neurologic deficits, worsening deformity, and increased levels of pain.[65] The rate of PJK varies in the literature between 17% and 39% in ASD surgery.[64,66–68] There are multiple risk factors for the development of PJK, including patient age, osteoporosis, anterior or posterior fusion, fusion to sacrum, sagittal plane deformity, and magnitude of lumbar lordosis correction (>30°).[69]

Multiple strategies are available to attempt to minimize the rate of PJK, including the preservation of the supraspinous ligament between UIV and UIV+1, preservation of the facet suprajacent to the UIV, avoiding over- or undercorrection, prophylactic vertebroplasty, transverse process hooks, sublaminar banding, terminal rod contouring, ligament augmentation with proximal tethering, and using a less stiff rod construct.[64,65]

Of the many strategies advocated for PJK prevention, vertebroplasty is frequently discussed. Zygourakis and colleagues[70] proposed a novel, CT-guided fluoroscopy-free vertebroplasty which decreased historical levels of PJK from 40% to 14%. However, Han and colleagues[71] did not find a significant difference in PJK in patients who underwent prophylactic vertebroplasty. Similarly, Raman and colleagues[72] performed a prospective study evaluating patients who received two-level prophylactic vertebroplasty at the upper instrumented and supra-adjacent vertebrae at the time of the initial fusion, which did not demonstrate significant differences in the development of PJK at 5 years postoperative. Ultimately, larger prospective trials will need to be completed to determine the benefit of vertebroplasty in preventing PJK.

In a large, multi-institutional, international study utilizing a propensity score-matched cohort, Line and colleagues[73] found that the use of transverse process hooks at the upper instrumented level resulted in significantly less PJK compared to patients without the hook augmentation (7.0% vs 20.3%, P < .05). While Matsumura and colleagues[74] did not significantly demonstrate a difference in PJK rate with transverse process hooks compared to pedicle screw only instrumentation (17.6% vs 27.3%, P = .47), they did find that the changes in proximal junctional angle were significantly higher in the pedicle screw only group compared to the transverse process hook group (19.0° vs 5.0°, P = .04).

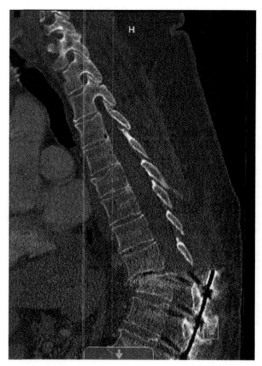

Fig. 3. Sagittal CT image demonstrating proximal junctional kyphosis/failure.

A re-emerging surgical strategy to reduce PJK is the use of sublaminar or spinous process band placement at the UIV+1 or UIV+2. Viswanathan and colleagues[75] performed a biomechanical study that demonstrated that sublaminar banding reduced flexibility at the proximal segment of the construct that was at risk for PJK, expanding the transition zone between construct and natural spinal motion, ultimately decreasing stress. A second biomechanical study was performed that similarly stated that sublaminar banding can help modulate biomechanical flexion range of motion to decrease the incidence of PJK.[76] Viswanathan and colleagues[77] then performed a prospective analysis that demonstrated that sublaminar band placement was safe and did not increase the rate of PJK. No patients developed PJF. In another study, Safaee and colleagues[78] described a technique to minimize PJK referred to as ligament augmentation, which consisted of passing a soft sublaminar cable through holes drilled in the spinous processes at the UIV, UIV+1, and UIV-1 levels to decrease junctional stress at those levels. When compared to a historical cohort, they found that the use of ligament augmentation significantly decreased the rates of PJK and PJF.[78] Of note, the potential benefits of these techniques must be weighed against the morbidity of increasing

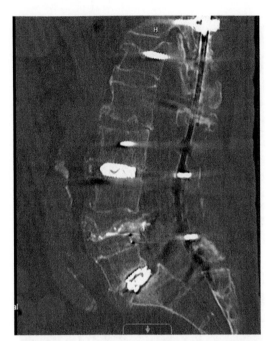

Fig. 4. Sagittal CT image showing L5-S1 pseudarthrosis after TLIF in patient who had T10-ilium deformity corrective surgery.

soft tissue dissection to these proximal levels including: possible disruption of suprajacent facets, disruption of muscular attachments, and increased blood loss.

Pseudarthrosis

Pseudarthrosis is a relatively common complication following ASD surgery, with some literature claiming that symptomatic pseudarthrosis occurs in up to 24% of patients who undergo ASD surgery **(Fig. 4)**.[79,80] Symptomatic pseudarthrosis can be devastating for patients due to the possible need for revision surgery, increased pain, and worse outcomes.[81,82] Given the biomechanical stress at the lumbosacral junction, pseudarthrosis at this level is most common.[83,84] Occasionally, pseudarthrosis is asymptomatic and is detected radiographically due to haloing around screws or unilateral rod fractures but without a clinical correlate.[80]

In order to minimize the incidence of pseudarthrosis, especially at the lumbosacral junction, surgeons should utilize interbody arthrodesis with meticulous endplate preparation, incorporate pelvic fixation, place supplemental rods, and incorporate biologics into the construct. The addition of interbody cages increases the potential surface area for arthrodesis. Among interbody techniques, it is generally accepted that ALIF is the most

effective option to obtain arthrodesis. The use of outrigger or kickstand rods can also potentially increase the rigidity of the construct, minimizing the risk of pseudarthrosis, though large studies have not been conducted to demonstrate that claim.[50,85] Although there are a host of graft options, it is generally accepted that bone morphogenetic proteins are most effective. Annis and colleagues[86] performed a retrospective case series which demonstrated a lower L5-S1 pseudarthrosis rate for patients that utilized low-dose BMP-2 with pelvic fixation.

Surgical Site Infection

Surgical site infections (SSI) for ASD surgery are fairly infrequent, ranging from 1.9% to 4.4%, but can significantly increase morbidity and mortality for patients.[87,88] Additionally, some studies have suggested that costs are increased by 2.3–3.1 times for patients with an SSI compared to patients without a postoperative infection.[89] Risk factors for SSI after ASD surgery include obesity and previous history of an SSI.[90,91] There are multiple methods for preventing SSI, including: precleansing of the patient before presenting to the hospital on the morning of surgery, thorough prep with chlorhexidine gluconate or iodine intraoperatively, prophylaxtic antibiotics, meticulous hemostasis, care in handling the soft tissues during the operation, irrigation following instrumentation, possibly the use of vancomycin powder, ideally pulling any subfascial drains within 3 days of the operation, and consideration of skin glue for closure.[88] Of these listed methods to minimize SSI, removal of drains within 3 days of surgery may not be practical given the high output of subfascial drains after most open deformity operations. Vancomycin powder is also a more recent and widely discussed modality. The literature, however, is inconsistent regarding the effectiveness of vancomycin powder, with some studies demonstrating a significant reduction in deep infection rates[92–95] and others not showing a significant reduction.[96,97]

MEDICAL COMPLICATIONS

Medical complications make up a significant contribution to the complication burden of ASD surgery. One multi-center study described a medical complication rate as high as 26.8%.[98] Dinizo and colleagues[45,98] found that 8.2% of their cohort developed a medical complication, with the most common being ileus and pulmonary embolism. Risk factors for medical complications included preoperative smoking, high ASA score, hypertension, and the number of years a patient had their spine problems. In another review, multiple modifiable risk factors were reported, including obesity, nutritional status, diabetes, preoperative anemia, nicotine use, and opioid use.[99]

To reduce the risk of medical complication, Maitra and colleagues recommended a nutritionist referral to help reduce BMI less than 35 and increase serum albumin greater than 3.5 g/dL; an endocrinology referral to lower HbA1c <7%, raise vitamin D > 30 ng/mL, and increase DEXA score greater than -2.5; and a hematology referral to raise hemoglobin greater than 12 g/dL for females and greater than 13 g/dL for males.[99] Smith and colleagues[100] recommended the use of enhanced recovery after surgery protocols, which had a significant reduction in postoperative opioid and antiemetic use.

Ultimately, preoperative patient selection is key in minimizing medical complications. High-risk preoperative clinics should be utilized, if available, to medically optimize patients. In these situations, extra care should be given when discussing consent for surgery to appropriately set postoperative expectations and risks. Despite the use of high-risk preoperative clinics, some patients will still not be appropriate surgical candidates due to severe medical comorbidities, even in the setting of significant, symptomatic spinal deformity.

SUMMARY

Perioperative and postoperative complications with ASD surgery are frequent given the complex nature of the surgical procedure and the typical comorbidity burden in patients with ASD. Given this high complication rate, it is crucial to recognize and treat the most common surgical and medical complications. As outlined in this article, comprehensive optimization is crucial as are the perioperative strategies to avoid, mitigate and/or treat complications as highlighted in this article.

CLINICS CARE POINTS

- Adult spinal deformity surgery has a high complication rate in the perioperative and postoperative periods.
- Intraoperative cerebrospinal fluid leak can be repaired with a combination of 1) primary closure with suture only, 2) sealant only, 3) fat or muscle graft only, 4) suture + sealant, 5) suture + fat or muscle graft, 6) fat or muscle graft + sealant, or 7) suture + fat or muscle graft + sealant, depending on the size and extent of the tear.

- High intraoperative blood loss can be mitigated by the use of bipolar sealer devices, Cell Saver, or the administration of tranexamic acid.
- New neurologic deficits can be identified early and possibly reversed with the use of intraoperative neuromonitoring.
- Risk of hardware malposition may be reduced with the use of navigation or robotic assistance. Rod fracture can be minimized with the use of multi-rod contructs.
- Cement augmentation can increase screw purchase.
- Proximal junctional kyphosis is common but can be potentially reduced by appropriate realignment, prophylactic vertebroplasty, transverse process hooks, terminal rod contouring, ligament augmentation, and a less stiff rod construct.

DISCLOSURE

Paul Park is a consultant for Globus, NuVasive, Medtronic, Depuy, Accelus and receives royalties from Globus. The othere authors have nothing to disclose.

REFERENCES

1. Bess S, Line B, Fu KM, et al. The health impact of symptomatic adult spinal deformity: Comparison of deformity types to United States population norms and chronic diseases. Spine 2016;41(3):224–33.
2. Bridwell KH, Glassman S, Horton W, et al. Does treatment (nonoperative and operative) improve the two-year quality of life in patients with adult symptomatic lumbar scoliosis: a prospective multicenter evidence-based medicine study. Spine 2009;34(20):2171–8.
3. Scheer JK, Smith JS, Clark AJ, et al. Comprehensive study of back and leg pain improvements after adult spinal deformity surgery: analysis of 421 patients with 2-year follow-up and of the impact of the surgery on treatment satisfaction. J Neurosurg Spine 2015;22(5):540–53.
4. Glassman SD, Hamill CL, Bridwell KH, et al. The impact of perioperative complications on clinical outcome in adult deformity surgery. Spine 2007; 32(24):2764–70.
5. Núñez-Pereira S, Vila-Casademunt A, Domingo-Sabat M, et al. Impact of early unanticipated revision surgery on health-related quality of life after adult spinal deformity surgery. Spine J 2018; 18(6):926–34.
6. Smith JS, Klineberg E, Lafage V, et al. Prospective multicenter assessment of perioperative and

minimum 2-year postoperative complication rates associated with adult spinal deformity surgery. J Neurosurg Spine 2016;25(1):1–14.

7. McCarthy IM, Hostin RA, Ames CP, et al. Total hospital costs of surgical treatment for adult spinal deformity: an extended follow-up study. Spine J 2014;14(10):2326–33.

8. Suk SI, Kim WJ, Lee SM, et al. Thoracic pedicle screw fixation in spinal deformities: are they really safe? Spine 2001;26(18):2049–57.

9. Kim YJ, Lenke LG, Bridwell KH, et al. Free hand pedicle screw placement in the thoracic spine: is it safe? Spine 2004;29(3):333–42. ; discussion 342.

10. Di Silvestre M, Parisini P, Lolli F, et al. Complications of thoracic pedicle screws in scoliosis treatment. Spine 2007;32(15):1655–61.

11. Di Silvestre M, Bakaloudis G, Lolli F, et al. Posterior fusion only for thoracic adolescent idiopathic scoliosis of more than 80 degrees: pedicle screws versus hybrid instrumentation. Eur Spine J 2008; 17(10):1336–49.

12. Feng B, Shen J, Zhang J, et al. How to deal with cerebrospinal fluid leak during pedicle screw fixation in spinal deformities surgery with intraoperative neuromonitoring change. Spine 2014;39(1):E20–5.

13. Bosacco SJ, Gardner MJ, Guille JT. Evaluation and treatment of dural tears in lumbar spine surgery: a review. Clin Orthop Relat Res 2001;389:238–47.

14. Fang Z, Tian R, Jia YT, et al. Treatment of cerebrospinal fluid leak after spine surgery. Chin J Traumatol 2017;20(2):81–3.

15. Choi EH, Chan AY, Brown NJ, et al. Effectiveness of repair techniques for spinal dural tears: A systematic review. World Neurosurg 2021;149:140–7.

16. Fang Z, Jia YT, Tian R, et al. Subfascial drainage for management of cerebrospinal fluid leakage after posterior spine surgeryd—A prospective study based on Poiseuille's law. Chin J Traumatol 2016; 19(1):35–8.

17. Hughes SA, Ozgur BM, German M, et al. Prolonged Jackson-Pratt drainage in the management of lumbar cerebrospinal fluid leaks. Surg Neurol 2006;65(4):410–4. discussion 414-415.

18. Lotfinia I, Sayyahmelli S. Incidental durotomy during lumbar spine surgery. Neurosurg Quart 2012; 22(2):105–12.

19. Grannum S, Patel MS, Attar F, et al. Dural tears in primary decompressive lumbar surgery. Is primary repair necessary for a good outcome? Eur Spine J 2014;23(4):904–8.

20. White SJW, Cheung ZB, Ye I, et al. Risk factors for perioperative blood transfusions in adult spinal deformity surgery. World Neurosurg 2018;115: e731–7.

21. Raad M, Amin R, Jain A, et al. Multilevel arthrodesis for adult spinal deformity: When should we anticipate major blood loss? Spine Deform 2019; 7(1):141–5.

22. Kleinman S, Caulfield T, Chan P, et al. Toward an understanding of transfusion-related acute lung injury: statement of a consensus panel. Transfusion 2004;44(12):1774–89.

23. Vamvakas EC, Blajchman MA. Transfusion-related mortality: the ongoing risks of allogeneic blood transfusion and the available strategies for their prevention. Blood 2009;113(15):3406–17.

24. Alam A, Lin Y, Lima A, et al. The prevention of transfusion-associated circulatory overload. Transfus Med Rev 2013;27(2):105–12.

25. Pong RP, Leveque JA, Edwards A, et al. Effect of tranexamic acid on blood loss, D-dimer, and fibrinogen kinetics in adult spinal deformity surgery. J Bone Joint Surg Am 2018;100(9):758–64.

26. Wang X, Sun G, Sun R, et al. Bipolar sealer device reduces blood loss and transfusion requirements in posterior spinal fusion for degenerative lumbar scoliosis: A randomized control trial. Clin Spine Surg 2016;29(2):E107–11.

27. Gum JL, Carreon LY, Kelly MP, et al. Cell Saver for adult spinal deformity surgery reduces cost. Spine Deform 2017;5(4):272–6.

28. Peters A, Verma K, Slobodyanyuk K, et al. Antifibrinolytics reduce blood loss in adult spinal deformity surgery: a prospective, randomized controlled trial. Spine 2015;40(8):E443–9.

29. Clohisy JCF, Lenke LG, Dafrawy MHE, et al. Randomized, controlled trial of two tranexamic acid dosing protocols in adult spinal deformity surgery. Spine Deform 2022;10(6):1399–406.

30. Wong J, El Beheiry H, Rampersaud YR, et al. Tranexamic acid reduces perioperative blood loss in adult patients having spinal fusion surgery. Anesth Analg 2008;107(5):1479–86.

31. Hariharan D, Mammi M, Daniels K, et al. The safety and efficacy of tranexamic acid in adult spinal deformity surgery: A systematic review and meta-analysis. Drugs 2019;79(15):1679–88.

32. Boachie-Adjei O, Ferguson JA, Pigeon RG, et al. Transpedicular lumbar wedge resection osteotomy for fixed sagittal imbalance: surgical technique and early results. Spine 2006;31(4):485–92.

33. Buchowski JM, Bridwell KH, Lenke LG, et al. Neurologic complications of lumbar pedicle subtraction osteotomy: a 10-year assessment. Spine 2007;32(20):2245–52.

34. Kelly MP, Lenke LG, Shaffrey CI, et al. Evaluation of complications and neurological deficits with three-column spine reconstructions for complex spinal deformity: a retrospective Scoli-RISK-1 study. Neurosurg Focus 2014;36(5):E17.

35. Kelly MP, Lenke LG, Godzik J, et al. Retrospective analysis underestimates neurological deficits in

complex spinal deformity surgery: a Scoli-RISK-1 Study. J Neurosurg Spine 2017;27(1):68–73.

36. Iorio JA, Reid P, Kim HJ. Neurological complications in adult spinal deformity surgery. Curr Rev Musculoskelet Med 2016;9(3):290–8.

37. Czerwein JK Jr, Thakur N, Migliori SJ, et al. Complications of anterior lumbar surgery. J Am Acad Orthop Surg 2011;19(5):251–8.

38. Bianco K, Norton R, Schwab F, et al. Complications and intercenter variability of three-column osteotomies for spinal deformity surgery: a retrospective review of 423 patients. Neurosurg Focus 2014; 36(5):E18.

39. Daubs MD, Lenke LG, Cheh G, et al. Adult spinal deformity surgery: complications and outcomes in patients over age 60. Spine 2007;32(20):2238–44.

40. Kim SS, Cho BC, Kim JH, et al. Complications of posterior vertebral resection for spinal deformity. Asian Spine J 2012;6(4):257–65.

41. Devlin VJ, Schwartz DM. Intraoperative neurophysiologic monitoring during spinal surgery. J Am Acad Orthop Surg 2007;15(9):549–60.

42. Rao RD, Gourab K, David KS. Operative treatment of cervical spondylotic myelopathy. J Bone Joint Surg Am 2006;88(7):1619–40.

43. Schwartz DM, Auerbach JD, Dormans JP, et al. Neurophysiological detection of impending spinal cord injury during scoliosis surgery. J Bone Joint Surg Am 2007;89(11):2440–9.

44. Ziewacz JE, Berven SH, Mummaneni VP, et al. The design, development, and implementation of a checklist for intraoperative neuromonitoring changes. Neurosurg Focus 2012;33(5):E11.

45. Dinizo M, Dolgalev I, Passias PG, et al. Complications after adult spinal deformity surgeries: All are not created equal. Int J Spine Surg 2021;15(1): 137–43.

46. Matur AV, Palmisciano P, Duah HO, et al. Robotic and navigated pedicle screws are safer and more accurate than fluoroscopic freehand screws: a systematic review and meta-analysis. Spine J 2023; 23(2):197–208.

47. Baky FJ, Milbrandt T, Echternacht S, et al. Intraoperative computed tomography-guided navigation for pediatric spine patients reduced return to operating room for screw malposition compared with freehand/fluoroscopic techniques. Spine Deform 2019;7(4):577–81.

48. Smith JS, Shaffrey E, Klineberg E, et al. Prospective multicenter assessment of risk factors for rod fracture following surgery for adult spinal deformity. J Neurosurg Spine 2014;21(6):994–1003.

49. Hyun SJ, Lenke LG, Kim YC, et al. Comparison of standard 2-rod constructs to multiple-rod constructs for fixation across 3-column spinal osteotomies. Spine 2014;39(22):1899–904.

50. Palumbo MA, Shah KN, Eberson CP, et al. Outrigger rod technique for supplemental support of posterior spinal arthrodesis. Spine J 2015; 15(6):1409–14.

51. Hallager DW, Gehrchen M, Dahl B, et al. Use of supplemental short pre-contoured accessory rods and cobalt chrome alloy posterior rods reduces primary rod strain and range of motion across the pedicle subtraction osteotomy level: An in vitro biomechanical study. Spine 2016;41(7):E388–95.

52. Gupta S, Eksi MS, Ames CP, et al. A novel 4-rod technique offers potential to reduce rod breakage and pseudarthrosis in pedicle subtraction osteotomies for adult spinal deformity correction. Oper Neurosurg (Hagerstown) 2018;14(4):449–56.

53. Lyu Q, Lau D, Haddad AF, et al. Multiple-rod constructs and use of bone morphogenetic protein-2 in relation to lower rod fracture rates in 141 patients with adult spinal deformity who underwent lumbar pedicle subtraction osteotomy. J Neurosurg Spine 2021;1–11.

54. Smith JS, Shaffrey CI, Ames CP, et al. Assessment of symptomatic rod fracture after posterior instrumented fusion for adult spinal deformity. Neurosurgery 2012;71(4):862–7.

55. Gupta A, Cha T, Schwab J, et al. Osteoporosis increases the likelihood of revision surgery following a long spinal fusion for adult spinal deformity. Spine J 2021;21(1):134–40.

56. Deshpande N, Hadi MS, Lillard JC, et al. Alternatives to DEXA for the assessment of bone density: a systematic review of the literature and future recommendations. J Neurosurg Spine 2023;38(4): 436–45.

57. Zhang AS, Khatri S, Balmaceno-Criss M, et al. Medical optimization of osteoporosis for adult spinal deformity surgery: a state-of-the-art evidence-based review of current pharmacotherapy. Spine Deform 2022. https://doi.org/10.1007/s43390-022-00621-6.

58. Yagi M, Ohne H, Konomi T, et al. Teriparatide improves volumetric bone mineral density and fine bone structure in the UIV+1 vertebra, and reduces bone failure type PJK after surgery for adult spinal deformity. Osteoporos Int 2016;27(12):3495–502.

59. Chang MC, Liu CL, Chen TH. Polymethylmethacrylate augmentation of pedicle screw for osteoporotic spinal surgery: a novel technique. Spine 2008; 33(10):E317–24.

60. Kolz JM, Pinter ZW, Sebastian AS, et al. Postoperative and intraoperative cement augmentation for spinal fusion. World Neurosurg 2022;160:e454–63.

61. Park P, Lau D, Brodt ED, et al. Electrical stimulation to enhance spinal fusion: a systematic review. Evid Based Spine Care J 2014;5(2):87–94.

62. Akhter S, Qureshi AR, Aleem I, et al. Efficacy of electrical stimulation for spinal fusion: A systematic

review and meta-analysis of randomized controlled trials. Sci Rep 2020;10(1):4568.

63. Lau D, Funao H, Clark AJ, et al. The clinical correlation of the Hart-ISSG proximal junctional kyphosis severity scale with health-related quality-of-life outcomes and need for revision surgery. Spine 2016; 41(3):213–23.

64. Safaee MM, Osorio JA, Verma K, et al. Proximal junctional kyphosis prevention strategies: A video technique guide. Oper Neurosurg (Hagerstown) 2017;13(5):581–5.

65. Shlobin NA, Le N, Scheer JK, et al. State of the evidence for proximal junctional kyphosis prevention in adult spinal deformity surgery: A systematic review of current literature. World Neurosurg 2022; 161:179–189 e171.

66. Glattes RC, Bridwell KH, Lenke LG, et al. Proximal junctional kyphosis in adult spinal deformity following long instrumented posterior spinal fusion: incidence, outcomes, and risk factor analysis. Spine 2005;30(14):1643–9.

67. Kim HJ, Lenke LG, Shaffrey CI, et al. Proximal junctional kyphosis as a distinct form of adjacent segment pathology after spinal deformity surgery: a systematic review. Spine 2012;37(22 Suppl): S144–64.

68. Yoshida G, Ushirozako H, Hasegawa T, et al. Preoperative and postoperative sitting radiographs for adult spinal deformity surgery: Upper instrumented vertebra selection using sitting C2 plumb line distance to prevent proximal junctional kyphosis. Spine 2020;45(15):E950–8.

69. Spina NT, Abiola R, Lawrence BD. Proximal junctional failure in adult spinal deformity surgery: Incidence, risk factors, and management. Oper Tech Orthop 2017;27(4):251–9.

70. Zygourakis CC, DiGiorgio AM, Crutcher CL 2nd, et al. The safety and efficacy of CT-guided, fluoroscopy-free vertebroplasty in adult spinal deformity surgery. World Neurosurg 2018;116: e944–50.

71. Han S, Hyun SJ, Kim KJ, et al. Effect of vertebroplasty at the upper instrumented vertebra and upper instrumented vertebra +1 for prevention of proximal junctional failure in adult spinal deformity surgery: A comparative matched-cohort study. World Neurosurg 2019. https://doi.org/10.1016/j.wneu.2018.12.113.

72. Raman T, Miller E, Martin CT, et al. The effect of prophylactic vertebroplasty on the incidence of proximal junctional kyphosis and proximal junctional failure following posterior spinal fusion in adult spinal deformity: a 5-year follow-up study. Spine J 2017;17(10):1489–98.

73. Line BG, Bess S, Lafage R, et al. Effective prevention of proximal junctional failure in adult spinal deformity surgery requires a combination of

surgical implant prophylaxis and avoidance of sagittal alignment overcorrection. Spine 2020; 45(4):258–67.

74. Matsumura A, Namikawa T, Kato M, et al. Effect of different types of upper instrumented vertebrae instruments on proximal junctional kyphosis following adult spinal deformity surgery: Pedicle screw versus transverse process hook. Asian Spine J 2018;12(4):622–31.

75. Viswanathan VK, Ganguly R, Minnema AJ, et al. Biomechanical assessment of proximal junctional semi-rigid fixation in long-segment thoracolumbar constructs. J Neurosurg Spine 2018;30(2): 184–92.

76. Cho SK, Caridi J, Kim JS, et al. Attenuation of proximal junctional kyphosis using sublaminar polyester tension bands: A biomechanical study. World Neurosurg 2018;120:e1136–42.

77. Viswanathan VK, Kukreja S, Minnema AJ, et al. Prospective assessment of the safety and early outcomes of sublaminar band placement for the prevention of proximal junctional kyphosis. J Neurosurg Spine 2018;28(5):520–31.

78. Safaee MM, Deviren V, Dalle Ore C, et al. Ligament augmentation for prevention of proximal junctional kyphosis and proximal junctional failure in adult spinal deformity. J Neurosurg Spine 2018;28(5): 512–9.

79. Kim YJ, Bridwell KH, Lenke LG, et al. Pseudarthrosis in long adult spinal deformity instrumentation and fusion to the sacrum: prevalence and risk factor analysis of 144 cases. Spine 2006;31(20): 2329–36.

80. Lertudomphonwanit T, Kelly MP, Bridwell KH, et al. Rod fracture in adult spinal deformity surgery fused to the sacrum: prevalence, risk factors, and impact on health-related quality of life in 526 patients. Spine J 2018;18(9):1612–24.

81. Daniels AH, DePasse JM, Durand W, et al. Rod fracture after apparently solid radiographic fusion in adult spinal deformity patients. World Neurosurg 2018;117:e530–7.

82. Patel SA, McDonald CL, Reid DBC, et al. Complications of thoracolumbar adult spinal deformity surgery. JBJS Rev 2020;8(5):e0214.

83. Kornblatt MD, Casey MP, Jacobs RR. Internal fixation in lumbosacral spine fusion. A biomechanical and clinical study. Clin Orthop Relat Res 1986; 203:141–50.

84. Cleveland M, Bosworth DM, Thompson FR. Pseudarthrosis in the lumbosacral spine. J Bone Joint Surg Am 1948;30A(2):302–12.

85. Safaee MM, Maloney PR, Deviren V, et al. Kickstand rod with asymmetric pedicle subtraction osteotomy for treatment of adult kyphoscoliosis with severe coronal imbalance. Oper Neurosurg (Hagerstown) 2022;22(6):e245–50.

86. Annis P, Brodke DS, Spiker WR, et al. The fate of L5-S1 with low-dose BMP-2 and pelvic fixation, with or without interbody fusion, in adult deformity surgery. Spine 2015;40(11):E634–9.

87. Schuster JM, Rechtine G, Norvell DC, et al. The influence of perioperative risk factors and therapeutic interventions on infection rates after spine surgery: a systematic review. Spine 2010;35(9 Suppl):S125–37.

88. Sawires AN, Park PJ, Lenke LG. A narrative review of infection prevention techniques in adult and pediatric spinal deformity surgery. J Spine Surg 2021; 7(3):413–21.

89. Yeramaneni S, Robinson C, Hostin R. Impact of spine surgery complications on costs associated with management of adult spinal deformity. Curr Rev Musculoskelet Med 2016;9(3):327–32.

90. Pull ter Gunne AF, van Laarhoven CJ, Cohen DB. Incidence of surgical site infection following adult spinal deformity surgery: an analysis of patient risk. Eur Spine J 2010;19(6):982–8.

91. Soroceanu A, Burton DC, Diebo BG, et al. Impact of obesity on complications, infection, and patient-reported outcomes in adult spinal deformity surgery. J Neurosurg Spine 2015;23(5):656–64.

92. Sweet FA, Roh M, Sliva C. Intrawound application of vancomycin for prophylaxis in instrumented thoracolumbar fusions: efficacy, drug levels, and patient outcomes. Spine 2011;36(24):2084–8.

93. O'Neill KR, Smith JG, Abtahi AM, et al. Reduced surgical site infections in patients undergoing posterior spinal stabilization of traumatic injuries using vancomycin powder. Spine J 2011;11(7): 641–6.

94. Molinari RW, Khera OA, Molinari WJ 3rd. Prophylactic intraoperative powdered vancomycin and postoperative deep spinal wound infection: 1,512 consecutive surgical cases over a 6-year period. Eur Spine J 2012;21(Suppl 4):S476–82.

95. Strom RG, Pacione D, Kalhorn SP, et al. Decreased risk of wound infection after posterior cervical fusion with routine local application of vancomycin powder. Spine 2013;38(12):991–4.

96. Martin JR, Adogwa O, Brown CR, et al. Experience with intrawound vancomycin powder for spinal deformity surgery. Spine 2014;39(2):177–84.

97. Xiong G, Fogel H, Tobert D, et al. Vancomycin-impregnated calcium sulfate beads compared with vancomycin powder in adult spinal deformity patients undergoing thoracolumbar fusion. N Am Spine Soc J 2021;5:100048.

98. Soroceanu A, Burton DC, Oren JH, et al. Medical complications after adult spinal deformity surgery: Incidence, risk factors, and clinical impact. Spine 2016;41(22):1718–23.

99. Maitra S, Mikhail C, Cho SK, et al. Preoperative maximization to reduce complications in spinal surgery. Global Spine J 2020;10(1 Suppl):45S–52S.

100. Smith J, Probst S, Calandra C, et al. Enhanced recovery after surgery (ERAS) program for lumbar spine fusion. Perioper Med (Lond) 2019;8:4.

Enhanced Recovery After Surgery Protocols and Spinal Deformity

Omar Sorour, MD, Mohamed Macki, MD, MPH, Lee Tan, MD*

KEYWORDS

- ERAS • Enhanced recovery after surgery • Spinal deformity • Scoliosis • Flatback syndrome

KEY POINTS

- Provide an overview of preoperative, intraoperative, and postoperative considerations surrounding adult spinal deformity.
- Review the importance of pre-operative imaging, hemoglobin A1c levels before spine surgery, osteoporosis management, and prehabilitation.
- Review intraoperative management include the use of peri-operative antibiotics, liposomal bupivacaine, and Foley catheters.
- Review postoperative questions surrounding analgesia, nausea and vomiting, thromboembolic prophylaxis, and early mobilization.
- Discuss incorporating enhanced recovery after surgery protocols in spinal deformity to optimizing surgical outcomes.

INTRODUCTION/HISTORY/DEFINITIONS/BACKGROUND

In 1997, Professor Kehlet from Denmark first described a multimodal approach to optimize postoperative care.[1] Initially described as a multimodal rehabilitation program, Kehlet proposed various interventions to decrease length of stay after open sigmoidectomy.[2] The concept later became known as enhanced recovery after surgery (ERAS), which is centered on three key concepts includingoptimizing the patient for surgery, executing best practice in management and safety intraoperatively, and ensuring highest standards of postoperative care and rehabilitation.[3] In this article, we aim to review ERAS protocols relevant for spinal deformity surgery.

PREOPERATION
Imaging

Despites its name "after surgery," ERAS programs begin before surgery. Before any surgical decisions, all patients should complete adquate imaging studies to evalute the spinal deformity, which typcially include full length scoliosis xrays, lumbar and/or cervical flexion/extension films, and either a MRI + computed tomography (CT) or CT myelogram of the spinal region of interest. MRI can be very helpful in demonstrating regions of neural compression.[4] The EOS system si also very useful since it allows simultaneous lateral and anteroposterior 2D images of the whole body, which is very helpful in surgical planning. Stereoradiography subsequently generates 3D reconstructions of the spine to further help surgeons to understsand the spinal deformity.[5]

Hemoglobin A1c

Hemoglobin A1c (Hb A1c) is a risk factor for the development of surgical site infections (SSIs) in patients undergoing spinal surgery.[6] Reviews in the literature show that diabetes mellitus increases the proportion of SSIs upward of 53%.[7] Uncontrolled A1c levels were also associated with

Department of Neurosurgery, University of California, San Francisco, 505 Parnassus Avenue – Office M779, San Francisco, CA 94143, USA
* Corresponding author. 400 Parnassus Avenue, Room A2300, San Francisco, CA 94920.
E-mail address: Lee.Tan@ucsf.edu

Neurosurg Clin N Am 34 (2023) 677–687
https://doi.org/10.1016/j.nec.2023.05.003
1042-3680/23/© 2023 Elsevier Inc. All rights reserved.

patient-reported outcomes, including higher visual analog scale (VAS) scores and Oswestry Disability Index (ODI) scores.

Among patients undergoing a single-level lumbar interbody fusion, hemoglobin (Hgb) A1c greater than 7.5% is associated with an increased risk of infection or reoperation after spine surgery.[8] Another study similarly described an Hgb A1c cutoff of 7%. Among diabetic patients undergoing thoracic and lumbar instrumentation, none with an Hgb A1c less than 7% experienced an SSI, whereas 35.3% developed SSIs when Hgb A1c was greater than 7%.[9] Other studies examined outcomes after poor glycemic control. For instance, Lim and colleagues determined that an Hb A1c greater than 8% was associated with a longer hospital stay, higher readmission rate, and higher frequency of postoperative complications after lumbar spine surgery.[10] In summary, Hgb A1c levels provide a critical screening tool for mitigating patients risk factors, and Hgb A1c level should be optimize to less than 7% to decrease complications from spinal deformity surgery.[11]

Osteoporosis

Over 10 million people in the United States have osteoporosis and are more common among the elderly with degenerative spine conditions. One study found that the incidence of postoperative pseudoarthrosis and revision surgery is higher in patients with osteopenia and osteoporosis who undergo single-level lumbar fusions.[12] Decreased bone mineral density has been associated with suboptimal screw fixation.[13] This is even more important with osteoporosis in deformity correction, which carries a high risk of both revision surgeries[14] and proximal junctional failure (PJF).[15,16]

Rates of vitamin D deficiency are unexpectedly high in many parts of the world. This is also the case in up to 40% of patients undergoing orthopedic procedures.[17] In one study, vitamin D was found to be deficient in 23% of patients undergoing spinal fusion.[18] These patients were more likely to suffer from nonunion even when adjusted for several variables including smoking and bone morphogenic protein use. Time to fusion was also significantly longer in patients with vitamin D deficiency.[18] One set of evidence-based clinical guidelines suggests that serum vitamin D3 levels less than 20 ng/mL are associated with an increased risk of osteoporosis complications after spine surgery.[19] Recently, intermittently dosed parathyroid hormone (PTH) analogs, such as teriparatide, have been shown to effectively treat osteoporosis.[20] Teriparatide is a recombinant human amino acid containing a biologically active component of native PTH, promoting bone formation without resorption.[21] Although teriparatide is relatively expensive,[22] it significantly improves functional, patient-reported, and radiographic outcomes compared with vitamin D in patients with distal end radius fractures.[21] Teriparatide increased the rate of bone union compared with risedronate, an osteoclast inhibitor, in postmenopausal women undergoing instrumented lumbar posterolateral fusion.[23] Teriparatide has also shown to increase the insertional torque of pedicle screws in postmenopausal osteoporotic patients.[20] In one study examining adult spinal deformity fusions, prophylactic teriparatide decreased the rate of proximal junctional kyphosis associated with vertebral fractures while increasing both bone mineral density and bone quality.[16] According to a systematic review, teriparatide was more efficacious in reducing the incidence of PJF and Proximal Junctional Kyphosis (PJK) compared with other interventions such as multi-rod constructs, cement augmentation, and sublaminar tethers or banding.[24] **Table 1** shows the comparison of the various osteoporosis medications that could be used to treat osteoporosis in patients who need spine surgery.[25]

Prehabilitation

Prehabilitation, otherwise known as "prehab," is a process that prepares a patient cognitively and physically for an upcoming operation.[26] This intervention is useful in optimizing the functional capacity of patients to combat stressors of postoperative inactivity.[26] Ideal prehabilitation programs involve both cognitive and physical components, such as warm-up, cardiovascular training, a functional task component, and resistance training.[26] In one randomized control trial (RCT) by Rolving and colleagues, patients who engaged in perioperative cognitive behavior therapy (CBT) therapy had lower ODI scores at 3 months after surgery, compared with those who did not.[26,27] At 1 year, the CBT group had higher Quality-Adjusted Life Years than the control group.[28] Patients who were educated on radicular pain before lumbar spine surgery used less health care resources—such as imaging and physical therapy—at 1 year postoperatively, compared with those who received a conventional preoperative education.[26,29] In addition, recovery time, hospital length of stay, and pain levels were lower in patients who underwent prehab.[26,30]

INTRAOPERATION
Peri-operative Antibiotics

The North American Spine Society (NASS) published evidence-based clinical guidelines in 2013

Table 1
Osteoporosis medications in spine surgery

Drug Class	Mechanism of Action	Generic Name (Brand Name)	Evidence in Spine Surgery
Parathyroid hormone (PTH) analogs	Directly stimulates bone formation by osteoblasts. Indirectly increases calcium absorption in intestines and kidney.	Teriparatide (Forteo)	Randomized clinical trials demonstrated superior efficacy in spinal fusion.
		Abaloparatide (Tymlos)	Efficacy for spinal fusion is limited to RCT in animals. Ongoing Phase II trial with abaloparatide vs placebo.
Nitrogen-containing bisphosphonates	Inhibiting farnesyl pyrophosphate synthase, thereby promoting detachment of osteoclasts from bone and halting resorption.	Alendronate (Fosamax)	Conflicting efficacy with respect to fusion rates. Animal models have demonstrated screw loosening.
		Zoledronate (Zometa, Reclast)	Randomized clinical trials demonstrated improved fusion rate and reduced incidence of subsequent adjacent vertebral compression fractures and pedicle screw loosening. Some studies show no difference in spinal fusion.
		Risedronate (Actonel)	Extent of pedicle screw loosening in risedronate group did not differ significantly from no medications.
		Ibandronate (Boniva)	Limited evidence in spinal fusion suggests that ibandronate decreases cage subsidence and increase interbody fusion.
		Pamidronate (Aredia)	Possible efficacy for spinal fusion rates is limited to RCT in rabbits.
Receptor activator of nuclear factor kappa-B ligand (RANK-L) inhibitors	Human monoclonal antibody that inhibits osteoclast-mediated bone destruction	Denosumab (Xgeva, Prolia)	Evidence is limited in combination with teriparatide. Ongoing Phase IV trial with denosumab vs calcium + vitamin D.

(*continued on next page*)

Table 1 (continued)			
Drug Class	**Mechanism of Action**	**Generic Name (Brand Name)**	**Evidence in Spine Surgery**
Sclerostin-inhibitors	Humanized monoclonal antibody inhibits sclerostin: a bone morphogenetic protein osteoblast antagonist.	Romosozumab (Evenity)	Although Romosozumab improves lumbar bone mineral density, efficacy in lumbar fusion limited to preclinical trials.

Modified and adapted from Sorour O, Macki M, Jamieson A, Mummaneni P. Pharmacology of Antithrombotics, Antifibrinolytics, and Osteoporosis Medications. In: Baaj A, Mummaneni P, Uribe J, Vaccaro A, Greenberg M, eds. *Handbook of Spine Surgery.* Thieme; 2023.

that addressed prophylactic antibiotic use in spine surgery based on a series of trials and meta-analyses. NASS recommended a single preoperative dose of prophylactic antibiotics for patients undergoing uncomplicated laminectomies and discectomies.

The most studied antibiotic is cefazolin. In a prospective randomized controlled trial, 1 g dose of cefazolin approximately 2 hours before surgery compared with a placebo group reduces the risk of wound or urinary tract infections.[31] At the very least, administering prophylactic antibiotics within 60 minutes of surgery is still favorable according to the general preoperative guidelines. With respect to spinal surgery, in particular, prophylaxis is recommended 30 to 60 minutes before skin incision.[32]

The duration of postoperative antibiotics in spine surgery is contentious. Current guidelines suggest that postoperative antibiotics should be discontinued within 24 hours after spinal surgery.[33] Another study found no difference in infection rates in discontinuing antibiotics 24 hours postoperatively versus an extended 72 hours postoperatively. This also included a subset of patients who received instrumented spinal surgery.[34] Other studies corroborated the concept that 1-day versus 3-day prophylactic dosages did not differ in instrumented spinal fusion surgeries.[35] Macki and colleagues similarly found that compared with no postoperative antimicrobial prophylaxis, both short-term (<24 hours) and long-term (>24 hours) postoperative antibiotics equally decreased the risk of deep SSIs. Interestingly, postoperative antibiotics did not impact superficial SSIs. This suggests that antibiotics prevent subfascial wound infections, whereas superficial SSIs are attributable to other factors, such as meticulous wound closures.[36]

With regard to more complex spine surgeries, cefazolin is still used. However, studies demonstrate that in, for instance, pediatric patients with high-risk instrumented spine surgeries, gram-negative bacilli are more commonplace. In adults, one study demonstrated that gram-negative and methicillin-resistant organisms composed 30.5% and 34.3% of all SSIs, respectively.[37] Of these gram-negative organisms, 61.6% of them were cefazolin-resistant. These organisms composed 18.8% of all SSIs.[37] Although one recommendation is to continue cefazolin to cover gram-positive cocci and coagulase-negative staphylococci while also adding prophylaxis for these gram-negative organisms, these studies increasingly illustrate the importance of accounting for other microbial flora that are more prevalent than previously assumed.[38] Regardless of the class of antibiotics, there is less evidence supporting the use of prolonged antibiotic regimens. For instance, the NASS provides a Grade C recommendation that prolonged postoperative antibiotic regimens can be considered in patients with comorbidities such as spinal cord injury or diabetes. Further studies need to examine postoperative regimens in more complex spinal deformity cases.

Liposomal Bupivacaine

The use of liposomal bupivacaine[39] has recently been shown to improve outcomes while obtaining adequate operative analgesia.[40] In our institution, liposomal bupivacaine is used for spine surgery with conscious sedation and spinal anesthetic (no intubation), also known as "awake spine surgery." The formulation may be mixed with 0.5% or 0.25% bupivacaine HCl. At the beginning of the case, the mixture is injected widely around the plane of the planned incision for a minimally invasive decompression. At the end of the case, more solution is injected into the small, surgical field at the level of the deep dermis and muscle tissue. For minimally invasive transforaminal lumbar interbody fusions, an erector spinae block is pursued; the needle is advanced down to the level of the transverse process, with a trajectory estimated by the intraoperative navigation. The anesthetic is injected gently, as the needle is slowly raised to the superficial tissue.[40] This technique is demonstrated in **Fig. 1**.

Foley Catheters

Patients undergoing spine surgery are at an increased risk for postoperative urinary retention given the relatively long durations of their surgeries under anesthesia, which has been shown to affect bladder function.[41,42] Reflexes at both the central and peripheral nervous system alter signaling in the pontine micturition center, sacral spinal cord, and detrusor muscle. The prevalence of postoperative urinary retention in patients undergoing spine surgery is not exact, ranging from 5.6% to 27.1%.[41,43]

The decision of whether to insert a catheter postoperatively depends on several factors. In one study, catheters were placed in patients who underwent surgeries longer than 3 hours or with larger volume shifts (eg,., blood loss)[44] Another study demonstrated that in addition to surrogate markers of surgery time, preoperative patient mobility must be considered.[45] Earlier postoperative mobilization correlates with a lower incidence of postoperative urinary retention, irrespective of when the intraoperative catheter was trialed for removal. This speaks to the importance of early postoperative ambulation in ERAS protocols. To support the relationship between postoperative

urinary retention and ambulation, performing a trial of void during the day, when patients are mobilized, reduces the incidence of postoperative urinary retention, compared with patients resting at night. Moreover, patients with poor baseline ambulation preoperatively may have a concomitant neurogenic bladder. These patients who self-catheterize may benefit from a prolonged Foley catheter postoperatively. Before spinal deformity correction, urodynamic testing[46] may assess the risk of worsening urinary retention after surgery.

The prevalence of postoperative urinary retention and straight catheterization to address voiding issues was examined in more complex spinal deformity cases. One study, for instance, published that 33% ($n = 53$) of patients with adolescent idiopathic scoliosis (AIS) who underwent posterior spinal fusion (PSF) experienced postoperative urinary retention after catheter removal; 49% of these patients required straight catheterization more than 24 hours after catheter removal. Sixteen of these 53 patients required intermittent catheterization once, whereas the remainder required more than one.[47] This likely reflects the duration of complex spinal fusions, for which surgeons should have a lower threshold to continue the Foley catheter postoperatively.

However, guidelines for the number of straight catheterizations after failing trial of void is not clearly established. In one study involving thoracolumbar spinal fusion patients, the intraoperative catheter was removed between 1 and 2 days after surgery. Straight catheterizations were limited to

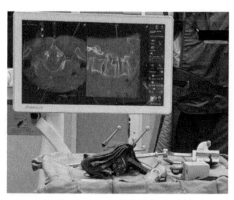
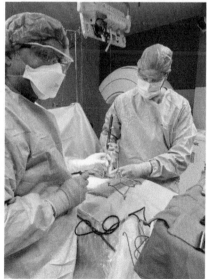

Fig. 1. The use of navigation to inject liposomal bupivacaine through spinal needle in awake minimally invasive transforaminal lumbar interbody fusion.

bladder scans greater than 300 mL after a 4-h trial of void. If the patient failed trial of void three times, a Foley catheter was placed, and tamsulosin was administered. Continued symptoms after Foley placement required an outpatient urology consultation.[48] This study suggests that a well-defined protocol may help stratify risk for long-term Foley placement in patients with postoperative urinary retention.

POSTOPERATION
Analgesia

Spinal surgeries carry considerable pain lasting several days. In addition, orthopedic and neurosurgery procedures have higher incidences of opioid use perioperatively, making pain management after spine surgery a particularly complex task.[49] There has been debate about optimal pain control methods for spine surgery patients. One such debate is whether patient-controlled analgesia (PCA) is an effective modality. Several reports demonstrate that intravenous (IV) PCA offers better pain control than IV, intramuscular, or subcutaneous opioids as needed.[50,51] The most common IV opioids for postoperative pain are morphine, hydromorphone, and fentanyl. All these drugs can be administered through the PCA pump[52]; however, morphine[53,54] and hydromorphone are the most common.[55] Morphine has a rapid onset of action and peak within minutes of administration.[56]

Side effects of PCA such as nausea, vomiting, and pruritus are relatively common, but more serious complications include respiratory depression[57] and patient dependence. Therefore, PCAs should be expeditiously transitioned to oral pain medications to mitigate the risks of these issues. One solution is to combine PCAs with local anesthetics, as this lowers the concentration of opioids.[58] Adding lidocaine to morphine in PCA formulations has been shown by Alebouyeh and colleagues to be efficacious in reducing opioid demand.[59] Another solution is to consider other opioid drugs. For instance, Schenk and colleagues found that patient-controlled epidural analgesia with ropivacaine and sufentanil placed intraoperatively during spinal fusion resulted in better pain control and better patient satisfaction compared with IV PCA with morphine.[60]

There is also debate over what *type* of PCA is best suited postoperatively for spine patients. One study compared patient-controlled epidural analgesia to IV PCA for opioid medication delivery.[61] Epidural analgesia was superior to IV PCA in managing postoperative pain, both at rest and with activity. This finding was true at 1, 2, and 3 days postoperatively. However, the greater efficacy of epidural analgesia should be weighed with the risks of respiratory depression, given the diffusion of opioids within the cerebrospinal fluid.[62] Epidural catheters are also arguably more difficult to place than the standard IV access. One solution to maximize the benefit of epidural analgesia is to include a single preoperative injection of intrathecal opioids + a postoperative IV PCA. This lowered postoperative pain scores while decreasing the rate of adverse events, in a comparative study by Milbrandt and colleagues on AIS who underwent PSF.[63] In addition, those who received only the single IT injection used less morphine compared with those who received only PCA. These findings suggest that complex spinal cases may benefit from exploring other options besides PCA for pain medication delivery.

Furthermore, epidural PCAs containing hydrophilic versus lipophilic-only opioid regimens have been compared. Interestingly, VAS scores for patients who received hydrophilic opioid epidural PCAs were significantly higher than those who received lipophilic opioid regimens. This suggests that hydrophilic opioid-only epidural PCA regimens should be avoided if possible.[61]

There is also the question of whether PCA regimens should incorporate an additional continuous background infusion. The evidence surrounding whether it provides better analgesia than a PCA regimen without a background infusion is inconclusive.[64] However, the risk of respiratory depression is increased when a background infusion is used.[65-67] Therefore, it is not routinely recommended to use a background infusion in most cases.[65]

Nausea and Vomiting

The *Fourth Consensus Guidelines for the Management of Postoperative Nausea and Vomiting (PONV)* recommends PONV medication prophylaxis in adult patients who exhibit one or two risk factors: female sex, age, history of PONV, duration of surgery, and postoperative opioids.[68]

Ondansetron, a serotonin antagonist, has been the "gold standard" for adult and pediatric patients with PONV.[69] Guidelines recommend a 4-mg IV dose or an 8 mg oral disintegrating tablet.[70] Although some studies claim ondansetron is more effective in reducing postoperative nausea than vomiting,[69] a meta-analysis in spine surgery recommends the alternative use of ramosetron—another serotonin antagonist—which is more successful in reducing both postoperative nausea and vomiting. Ramosetron limited the use of other breakthrough antiemetic medications compared with its ondansetron counterpart.[71] Other studies showed equal efficacy between ramosetron and ondansetron.[72] These conflicting results should not be weighed heavily considering the ubiquity of ondansetron in hospital systems.

With respect to IV versus oral formulations of antiemetics, patients with emesis may not be able to digest oral pills. The effects of anesthesia may alter gastrointestinal motility and therefore an oral formulation's bioavailability.[73] In one alternative, administering an oral dose 1 hour preoperatively may provide long-lasting relief postoperatively, given its plasma half-life of 3 to 4 hours. Orally disintegrating pills can be considered because of the ease of digestion and rapid onset of action.[73]

Oral formulations may be less convenient in deformity surgeries, where recovery may be prolonged. Patients may continue to experience nausea and require high doses of opioids well after 24 hours postoperatively. These factors render IV antiemetic formulations more convenient in complex spinal operations. In addition, in patients who have delayed emergence of anesthesia, decreased levels of consciousness as well as the subsequent risk of aspiration support the use of IV antiemetics.

Prophylaxis Against Thromboembolism

The incidence of venous thromboembolic events (VTEs), such as deep venous thromboses and pulmonary emboli, with prolonged immobilization after spine surgery may reach as high as 2% to 4%.[74] The optimal thromboprophylaxis patterns are difficult to discern because of the paucity of randomized clinical trials and wide practice variations. However, one intervention, early ambulation, cannot be overstated. All patients should be encouraged to ambulate, at the very least, on postoperative day 1, if not the day of surgery.[75,76]

Mechanoprophylaxis, including compression stockings and intermittent pneumatic compression, is a staple in any postoperative regimen, given the relatively low cost and low complication rates with proven efficacy.[77,78]

Chemoprophylaxis entails subcutaneous injections of smaller doses of anticoagulants, typically low-molecular-weight heparin (LMWH) or unfractionated heparin (UFH). Several reports published in anesthesia have described the risk of spinal hematomas with epidural catheters in patients anticoagulated on LMWH.[79–81] The pharmaceutical company Sanofi subsequently released a black box warning for their drug, enoxaparin, in the setting of neuroanesthesia. Although these cautionary measures were intended for therapeutic doses of LMWH, spine surgeons still became apprehensive with prophylactic doses after spine surgeries that often include a subfascial drain. Although a large number of spine practices largely favor the more historical UFH, the Prophylactic LMWH versus UFH in Spine Surgery project has shined new light on the selection of chemoprophylaxis in ERAS protocols.[79–81] The choice of LMWH versus UFH failed to predict VTE or epidural hematomas, suggesting that both chemoprophylaxis drugs are safe after spine surgery.

Early Mobilization

Barring any restrictions, patients should be encouraged to ambulate early in the postoperative course to prevent the unfavorable physiological effects of protracted immobilization (muscle atrophy, insulin resistance, tissue deoxygenation, VTEs, pulmonary dysfunction).[82] In a randomized clinical trial, early postoperative ambulation decreased length of inpatient stay. In fact, early ambulation as soon as postoperative day #0 decreases length of stay and rehab discharges as well as 90-day complications, such as urinary tract infections, ileus, and urinary retention among patient undergoing elective lumbar spine surgery.[76] The distance ambulated has also been correlated with decreased length of stay.[83] Some studies have suggested that a threshold of at least 30 feet on the day of surgery will decrease length of stay.[84]

The "fear avoidance" model describes emotional, physical, behavioral, and cognitive constructs that have been associated with lumbar surgery outcomes.[85] Passive pain coping, negative outcome expectancies, fear of movement/(re)injury all contribute to postoperative disability.[86] Patient-reported outcomes on disability and pain after surgery worsen in postoperative patients who fear that ambulation would cause physical injury and pain.[83] This kinesiophobia is especially prominent in chronic back pain patients and results in prolonged inactivity following lumbar spinal fusion.[87] Therefore, before surgery, patients should be educated on the expectations with ambulation immediately after surgery, as stair climbing and independent transfer should be achieved before discharge.

CLINICS CARE POINTS

- Preoperatively:
  - Imaging: Before spinal deformity surgery, patients should complete complete adquate imaging evaluation including scoliosis x-rays, MRI and CT or CT myelogram to help

surgeons to formutate a sound surgical plan.

○ HgbA1c: Uncontrolled A1c levels have been associated with increased surgical site infections, increased rate of reoperationand worsened patient-reported outcomes; ideally pre-op HgbA1c should be <7%.

○ Osteoporosis: Teriparatide treatment is useful in improving bone mineral density, bone quality, and fusion in osteoporotic patients who are planning undergoing spinal deformitysurgery.

○ Prehabilitation: Prehabilitation can improve recovery time, decrease hospital length of stay andpain levels, and increase quality-adjusted life years.

- Intraoperatively:

○ Antibiotics: Cefazolin is the most studied and used prophylactic antibiotic in spine surgery. Some studies show that short-term (<24 hours) versus long-term (>24 hours) antibiotics equally decreased the risk of deep surgical site infections. Shorter duration of antibiotic usage may be preferrable in decreaseing antibiotic resistence.

○ Liposomal bupivacaine: utilization of liposomal bupivacaine intraoperatively may decrease overal postoperative analgesia requirements.

○ Foley catheters: As the incidence of postoperative urinary retention is relatively high in complex spinal deformity patients, a well-defined management protocol may help stratify risk for long-term Foley placement.

- Postoperatively:

○ Analgesia: The possible superiority of epidural patient-controlled analgesia (PCA) analgesia as compared with IV PCA in reducing postoperative pain must be carefully weighed against the increased risk of respiratory depression. Complex spinal cases may benefit from exploring other options besides PCA alone, such as combination formulations with local anesthetics.

○ Nausea and vomiting: Postoperative nausea and vomiting medication prophylaxis is strongly recommended in spinal deformity patients. Intravenous ondansetron is the gold standard; however, debate exists as to whether other medications such as ramosetron are more efficacious.

○ Prophylaxis against thromboembolism: The prophylactic low-molecular-weight heparin versus unfractionated heparin in spine surgery demonstrated that both unfractionated and low-molecular-weight heparins are safe for spine surgery patients.

○ Early mobilization: Ambulation is strongly recommended in all patients as soon after surgery as possible. In addition, patients should be educated on the expectations for ambulation postoperatively to reduce fear avoidance habits that many patients may exhibit.

DISCLOSURE

The authors have no relevant conflict of interest to disclose.

REFERENCES

1. Kehlet H. Multimodal approach to control postoperative pathophysiology and rehabilitation. Br J Anaesth 1997;78(5):606–17.
2. Kehlet H, Mogensen T. Hospital stay of 2 days after open sigmoidectomy with a multimodal rehabilitation programme. Br J Surg 1999;86(2):227–30.
3. Angus M, Jackson K, Smurthwaite G, et al. The implementation of enhanced recovery after surgery (ERAS) in complex spinal surgery. J Spine Surg 2019;5(1):116–23.
4. Mummaneni PV, Kaiser MG, Matz PG, et al. Preoperative patient selection with magnetic resonance imaging, computed tomography, and electroencephalography: does the test predict outcome after cervical surgery? J Neurosurg Spine 2009;11(2):119–29.
5. Melhem E, Assi A, el Rachkidi R, et al. EOS(®) biplanar X-ray imaging: concept, developments, benefits, and limitations. J Child Orthop 2016; 10(1):1–14.
6. Hwang JU, Son DW, Kang KT, et al. Importance of Hemoglobin A1c Levels for the Detection of Post-Surgical Infection Following Single-Level Lumbar Posterior Fusion in Patients with Diabetes. Korean J Neurotrauma 2019;15(2):150.
7. Martin ET, Kaye KS, Knott C, et al. Diabetes and Risk of Surgical Site Infection: A systematic review and meta-analysis. Infect Control Hosp Epidemiol 2016; 37(1):88.
8. Harrop JS, Mohamed B, Bisson EF, et al. Congress of Neurological Surgeons Systematic Review and Evidence-Based Guidelines for Perioperative Spine: Preoperative Surgical Risk Assessment. Neurosurgery 2021;89(Suppl 1):S9–18.
9. Hikata T, Iwanami A, Hosogane N, et al. High preoperative hemoglobin A1c is a risk factor for surgical site infection after posterior thoracic and lumbar spinal instrumentation surgery. J Orthop Sci 2014; 19(2):223–8.
10. Lim S, Yeh HH, Macki M, et al. Preoperative HbA1c > 8% Is Associated with Poor Outcomes in Lumbar Spine Surgery: A Michigan Spine Surgery

Improvement Collaborative Study. Neurosurgery 2021;89(5):819–26.

11. Suresh Kv, Wang K, Sethi I, et al. Spine Surgery and Preoperative Hemoglobin, Hematocrit, and Hemoglobin A1c: A Systematic Review. Global Spine J 2022;12(1):155.

12. Khalid SI, Nunna RS, Maasarani S, et al. Association of osteopenia and osteoporosis with higher rates of pseudarthrosis and revision surgery in adult patients undergoing single-level lumbar fusion. Neurosurg Focus 2020;49(2):E6.

13. Rometsch E, Spruit M, Zigler JE, et al. Screw-Related Complications After Instrumentation of the Osteoporotic Spine: A Systematic Literature Review With Meta-Analysis. Global Spine J 2020;10(1): 69–88.

14. Puvanesarajah V, Shen FH, Cancienne JM, et al. Risk factors for revision surgery following primary adult spinal deformity surgery in patients 65 years and older. J Neurosurg Spine 2016;25(4):486–93.

15. Park SJ, Lee CS, Chung SS, et al. Different Risk Factors of Proximal Junctional Kyphosis and Proximal Junctional Failure Following Long Instrumented Fusion to the Sacrum for Adult Spinal Deformity: Survivorship Analysis of 160 Patients. Neurosurgery 2017;80(2):279–86.

16. Yagi M, Ohne H, Konomi T, et al. Teriparatide improves volumetric bone mineral density and fine bone structure in the UIV+1 vertebra, and reduces bone failure type PJK after surgery for adult spinal deformity. Osteoporos Int 2016;27(12):3495–502.

17. Bogunovic L, Kim AD, Beamer BS, et al. Hypovitaminosis D in patients scheduled to undergo orthopaedic surgery: a single-center analysis. J Bone Joint Surg Am 2010;92(13):2300–4.

18. Ravindra VM, Godzik J, Dailey AT, et al. Vitamin D Levels and 1-Year Fusion Outcomes in Elective Spine Surgery: A Prospective Observational Study. Spine (Phila Pa 1976) 2015;40(19):1536–41.

19. Dimar J, Bisson EF, Dhall S, et al. Congress of Neurological Surgeons Systematic Review and Evidence-Based Guidelines for Perioperative Spine: Preoperative Osteoporosis Assessment. Neurosurgery 2021;89(Suppl 1):S19–25.

20. Inoue G, Ueno M, Nakazawa T, et al. Teriparatide increases the insertional torque of pedicle screws during fusion surgery in patients with postmenopausal osteoporosis. J Neurosurg Spine 2014;21(3): 425–31.

21. Samant PD, Sane RM, Butala RR, et al. Comparison of functional outcomes between teriparatide and vitamin D3 in distal end radius fractures of osteoporotic patients. undefined 2021;05(01):35–40.

22. Liu H, Michaud K, Nayak S, et al. The Cost-effectiveness of Therapy With Teriparatide and Alendronate in Women With Severe Osteoporosis. Arch Intern Med 2006;166(11):1209–17.

23. Ohtori S, Inoue G, Orita S, et al. Teriparatide accelerates lumbar posterolateral fusion in women with postmenopausal osteoporosis: prospective study. Spine (Phila Pa 1976) 2012;37(23). https://doi.org/10.1097/BRS.0B013E31826CA2A8.

24. Echt M, Ranson W, Steinberger J, et al. A Systematic Review of Treatment Strategies for the Prevention of Junctional Complications After Long-Segment Fusions in the Osteoporotic Spine. Global Spine J 2021;11(5):792–801.

25. Sorour O, Macki M, Jamieson A, et al. Pharmacology of antithrombotics, antifibrinolytics, and osteoporosis medications. In: Baaj A, Mummaneni P, Uribe J, et al, editors. Handbook of spine surgery. Thieme; 2023. p. 387–91.

26. Gometz A, Maislen D, Youtz C, et al. The Effectiveness of Prehabilitation (Prehab) in Both Functional and Economic Outcomes Following Spinal Surgery: A Systematic Review. Cureus 2018;10(5). https://doi.org/10.7759/CUREUS.2675.

27. Rolving N, Nielsen CV, Christensen FB, et al. Does a preoperative cognitive-behavioral intervention affect disability, pain behavior, pain, and return to work the first year after lumbar spinal fusion surgery? Spine (Phila Pa 1976) 2015;40(9):593–600.

28. Rolving N, Sogaard R, Nielsen CV, et al. Preoperative Cognitive-Behavioral Patient Education Versus Standard Care for Lumbar Spinal Fusion Patients: Economic Evaluation Alongside a Randomized Controlled Trial. Spine (Phila Pa 1976) 2016;41(1): 18–25.

29. Louw A, Diener I, Landers MR, et al. Preoperative pain neuroscience education for lumbar radiculopathy: a multicenter randomized controlled trial with 1-year follow-up. Spine (Phila Pa 1976) 2014; 39(18):1449–57.

30. Nielsen PR, Jørgensen LD, Dahl B, et al. Prehabilitation and early rehabilitation after spinal surgery: randomized clinical trial. Clin Rehabil 2010;24(2): 137–48.

31. Perioperative prophylactic cephazolin in spinal surgery. A double-blind placebo-controlled trial - PubMed. Available at: https://pubmed.ncbi.nlm.nih.gov/8300691/. Accessed September 7, 2022.

32. SIGN Guideline 58: safe sedation of children undergoing diagnostic and therapeutic procedures. Paediatr Anaesth 2008;18(1):11–2.

33. Crader MF, Varacallo M. Preoperative Antibiotic Prophylaxis. StatPearls. Published online June 1, 2022. Available at: https://www.ncbi.nlm.nih.gov/books/NBK442032/. Accessed September 8, 2022.

34. Kim B, Moon SH, Moon ES, et al. Antibiotic Microbial Prophylaxis for Spinal Surgery: Comparison between 48 and 72-Hour AMP Protocols. Asian Spine J 2010;4(2):71.

35. Marimuthu C, Abraham VT, Ravichandran M, et al. Antimicrobial Prophylaxis in Instrumented Spinal

Fusion Surgery: A Comparative Analysis of 24-Hour and 72-Hour Dosages. Asian Spine J 2016;10(6):1018.

36. Macki M, Hamilton T, Lim S, et al. The role of postoperative antibiotic duration on surgical site infection after lumbar surgery. J Neurosurg Spine 2021;36(2):254–60.

37. Abdul-Jabbar A, Berven SH, Hu SS, et al. Surgical site infections in spine surgery: identification of microbiologic and surgical characteristics in 239 cases. Spine (Phila Pa 1976) 2013;38(22).

38. Piantoni L, Tello CA, Remondino RG, et al. Antibiotic prophylaxis in high-risk pediatric spine surgery: Is cefazolin enough? Spine Deform 2020;8(4):669–76.

39. Reduce or eliminate opioids for postsurgical pain | EXPAREL.com. Available at: https://www.exparel.com/hcp/about-exparel/exparel-liposomal-bupivacaine. Accessed March 11, 2023.

40. Chan AKH, Choy W, Miller CA, et al. A novel technique for awake, minimally invasive transforaminal lumbar interbody fusion: technical note. Neurosurg Focus 2019;46(4). https://doi.org/10.3171/2019.1.FOCUS18510.

41. Lee S, Kim CH, Chung CK, et al. Risk factor analysis for postoperative urinary retention after surgery for degenerative lumbar spinal stenosis. Spine J 2017;17(4):469–77.

42. Aiyer SN, Kumar A, Shetty AP, et al. Factors Influencing Postoperative Urinary Retention Following Elective Posterior Lumbar Spine Surgery: A Prospective Study. Asian Spine J 2018;12(6):1100.

43. Gandhi SD, Patel SA, Maltenfort M, et al. Patient and surgical factors associated with postoperative urinary retention after lumbar spine surgery. Spine (Phila Pa 1976) 2014;39(22):1905–9.

44. Leitner L, Wanivenhaus F, Bachmann LM, et al. Bladder management in patients undergoing spine surgery: An assessment of care delivery. North American Spine Society Journal 2021;6:100059.

45. Tan CMP, Kaliya-Perumal AK, Ho GWK, et al. Postoperative Urinary Retention Following Thoracolumbosacral Spinal Fusion: Prevalence, Risk Factors, and Outcomes. Cureus 2021;13(11). https://doi.org/10.7759/CUREUS.19724.

46. SELIUS BA, SUBEDI R. Urinary Retention in Adults: Diagnosis and Initial Management. Am Fam Physician 2008;77(5):643–50. Available at: https://www.aafp.org/pubs/afp/issues/2008/0301/p643.html. Accessed September 20, 2022.

47. Yrjälä T, Helenius L, Taittonen M, et al. Predictors of postoperative urinary retention after posterior spinal fusion for adolescent idiopathic scoliosis. Eur Spine J 2021;30(12):3557–62.

48. Strickland AR, Farooq Usmani M, Camacho JE, et al. Evaluation of Risk Factors for Postoperative Urinary Retention in Elective Thoracolumbar Spinal Fusion Patients. Global Spine J 2021. https://doi.org/10.1177/2192568220904681.

49. Hilliard PE, Waljee J, Moser S, et al. Prevalence of Preoperative Opioid Use and Characteristics Associated With Opioid Use Among Patients Presenting for Surgery. JAMA Surg 2018;153(10):929–37.

50. Walder B, Schafer M, Henzi I, et al. Efficacy and safety of patient-controlled opioid analgesia for acute postoperative pain. A quantitative systematic review. Acta Anaesthesiol Scand 2001;45(7):795–804.

51. Ballantyne JC, Carr DB, DeFerranti S, et al. The comparative effects of postoperative analgesic therapies on pulmonary outcome: cumulative meta-analyses of randomized, controlled trials. Anesth Analg 1998;86(3):598–612.

52. Garimella V, Cellini C. Postoperative Pain Control. Clin Colon Rectal Surg 2013;26(3):191.

53. Mann C, Ouro-Bang'na F, Eledjam J. Patient-controlled analgesia. Curr Drug Targets 2005;6(7):815–9.

54. Hong D, Flood P, Diaz G. The side effects of morphine and hydromorphone patient-controlled analgesia. Anesth Analg 2008;107(4):1384–9.

55. DiGiusto M, Bhalla T, Martin D, et al. Patient-controlled analgesia in the pediatric population: morphine versus hydromorphone. J Pain Res 2014;7:471.

56. Vahedi HSM, Hajebi H, Vahidi E, et al. Comparison between intravenous morphine versus fentanyl in acute pain relief in drug abusers with acute limb traumatic injury. World J Emerg Med 2019;10(1):27.

57. Pastino A, Lakra A. Patient Controlled Analgesia. StatPearls. Published online July 19, 2022. Available at: https://www.ncbi.nlm.nih.gov/books/NBK551610/. Accessed September 18, 2022.

58. Bajwa SJS. Rare and Serious Side Effects in Chronic Pain after Opioids. J Pain & Relief 2012;1(4):1–5.

59. Alebouyeh MR, Imani F, Rahimzadeh P, et al. Analgesic effects of adding lidocaine to morphine pumps after orthopedic surgeries. J Res Med Sci 2014;19(2):122. Available at: http://pmc/articles/PMC3999597/. Accessed September 18, 2022.

60. Schenk MR, Putzier M, Kügler B, et al. Postoperative analgesia after major spine surgery: Patient-controlled epidural analgesia versus patient-controlled intravenous analgesia. Anesth Analg 2006;103(5):1311–7.

61. Wu CL, Cohen SR, Richman JM, et al. Efficacy of Postoperative Patient-controlled and Continuous Infusion Epidural Analgesia versus Intravenous Patient-controlled Analgesia with OpioidsA Meta-analysis. Anesthesiology 2005;103(5):1079–88.

62. Bajwa SJS, Haldar R. Pain management following spinal surgeries: An appraisal of the available options. J Craniovertebr Junction Spine 2015;6(3):105.

63. Milbrandt TA, Singhal M, Minter C, et al. A comparison of three methods of pain control for posterior spinal fusions in adolescent idiopathic scoliosis. Spine (Phila Pa 1976) 2009;34(14): 1499–503.

64. Russell AW, Owen H, Ilsley AH, et al. Background infusion with patient-controlled analgesia: effect on postoperative oxyhaemoglobin saturation and pain control. Anaesth Intensive Care 1993;21(2):174–9.

65. Soffin EM, Liu SS. Patient-controlled analgesia. In: Benzon HT, Raja SN, Fishman SM, et al, editors. *Essentials of pain medicine*. 4th edition. Elsevier; 2018. p. 117–22.e2. https://doi.org/10.1016/B978-0-323-40196-8.00013-9.

66. Etches RC. Respiratory depression associated with patient-controlled analgesia: a review of eight cases. Can J Anaesth 1994;41(2):125–32.

67. Fleming BM, Coombs DW. A survey of complications documented in a quality-control analysis of patient-controlled analgesia in the postoperative patient. J Pain Symptom Manage 1992;7(8):463–9.

68. Ashp. Fourth consensus guidelines for the management of postoperative nausea and vomiting. Anesth Analg 2020. https://doi.org/10.1213/ANE.0000000000004833.

69. Tricco AC, Soobiah C, Blondal E, et al. Comparative safety of serotonin (5-HT3) receptor antagonists in patients undergoing surgery: a systematic review and network meta-analysis. BMC Med 2015;13(1). https://doi.org/10.1186/S12916-015-0379-3.

70. Apfel CC, Korttila K, Abdalla M, et al. An international multicenter protocol to assess the single and combined benefits of antiemetic interventions in a controlled clinical trial of a 2×2×2×2×2×2 factorial design (IMPACT). Control Clin Trials 2003;24(6): 736–51.

71. Lin Y, Tiansheng S, Zhicheng Z, et al. Effects of Ramosetron on Nausea and Vomiting Following Spinal Surgery: A Meta-Analysis. Curr Ther Res Clin Exp 2022;96:100666.

72. Choi YS, Shim JK, Ahn SH, et al. Efficacy comparison of ramosetron with ondansetron on preventing nausea and vomiting in high-risk patients following spine surgery with a single bolus of dexamethasone as an adjunct. Korean J Anesthesiol 2012;62(6):543.

73. Bhure A, Deshmukh S, Parate S. Comparative study of Oral Vs IV Ondansetron for reducing PONV in patients undergoing laparoscopic surgery under General anesthesia. International Journal of Pharmaceutical Science Invention ISSN 2015;4: 2319–670. Available at: www.ijpsi.org. Accessed September 6, 2022.

74. Cox JB, Weaver KJ, Neal DW, et al. Decreased incidence of venous thromboembolism after spine surgery with early multimodal prophylaxis. J Neurosurg Spine 2014;21(4):677–84.

75. Lim S, Bazydlo M, Macki M, et al. Validation of the Benefits of Ambulation Within 8 Hours of Elective Cervical and Lumbar Surgery: A Michigan Spine Surgery Improvement Collaborative Study. Neurosurgery 2022;91(3):505–12.

76. Zakaria HM, Bazydlo M, Schultz L, et al. Ambulation on Postoperative Day #0 Is Associated With Decreased Morbidity and Adverse Events After Elective Lumbar Spine Surgery: Analysis From the Michigan Spine Surgery Improvement Collaborative (MSSIC). Neurosurgery 2019;87(2):320–8.

77. Epstein NE. Intermittent Pneumatic Compression Stocking Prophylaxis Against Deep Venous Thrombosis in Anterior Cervical Spinal Surgery. Spine (Phila Pa 1976) 2005;30(22):2538–43.

78. Epstein NE. Efficacy of Pneumatic Compression Stocking Prophylaxis in the Prevention of Deep Venous Thrombosis and Pulmonary Embolism Following 139 Lumbar Laminectomies With Instrumented Fusions. J Spinal Disord Tech 2006;19(1): 28–31.

79. Macki M, Haddad Y, Suryadevara R, et al. Prophylactic Low-Molecular-Weight Heparin Versus Unfractionated Heparin in Spine Surgery (PLUSS). Neurosurgery 2021;89(6):1097–103.

80. Macki M, Fakih M, Anand SK, et al. A direct comparison of prophylactic low-molecular-weight heparin versus unfractionated heparin in neurosurgery: A meta-analysis. Surg Neurol Int 2019;10:202.

81. Macki M, Haider SA, Anand SK, et al. A Survey of Chemoprophylaxis Techniques in Spine Surgery Among American Neurosurgery Training Programs. World Neurosurg 2020;133:e428–33.

82. Debono B, Wainwright TW, Wang MY, et al. Consensus statement for perioperative care in lumbar spinal fusion: Enhanced Recovery After Surgery (ERAS) Society recommendations. Spine J 2021; 21(5):729–52.

83. Macki M, Zakaria HM, Massie LW, et al. The Effect of Physical Therapy on Time to Discharge After Lumbar Interbody Fusion. Clin Neurol Neurosurg 2020; 197:106157.

84. Ferrel J. Obstacles to Early Mobilization After Spinal Fusion and Effect on Hospital Length of Stay. Spine J 2013;13(9):S168.

85. Alodaibi FA, Fritz JM, Thackeray A, et al. The Fear Avoidance Model predicts short-term pain and disability following lumbar disc surgery. PLoS One 2018;13(3):e0193566.

86. den Boer JJ, Oostendorp RAB, Beems T, et al. Continued disability and pain after lumbar disc surgery: The role of cognitive-behavioral factors. Pain 2006;123(1):45–52.

87. Tarnanen SP, Neva MH, Häkkinen K, et al. Neutral Spine Control Exercises in Rehabilitation After Lumbar Spine Fusion. J Strength Cond Res 2014;28(7): 2018–25.

Measuring Outcomes in Spinal Deformity Surgery

Stephen M. Bergin, MD, PhD, Muhammad M. Abd-El-Barr, MD, PhD, Oren N. Gottfried, MD, C. Rory Goodwin, MD, PhD, Christopher I. Shaffrey, MD, Khoi D. Than, MD*

KEYWORDS

- Spinal deformity outcomes • Patient-reported outcomes • Surgery

KEY POINTS

- The SRS-22 classification system is a highly reliable and well-validated system for ASD.
- The importance of the sagittal plane in adult spinal deformity is a well-established cause of pain and disability. T1 spinopelvic inclination strongly correlates with health-related quality-of-life.
- Wearable technologies such as accelerometers are a promising, objective method to measure outcomes, but remain in development.

INTRODUCTION

Adult spinal deformity (ASD) causes severe functional disability, reduces a patient's quality of life, and imposes a substantial financial and societal burden.[1] ASD surgery can improve these outcomes, but there is no consensus on what defines a successful surgical outcome for deformity surgery. The goal of this narrative review is to provide a summary of spinal deformity outcomes research and relevant outcome measurements including clinical, radiographic, and functional outcomes.

Historically, ASD surgery outcomes have been measured using physician-based assessments such as curve correction with a focus on the achievement of spinal alignment. Outcome assessment in ASD has evolved from these physician-based assessments, to include a patient-centered perception of improvement and health-related quality-of-life (HRQOL) and patient-reported outcome measures (PROMs).[2] From 2004 to 2013 there was an increase in the frequency of studies using PROMs in ASD research, yet quality studies and standardization are lacking.[3,4] Other outcome metrics have been introduced into clinical practice including self-image questionnaires, functional mobility tests, and accelerometers. Financial instruments including cost/quality-adjusted life years (QALYs)

are also important metrics that assess cost-effectiveness of ASD surgery for patients. In this narrative review, we outline the major developments in assessing outcomes in ASD surgery, with a particular focus on evolving assessment tools.

METHODS

This narrative literature review was conducted to provide the synthesis of the available literature regarding ASD outcomes. Relevant studies and reviews published between January 1, 2012, and August 1, 2022, were identified using a PubMed search using the keywords "adult spinal deformity surgery" and "outcomes." From the 236 publications identified during this period, titles and abstracts were reviewed. The narrative review was then synthesized from selected full texts identified in this search. Additional references were identified through backward citations of obtained articles.

DISCUSSION
Patient-Reported Outcomes

The U.S. Food and Drug Administration defines a patient-reported outcome (PRO) as "any report of the status of a patient's health condition that comes directly from the patient, without the

Department of Neurosurgery, Division of Spine, Duke University, 2301 Erwin Road, Durham, NC 27710, USA
* Corresponding author. 3480 Wake Forest Road Suite 310, Raleigh, NC 27609.
E-mail address: Khoi.Than@duke.edu

Neurosurg Clin N Am 34 (2023) 689–696
https://doi.org/10.1016/j.nec.2023.06.013

interpretation of the patient's response by a clinician or anyone else."[5] PROs include information about the physical, psychological, and social factors that define a health-related quality of life (HRQOL). Along with the increasing demand for evidence-based medicine, the emphasis on PROs to guide decision-making for ASD treatment is increasing.[3] Therefore, a more relevant discussion of "outcomes" measures involves evaluating the quality of an outcome instrument, which depends on several features including content validity, construct validity, reliability, responsiveness, and ability to detect clinically important differences.[6] Content validity refers to the degree by which the assessment measures the intended outcome it is designed to measure. Construct validity refers to the expectation that HRQOL questionnaires will evaluate the domains considered significant in ASD. Reliability refers to an outcome measurement's stability over time and the accuracy with which it estimates the true effect of a treatment. Responsiveness refers to the sensitivity and ability to detect change, which allows the determination of the effect of a therapeutic intervention such as surgery. The concept of a minimum clinically important difference (MCID) helps researchers and clinicians to understand the context of PROMs scores by establishing clinically relevant thresholds for changes in PROMs values.[7] The MCID quantifies the smallest measurable change in an outcome score that will make a relevant difference to the patient.

Standardized PROMs questionnaires used in ASD studies include the 12-Item Short Form Health Survey (SF-12) and the longer 36-Item Short Form Health Survey (SF-36), Oswestry Disability Index (ODI), and the Scoliosis Research Society-22 Patient Questionnaire (SRS-22).[3] SF-12 and SF-36 are not disease-specific, whereas the ODI and SRS-22 are specific to spinal conditions. In general, based on a bibliometric analysis of usage, the ODI and SRS instruments have emerged as standards in ASD surgery.[3]

The ODI is a questionnaire that was developed to measure the degree of disability caused by spine-related pain.[8,9] The ODI questions focus on function; intensity of pain; lifting; ability to care for oneself; ability to walk, sit, and stand; sexual function; social life; sleep quality; and ability to travel. It correlates with the SF-36 score and is a widely used marker of overall health.[10] The ODI has been validated as a responsive measurement tool.[11] In one study of patients with ASD who underwent surgery, the ODI domains in which the greatest functional improvement occurred were those of lifting, walking, standing, and traveling.[12]

The SRS-22 was developed in 1999 by the Scoliosis Research Society as a disease-specific measure of clinical outcomes for idiopathic scoliosis.[13,14] The SRS-22 questionnaire contains 20 questions distributed in 4 domains (function/activity, pain, self-perceived image, and mental health) and 2 additional questions about the patient's satisfaction with the received treatment. Each dimension has five items, except for "satisfaction," which has 2 items. Each item is scored from 1 (worst possible) to 5 (best possible). Each dimension has a total sum score ranging from 5 to 25, except *satisfaction*, whose sum score ranges from 2 to 10. A subtotal sum score of the 4 scales with a range of 20 to 100 can be obtained, but the usual practice is to calculate the mean of each dimension. With the addition of the 2 questions on satisfaction, the overall score ranges from 22 to 110.[15] The SRS-22 has been modified with standardized methods to include a revised (SRS-22r) questionnaire and an extended version, the SRS-30, which includes questions about the patient's self-image as well as the perceived effect of treatment on the disease. The SRS-22 and SRS-22R are valid and reliable instruments for assessing patients with idiopathic scoliosis, and it is sensitive to changes following surgery.[16] In an analysis of 1321 patients with ASD undergoing surgery, the MCID was identified to be 0.4 for the SRS-22R pain domain, activity domain, subscore, and total.[17] Unlike the SRS-22, the SRS-30 has not been specifically validated, and it is unclear whether these additional questions correlate with the true treatment score changes on the main scale (SRS-22).

Other outcome measurements have been employed for spinal deformity surgery including The Core Outcome Measures Index for the back (COMI-back),[18] EuroQoL 5-dimension 5-level,[19] and Patient-Reported Outcomes Measurement Information System (PROMIS). The COMI-back and PROMIS scores correlate strongly with SRS-22 and show good construct validity and responsiveness to surgery.[18,20]

Numerical rating scale (NRS) and visual analog score (VAS) are quantifiable PROs that are used in ASD to define a patient's back and leg pain and may help to better predict patient outcome. For instance, one study found that after deformity surgery, patients with radiculopathy exhibited increased pain and disability when compared to patients without leg pain.[21] Another study demonstrated a higher correlation with HRQOL scores for back pain and a higher correlation with sagittal parameters for leg pain.[22]

The aforementioned PROMs have been extensively used in ASD research (**Table 1**). Overall

Table 1
Selected patient-reported outcome measures

Outcome Measurement	Scope
ODI	Identifies the disruption of activities of daily living due to chronic low back pain
SRS-22, SRS-22R, SRS-24	Disease-specific health-related quality of life questionnaire for spinal deformity patients. SRS-30 includes additional evaluation of self-image and perception of one's treatment.
SF-12, SF-36,	Generic health status to measure the quality of life
NRS -back, -leg	11-point scale that measures pain sensation and intensity
VAS	100mm horizontal line that measures "no pain" to "most severe pain imaginable"
COMI -back	Identifies the disruption of activities of daily living due to chronic back pain

Abbreviations: COMI, Core Outcome Measures IndexNRS; numeric rating scale, ODI; oswestry disability index, SF; short form, SRS; scoliosis research society, VAS; visual analog scale.

the ODI, SRS-22, SF-12, and SF-36 are the most widely used PROMs and have been translated and validated in more than 10 different languages, making them suitable for international use.[4] Three studies have evaluated the clinimetric properties of the SRS-22, SF-12, and ODI in the ASD population, and Pearson's correlations of 0.70 were found between the SRS-22, SF-12, and ODI, reflecting good criterion validity.[23–25]

Bridwell and colleagues[23] compared the SRS-22 with the ODI and SF-12. They found that the SRS-22 did as well or better in score distribution compared with the other instruments. Looking at the domains of pain, function, and mental health, the concurrent validity was high between the SRS-22 and the SF-12. Reliability was excellent in all domains, and internal consistencies were high in all domains except pain, where it was .67, which is still acceptable. Berven and colleagues analyzed the SRS-22 alongside the SF-36 to evaluate validity, reliability, and discrimination in an adult population.[24] They found the SRS-22 to have excellent psychometric properties, which is in line with other studies.[23,26] For function, the SRS function scale has better characteristics (based on the floor/ceiling response distribution) than the SF-12, and similar characteristics as the ODI with fewer questions.[23] A limitation of the SRS-22R includes that domain scores are found to be affected by demographic and socioeconomic factors.[27]

Radiographic

The association between spinopelvic parameters and HRQOL has been studied extensively, and HRQOL scores are associated with improvement in radiographic alignment.[28] Positive sagittal balance strongly correlates with poor clinical outcomes[29]; proper restoration of sagittal alignment is critical to improving clinical outcome and reducing pain.[30,31] The sagittal vertical axis (SVA) is the most used measurement to evaluate global sagittal alignment, but the T1 spinopelvic inclination (T1-SPi) and T1 pelvic angle (T1PA) also measure sagittal alignment and correlate with HRQOL.[30,32] T1PA was developed to account for postural compensation and pelvic retroversion, and is less affected by variations in standing compensation. T1PA correlates with ODI, SF-36, and SRS, and the MCID was found to be 4.1° on the ODI.[32] High values of pelvic tilt (PT), which represents compensatory pelvic retroversion for sagittal spinal malalignment, also strongly correlated to the HRQOL of patients.[33]

A general consensus has not been reached on which radiographic parameters best correlate with outcomes,[34,35] possibly due to the various subtypes of ASD.[36] One study reported that the most strongly correlated radiographic parameters for the ODI were PT, SVA, and pelvic incidence-lumbar lordosis (PI-LL).[37] In contrast, Chapman and colleagues reported only weak correlations between sagittal modifiers and SRS function in patients with lumbar scoliosis.[38] Takemoto and colleagues found no significant association between preoperative HRQOL and radiographic parameters but found a significant correlation with postoperative HRQOL and sagittal parameters.[34] The lack of association between spinopelvic parameters and HRQOL in these studies was thought to be due to the broad spectrum of scoliosis subtypes that were included. Faraj and colleagues performed a study composed of 74 patients with degenerative lumbar scoliosis to evaluate the impact of the surgical correction on scoliosis outcomes and found only weak correlations were found between SVA with ODI, NRS-back, and SRS pain domain.[35] Similarly, weak correlations between the ODI with T1PA (r = 0.137) and PI-LL (r = 0.137) were demonstrated in another study.[39] A Japanese study found a weak correlation between LL with lumbar function (r = 0.285), and moderate correlation between LL with VAS score for leg pain (r = 0.328).[40] The aforementioned studies suggest that at least a weak correlation between HRQOL and radiographic parameters is found in the degenerative scoliosis population.

Self-Image Outcome Measurements

In addition to PROMs and radiographic outcomes, a patient's perception of his or her own self-image has been recognized as negatively impacts preoperative health and life satisfaction for many patients with ASD.[13,41] A low degree of life satisfaction associated with physical disorders such as spinal deformity can have a serious psychological impact, leading to the deterioration of physical health and self-perceived quality of life. Importantly self-image consistently demonstrates improvement following surgery.[13,41] The SRS-22r scale recognizes the importance of the impact of self-image and includes a self-image domain,[42] but specific surveys for assessing appearance

have also been developed including the Spinal Appearance Questionnaire (SAQ) and the Trunk Appearance Perception Scale (TAPS) (**Table 2**). TAPS uses drawings of the torso to evaluate patients' perceptions of their trunk deformity in addition to self-image, but it has not been extensively studied.[43] SAQ was developed from the Walter Reed Visual Assessment Scale (WRVAS) to assess patients' perceptions of several aspects of their spinal deformity and their expectations regarding treatment.[44] The SAQ questions include body curve, rib and flank prominence, thoracic deformity, head position, shoulder, and scapular asymmetry. The SAQ has been validated, and one study found that the SAQ measured self-image with greater correlation to curve magnitude than SRS Appearance and Total Score. It also discriminated between patients who required surgery from those who did not.[44]

Functional Mobility Tests

The main evaluation of patients with ASD is based on PROMs or radiographic parameters derived from X-rays. However, due to their static nature, X-rays can be deficient in assessing dynamic functionalities including balance, gait, and the risk of falling.[38] Several assessment tools that evaluate the dynamic properties of patients with ASD include the Berg balance scale,[45] The Dubousset

Table 2
Selected self-image outcome measurements

Self-Image Outcome Measurements	Description
SRS-22R	Five questions scored from 1 to 5. Questions include • How do you look in clothes? • Which of the following best describes the appearance of your trunk? • Do you feel attractive with your current back condition? • If you had to spend the rest of your life with your back shape as it is right now, how would you feel about it? • Do you feel that your back condition affects your personal relationships?
Spinal Appearance Questionnaire	A 33-questions assessment that include body curve, rib and flank prominence, thoracic deformity, head position, shoulder, and scapular asymmetry. There are also 11 pictorial questions that the patient identifies what most looks like him or herself.
Trunk Appearance Perception Scale	Uses three sets of figures that depict the trunk from three viewpoints. Each drawing is scored from 1 (greatest deformity) to 5 (smallest deformity) and a mean score is obtained from the three drawings. Scores range from 1 to 15 with higher scores indicating a smaller self-perception of deformity
Walter Reed Visual Assessment Scale	A visual test including seven items that deal with various aspects of the deformity including spinal deformity, rib prominence, lumbar prominence, thoracic deformity, trunk imbalance, shoulder asymmetry, and scapular asymmetry. Each question has a set of five figures that represent the degrees of severity of the deformity.

Abbreviation: SRS, scoliosis research society.

Functional Test,[46] and kinetic models to measure dynamic spinal parameters.[47] Functional mobility tests (FMTs) have also been validated for the assessment of physical function, trunk and lower limb muscle integrity, and body balance.[48] FMTs should be simple, easy to perform, reproducible and not require special equipment. Therefore, FMTs may be useful in preoperatively assessing the functionalities of patients with ASD and anticipating their surgical outcomes. In one study of patients with either ASD or lumbar spinal stenosis, four FMTs including alternate step test (AST), six-m walk test (SMT), sit-to-stand test (STS), and timed up and go test (TUGT) were found to be significantly correlated with the ODI scores postoperatively in the ASD group, but not the lumbar spinal stenosis group.[48] Patients with ASD are at high risk of falls, and postural balance measurements have been shown to significantly differ between fallers and non-fallers.[49] Overall, FMTs are appropriate tools for assessing the dynamic functionalities of patients with ASD and might play a bridging role between static radiographic parameters and subjective PROs when assessing patients with ASD.

Accelerometers

Emerging technological advances provide an opportunity to objectively measure activity and disability.[50] Wearable technologies, including continuous physical activity monitors, or accelerometers, present an opportunity for the objective measurement of physical activity, as patient questionnaires have been shown to exaggerate physical activity levels compared to device-based measurements.[51] Accelerometers also provide real-time and longitudinal information about patient mobility and return of function. In a spinal surgery study that included of 17 of 22 patients who had undergone deformity surgery, a moderate preoperative correlation was found between greater mean total daily steps and lower ODI ($r = -0.61$) and higher SF-36 physical component ($r = 0.60$).[52] A small body of literature regarding the portable assessment of spine motion has found that wearable systems represent valid tools to track spine movement.[53] However, the use of these technologies is still confined to research studies and is in a preliminary stage of development, but represent a promising adjunct to measuring outcomes after scoliosis surgery.

FINANCIAL OUTCOMES

As the cost of spine care is high, surgery costs and return to work outcomes are important economic metrics for ASD care.[54,55] Cost-effectiveness research is conducted using the outcomes measure *cost/quality-adjusted life years (QALYs)*: the cost of the health intervention divided by the QALYs. A QALY measures the health state of an individual on a scale, with zero the equivalent of death and 1 equal to the optimal state for 1 year of life.[56] Traditionally, $100,000/QALY is accepted as the threshold in the US for cost effectiveness.[57] A data analysis of 541 patients who underwent ASD surgery found that the average cost/QALY at 5-year follow-up was $120,311.73, but that 40.7% of patients fell under the threshold of a cost/QALY of less than $100,000. Cost-effective patients had higher baseline ODI scores, lower baseline total SRS scores, and shorter fusions.[58] Of the most common instruments used to measure outcomes, only SF-36 is routinely used for cost-effectiveness studies,[3] which makes surgical cost-outcome decisions difficult. Overall, the financial impact of ASD surgery is an important outcome measurement.

Accounting for Risk Factors

Many of the PROMs used in clinical practice fail to account for patient-specific risk factors that influence outcomes. To develop a standardized set of PROMs for future clinical trials and registries, it is necessary to correct for patient risk factors to allow fair comparison of outcomes. Without correcting for patient risk factors, surgeons managing patients with more comorbidities would appear to have worse outcomes.[59] Several indices have been developed to risk-stratify and predict patient outcomes in patients, such as the general Charlson Comorbidity Index and scoliosis-specific indices including the Seattle Spine Score,[60] the Adult Spinal Deformity Frailty Index,[61] and the adult spinal deformity (ASD)-comorbidity scale (ASD-CS).[10] The ASD-CS index accounts for patient comorbidities, and this index was associated with PROMs (such as SRS22r) as well as postoperative complications.[10]

An adult spinal deformity-surgical and radiographical (ASD-SR) score has been developed, which predicts EBL and operative time.[62] Although some studies have indicated that complications do not significantly correlate with changes in ODI scores,[63] complications can significantly affect other outcome measurements such as length of hospital stay, 90-day readmission, and reoperation and can have a significant economic impact.[12,64] Despite a substantial complication rate in adult scoliosis surgery,[65] patient satisfaction is high with improved pain scale and ODI scores.[12] Further external validation of these indices with PROs would be beneficial.

SUMMARY

The SRS-22 and ODI are the predominantly used PRO measurements for deformity surgery. Correction of sagittal alignment correlates with improved PRO, and T1-SPI outperforms the SVA. Functional outcomes and accelerometer measurements represent newer methods of measuring outcomes that have not yet been widely adopted or validated. Further adoption of a minimum set of core outcome domains, PROs such as SRS-22, and contributing risk factors will help facilitate international comparisons and benchmarking, and ultimately enhance value-based healthcare.

CLINICS CARE POINTS

- The SRS-22 classification system is a highly reliable and well-validated system for ASD.
- The importance of the sagittal plane in adult spinal deformity is a well-established cause of pain and disability. T1-SPI strongly correlates with HRQOL and outperforms the SVA.

DISCLOSURE

Dr K. Than is a consultant for DePuy Synthes, NuVasive, Accelus, Bioventus, and Cerapedics, and receives honoraria from SI Bone. Dr M.M. Abd-El-Barr is a consultant for Spineology, DePuy Synthes, TrackX. He has received research funding from NIH, United States, Abbvie, United States, Dana and Christopher Reeve Foundation.

REFERENCES

1. Bess S, Line B, Fu KM, et al. The Health Impact of Symptomatic Adult Spinal Deformity: Comparison of Deformity Types to United States Population Norms and Chronic Diseases. Spine 2016;41(3): 224–33.
2. Gum JL, Carreon LY, Glassman SD. State-of-the-art: outcome assessment in adult spinal deformity. Spine Deformity 2021;9(1):1–11.
3. Cutler HS, Guzman JZ, Al Maaieh M, et al. Patient Reported Outcomes in Adult Spinal Deformity Surgery: A Bibliometric Analysis. Spine Deform 2015; 3(4):312–7.
4. Faraj S, van Hooff M, Holewijn R, et al. Measuring outcomes in adult spinal deformity surgery: a systematic review to identify current strengths, weaknesses and gaps in patient-reported outcome measures. Eur Spine J 2017;26:2084–93.
5. Patient-reported outcome measures: use in medical Product development to support labeling claims. Rockville, MD: Food and Drug Administration; 2009.
6. Bago J, Climent JM, Pineda S, et al. Further evaluation of the Walter Reed Visual Assessment Scale: correlation with curve pattern and radiological deformity. Scoliosis 2007;2(1):12.
7. Copay AG, Glassman SD, Subach BR, et al. Minimum clinically important difference in lumbar spine surgery patients: a choice of methods using the Oswestry Disability Index, Medical Outcomes Study questionnaire Short Form 36, and pain scales. Spine J 2008;8(6):968–74.
8. Fairbank J, Couper J, Davies J, et al. The Oswestry low back pain disability questionnaire. Physiotherapy 1980;66:271–3.
9. Leclaire R, Blier F, Fortin L, et al. A cross-sectional study comparing the Oswestry and Roland-Morris Functional Disability scales in two populations of patients with low back pain of different levels of severity. Spine 1997;22(1):68–71.
10. Sciubba D, Jain A, Kebaish KM, et al. Development of a Preoperative Adult Spinal Deformity Comorbidity Score That Correlates With Common Quality and Value Metrics: Length of Stay, Major Complications, and Patient-Reported Outcomes. Global Spine J 2019;11(2):146–53.
11. Fisher K, Johnston M. Validation of the Oswestry low back pain disability questionnaire. Article. Its sensitivity as a measure of change following treatment and its relationship with other aspects of the pain experience. Physiotherapy Theory and Practice 1997;13(1):67–80. https://doi.org/10.3109/09593989709036449.
12. Bridwell KH, Lewis SJ, Edwards C, et al. Complications and outcomes of pedicle subtraction osteotomies for fixed sagittal imbalance. Spine 2003; 28(18):2093–101.
13. Bridwell K, Berven S, Glassman S, et al. Is the SRS-22 instrument responsive to change in adult scoliosis patients having primary spinal deformity surgery? Spine 2007;32:2220–5.
14. Haher TR, Gorup JM, Shin TM, et al. Results of the Scoliosis Research Society instrument for evaluation of surgical outcome in adolescent idiopathic scoliosis. A multicenter study of 244 patients. Spine 1999;24(14):1435–40.
15. Asher MA, Lai SM, Glattes RC, et al. Refinement of the SRS-22 health-related quality of life questionnaire function domain. Spine 2006;31(5): 593–7.
16. Asher M, Lai SM, Burton D, et al. The reliability and concurrent validity of the scoliosis research society-22 patient questionnaire for idiopathic scoliosis. Spine 2003;28(1):63–9.
17. Crawford CH 3rd, Glassman SD, Bridwell KH, et al. The minimum clinically important difference in

SRS-22R total score, appearance, activity and pain domains after surgical treatment of adult spinal deformity. Spine 2015;40(6):377–81.

18. Mannion AF, Vila-Casademunt A, Domingo-Sàbat M, et al. The Core Outcome Measures Index (COMI) is a responsive instrument for assessing the outcome of treatment for adult spinal deformity. Eur Spine J 2016;25(8):2638–48.

19. Cheung PWH, Wong CKH, Samartzis D, et al. Psychometric validation of the EuroQoL 5-Dimension 5-Level (EQ-5D-5L) in Chinese patients with adolescent idiopathic scoliosis. Scoliosis and Spinal Disorders 2016;11(1):19.

20. Ibaseta A, Rahman R, Skolasky RL, et al. SRS-22r legacy scores can be accurately translated to PROMIS scores in adult spinal deformity patients. Spine J 2020;20(2):234–40.

21. Verma R, Lafage R, Scheer J, et al. Improvement in Back and Leg Pain and Disability Following Adult Spinal Deformity Surgery: Study of 324 Patients With 2-year Follow-up and the Impact of Surgery on Patient-reported Outcomes. Spine 2019;44(4): 263–9.

22. Cawley DT, Larrieu D, Fujishiro T, et al. NRS20: Combined Back and Leg Pain Score: A Simple and Effective Assessment of Adult Spinal Deformity. Spine 2018;43(17):1184–92.

23. Bridwell KH, Cats-Baril W, Harrast J, et al. The validity of the SRS-22 instrument in an adult spinal deformity population compared with the Oswestry and SF-12: a study of response distribution, concurrent validity, internal consistency, and reliability. Spine 2005;30(4):455–61.

24. Berven S, Deviren V, Demir-Deviren S, et al. Studies in the modified Scoliosis Research Society Outcomes Instrument in adults: validation, reliability, and discriminatory capacity. Spine 2003;28(18): 2164–9. ; discussion 2169.

25. Liu S, Schwab F, Smith JS, et al. Likelihood of reaching minimal clinically important difference in adult spinal deformity: a comparison of operative and nonoperative treatment. Ochsner J. Spring 2014; 14(1):67–77.

26. Asher M, Lai SM, Burton D, et al. Discrimination validity of the scoliosis research society-22 patient questionnaire: relationship to idiopathic scoliosis curve pattern and curve size. Spine 2003;28(1): 74–7.

27. Verma K, Lonner B, Hoashi JS, et al. Demographic factors affect Scoliosis Research Society-22 performance in healthy adolescents: a comparative baseline for adolescents with idiopathic scoliosis. Spine 2010;35(24):2134–9.

28. O'Neill KR, Lenke LG, Bridwell KH, et al. Factors associated with long-term patient-reported outcomes after three-column osteotomies. Spine J 2015;15(11):2312–8.

29. Glassman SD, Bridwell K, Dimar JR, et al. The impact of positive sagittal balance in adult spinal deformity. Spine 2005;30(18):2024–9.

30. Lafage V, Schwab F, Patel A, et al. Pelvic tilt and truncal inclination: two key radiographic parameters in the setting of adults with spinal deformity. Spine 2009;34(17):E599–606.

31. Lazennec JY, Ramaré S, Arafati N, et al. Sagittal alignment in lumbosacral fusion: relations between radiological parameters and pain. Eur Spine J 2000;9(1):47–55.

32. Protopsaltis TS, Lafage R, Smith JS, et al. The Lumbar Pelvic Angle, the Lumbar Component of the T1 Pelvic Angle, Correlates With HRQOL, PI-LL Mismatch, and it Predicts Global Alignment. Spine 2018;43(10):681–7.

33. Qiao J, Zhu F, Xu L, et al. T1 pelvic angle: a new predictor for postoperative sagittal balance and clinical outcomes in adult scoliosis. Spine 2014;39(25):2103–7.

34. Takemoto M, Boissière L, Vital J-M, et al. Are sagittal spinopelvic radiographic parameters significantly associated with quality of life of adult spinal deformity patients? Multivariate linear regression analyses for pre-operative and short-term post-operative health-related quality of life. Eur Spine J 2017; 26(8):2176–86.

35. Faraj SSA, De Kleuver M, Vila-Casademunt A, et al. Sagittal radiographic parameters demonstrate weak correlations with pretreatment patient-reported health-related quality of life measures in symptomatic de novo degenerative lumbar scoliosis: a European multicenter analysis. J Neurosurg Spine 2018; 28(6):573–80.

36. Gao A, Wang Y, Yu M, et al. Association Between Radiographic Spinopelvic Parameters and Health-related Quality of Life in De Novo Degenerative Lumbar Scoliosis and Concomitant Lumbar Spinal Stenosis. Spine 2020;45(16).E1013-e1019.

37. Schwab FJ, Blondel B, Bess S, et al. Radiographical spinopelvic parameters and disability in the setting of adult spinal deformity: a prospective multicenter analysis. Spine 2013;38(13):E803–12.

38. Chapman TM Jr, Baldus CR, Lurie JD, et al. Baseline Patient-Reported Outcomes Correlate Weakly With Radiographic Parameters: A Multicenter, Prospective NIH Adult Symptomatic Lumbar Scoliosis Study of 286 Patients. Spine 2016;41(22):1701–8.

39. Ha KY, Jang WH, Kim YH, et al. Clinical Relevance of the SRS-Schwab Classification for Degenerative Lumbar Scoliosis. Spine 2016;41(5):E282–8.

40. Iizuka Y, Iizuka H, Mieda T, et al. Epidemiology and associated radiographic spinopelvic parameters of symptomatic degenerative lumbar scoliosis: are radiographic spinopelvic parameters associated with the presence of symptoms or decreased quality of life in degenerative lumbar scoliosis? Eur Spine J 2016;25(8):2514–9.

41. Line B, Bess S, Lafage V, et al. Counseling Guidelines for Anticipated Postsurgical Improvements in Pain, Function, Mental Health, and Self-image for Different Types of Adult Spinal Deformity. Spine 2020;45(16):1118–27.

42. Baldus C, Bridwell KH, Harrast J, et al. Age-gender matched comparison of SRS instrument scores between adult deformity and normal adults: are all SRS domains disease specific? Spine 2008;33(20): 2214–8.

43. Bago J, Sanchez-Raya J, Perez-Grueso FJ, et al. The Trunk Appearance Perception Scale (TAPS): a new tool to evaluate subjective impression of trunk deformity in patients with idiopathic scoliosis. Scoliosis 2010;5:6.

44. Carreon LY, Sanders JO, Polly DW, et al. Spinal appearance questionnaire: factor analysis, scoring, reliability, and validity testing. Spine 2011;36(18): E1240–4.

45. Laratta JL, Glassman SD, Atanda AA, et al. The Berg balance scale for assessing dynamic stability and balance in the adult spinal deformity (ASD) population. Journal of Spine Surgery 2019;5(4):451–6.

46. Diebo BG, Challier V, Shah NV, et al. The Dubousset Functional Test is a Novel Assessment of Physical Function and Balance. Clin Orthop Relat Res 2019; 477(10):2307–15.

47. Severijns P, Overbergh T, Thauvoye A, et al. A subject-specific method to measure dynamic spinal alignment in adult spinal deformity. Spine J 2020; 20(6):934–46.

48. Lee HR, Park J, Ham DW, et al. functional mobility tests for evaluation of functionalities in patients with adult spinal deformity. BMC Musculoskelet Disord 2022;23(1):391.

49. Imagama S, Ito Z, Wakao N, et al. Influence of spinal sagittal alignment, body balance, muscle strength, and physical ability on falling of middle-aged and elderly males. Eur Spine J 2013;22(6): 1346–53.

50. Stienen MN, Rezaii PG, Ho AL, et al. Objective activity tracking in spine surgery: a prospective feasibility study with a low-cost consumer grade wearable accelerometer. Sci Rep 2020;10(1):4939.

51. Lee PH, Macfarlane DJ, Lam TH, et al. Validity of the international physical activity questionnaire short form (IPAQ-SF): A systematic review. Int J Behav Nutr Phys Activ 2011;8(1):115.

52. Scheer JK, Bakhsheshian J, Keefe MK, et al. Initial Experience With Real-Time Continuous Physical Activity Monitoring in Patients Undergoing Spine Surgery. Clinical spine surgery 2017;30(10): E1434-e1443.

53. Papi E, Koh WS, McGregor AH. Wearable technology for spine movement assessment: A systematic review. J Biomech 2017;64:186–97.

54. Zygourakis CC, Liu CY, Keefe M, et al. Analysis of National Rates, Cost, and Sources of Cost Variation in Adult Spinal Deformity. Neurosurgery 2018;82(3): 378–87.

55. Neuman BJ, Wang KY, Harris AB, et al. Return to work after adult spinal deformity surgery. Spine Deform 2022. https://doi.org/10.1007/s43390-022-00552-2.

56. Miyamoto JM. Quality-Adjusted Life Years (QALY) Utility Models under Expected Utility and Rank Dependent Utility Assumptions. J Math Psychol 1999;43(2):201–37.

57. Chapman RH, Berger M, Weinstein MC, et al. When does quality-adjusting life-years matter in cost-effectiveness analysis? Health Econ 2004;13(5): 429–36.

58. Terran J, McHugh BJ, Fischer CR, et al. Surgical treatment for adult spinal deformity: projected cost effectiveness at 5-year follow-up. Ochsner J. Spring 2014;14(1):14–22.

59. Spence RT, Mueller JL, Chang DC. A Novel Approach to Global Benchmarking of Risk-Adjusted Surgical Outcomes: Beyond Perioperative Mortality Rate. JAMA Surg 2016;151(6):501–2.

60. Buchlak QD, Yanamadala V, Leveque JC, et al. The Seattle spine score: Predicting 30-day complication risk in adult spinal deformity surgery. J Clin Neurosci 2017;43:247–55.

61. Miller EK, Neuman BJ, Jain A, et al. An assessment of frailty as a tool for risk stratification in adult spinal deformity surgery. Neurosurg Focus 2017;43(6):E3.

62. Neuman BJ, Ailon T, Scheer JK, et al. Development and Validation of a Novel Adult Spinal Deformity Surgical Invasiveness Score: Analysis of 464 Patients. Neurosurgery 2018;82(6):847–53.

63. Daubs MD, Lenke LG, Cheh G, et al. Adult Spinal Deformity Surgery: Complications and Outcomes in Patients Over Age 60. Spine 2007;32(20):2238–44.

64. Williamson TK, Owusu-Sarpong S, Imbo B, et al. An Economic Analysis of Early and Late Complications After Adult Spinal Deformity Correction. Global Spine J 2022. https://doi.org/10.1177/21925682221122762 21925682221122762.

65. Lee NJ, Kothari P, Kim JS, et al. Early Complications and Outcomes in Adult Spinal Deformity Surgery: An NSQIP Study Based on 5803 Patients. Global Spine J 2017;7(5):432–40.

UNITED STATES POSTAL SERVICE ®

Statement of Ownership, Management, and Circulation (All Periodicals Publications Except Requester Publications)

1. Publication Title	2. Publication Number	3. Filing Date
NEUROSURGERY CLINICS OF NORTH AMERICA	010 – 548	9/18/2023

4. Issue Frequency	5. Number of Issues Published Annually	6. Annual Subscription Price
JAN, APR, JUL OCT	4	$451.00

7. Complete Mailing Address of Known Office of Publication (Not printer) (Street, city, county, state, and ZIP+4®)

ELSEVIER INC.
230 Park Avenue, Suite 800
New York, NY 10169

Contact Person
Malathi Samayan
Telephone (Include area code)
91-44-4299-4507

8. Complete Mailing Address of Headquarters or General Business Office of Publisher (Not printer)

ELSEVIER INC.
230 Park Avenue, Suite 800
New York, NY 10169

9. Full Names and Complete Mailing Addresses of Publisher, Editor, and Managing Editor (Do not leave blank)

Publisher (Name and complete mailing address)

Dolores Meloni, ELSEVIER INC.
1600 JOHN F KENNEDY BLVD. SUITE 1600
PHILADELPHIA, PA 19103-2899

Editor (Name and complete mailing address)

STACY EASTMAN, ELSEVIER INC.
1600 JOHN F KENNEDY BLVD. SUITE 1600
PHILADELPHIA, PA 19103-2899

Managing Editor (Name and complete mailing address)

PATRICK MANLEY, ELSEVIER INC.
1600 JOHN F KENNEDY BLVD. SUITE 1600
PHILADELPHIA, PA 19103-2899

10. Owner (Do not leave blank. If the publication is owned by a corporation, give the name and address of the corporation immediately followed by the names and addresses of all stockholders owning or holding 1 percent or more of the total amount of stock. If not owned by a corporation, give the names and addresses of the individual owners. If owned by a partnership or other unincorporated firm, give its name and address as well as those of each individual owner. If the publication is published by a nonprofit organization, give its name and address.)

Full Name	Complete Mailing Address
WHOLLY OWNED SUBSIDIARY OF REED/ELSEVIER, US HOLDINGS	1600 JOHN F KENNEDY BLVD. SUITE 1600 PHILADELPHIA, PA 19103-2899

11. Known Bondholders, Mortgagees, and Other Security Holders Owning or Holding 1 Percent or More of Total Amount of Bonds, Mortgages, or Other Securities. If none, check box ► ☐ None

Full Name	Complete Mailing Address
N/A	

12. Tax Status (For completion by nonprofit organizations authorized to mail at nonprofit rates) (Check one)
The purpose, function, and nonprofit status of this organization and the exempt status for federal income tax purposes:
☒ Has Not Changed During Preceding 12 Months
☐ Has Changed During Preceding 12 Months (Publisher must submit explanation of change with this statement)

PS Form 3526, July 2014 [Page 1 of 4 (see instructions page 4)] PSN 7533-01-000-9931   PRIVACY NOTICE: See our privacy policy on www.usps.com.

---

13. Publication Title	14. Issue Date for Circulation Data Below
NEUROSURGERY CLINICS OF NORTH AMERICA	JULY 2023

15. Extent and Nature of Circulation		Average No. Copies Each Issue During Preceding 12 Months	No. Copies of Single Issue Published Nearest to Filing Date
a. Total Number of Copies (Net press run)		133	137
b. Paid Circulation (By Mail and Outside the Mail)	(1) Mailed Outside-County Paid Subscriptions Stated on PS Form 3541 (Include paid distribution above nominal rate, advertiser's proof copies, and exchange copies)	84	97
	(2) Mailed In-County Paid Subscriptions Stated on PS Form 3541 (Include paid distribution above nominal rate, advertiser's proof copies, and exchange copies)	0	0
	(3) Paid Distribution Outside the Mails Including Sales Through Dealers and Carriers, Street Vendors, Counter Sales, and Other Paid Distribution Outside USPS®	33	22
	(4) Paid Distribution by Other Classes of Mail Through the USPS (e.g., First-Class Mail®)	11	12
c. Total Paid Distribution (Sum of 15b (1), (2), (3), and (4))	►	128	131
d. Free or Nominal Rate Distribution (By Mail and Outside the Mail)	(1) Free or Nominal Rate Outside-County Copies included on PS Form 3541	4	5
	(2) Free or Nominal Rate In-County Copies Included on PS Form 3541	0	0
	(3) Free or Nominal Rate Copies Mailed at Other Classes Through the USPS (e.g., First-Class Mail)	0	0
	(4) Free or Nominal Rate Distribution Outside the Mail (Carriers or other means)	1	1
e. Total Free or Nominal Rate Distribution (Sum of 15d (1), (2), (3) and (4))	►	5	6
f. Total Distribution (Sum of 15c and 15e)	►	133	137
g. Copies not Distributed (See instructions to Publishers #4 (page #3))	►	0	0
h. Total (Sum of 15f and g)	►	133	137
i. Percent Paid (15c divided by 15f times 100)		96.24%	95.62%

* If you are claiming electronic copies, go to line 16 on page 3. If you are not claiming electronic copies, skip to line 17 on page 3.

16. Electronic Copy Circulation		Average No. Copies Each Issue During Preceding 12 Months	No. Copies of Single Issue Published Nearest to Filing Date
a. Paid Electronic Copies	►		
b. Total Paid Print Copies (Line 15c) + Paid Electronic Copies (Line 16a)	►		
c. Total Print Distribution (Line 15f) + Paid Electronic Copies (Line 16a)	►		
d. Percent Paid (Both Print & Electronic Copies) (16b divided by 16c × 100)	►		

☒ I certify that 50% of all my distributed copies (electronic and print) are paid above a nominal price.

17. Publication of Statement of Ownership

☒ If the publication is a general publication, publication of this statement is required. Will be printed
in the ___OCTOBER 2023___ issue of this publication.   ☐ Publication not required.

18. Signature and Title of Editor, Publisher, Business Manager, or Owner		Date
Malathi Samayan	Malathi Samayan - Distribution Controller	9/18/2023

I certify that all information furnished on this form is true and complete. I understand that anyone who furnishes false or misleading information on this form or who omits material or information requested on the form may be subject to criminal sanctions (including fines and imprisonment) and/or civil sanctions (including civil penalties).

PS Form 3526, July 2014 (Page 2 of 4)   PRIVACY NOTICE: See our privacy policy on www.usps.com